# Photodermatology

*Editor*

HENRY W. LIM

*Assistant Editor*

SO YEON PAEK

# DERMATOLOGIC CLINICS

www.derm.theclinics.com

*Consulting Editor*
BRUCE H. THIERS

July 2014 • Volume 32 • Number 3

**ELSEVIER**

1600 John F. Kennedy Boulevard • Suite 1800 • Philadelphia, Pennsylvania, 19103-2899

http://www.theclinics.com

**DERMATOLOGIC CLINICS Volume 32, Number 3**
**July 2014 ISSN 0733-8635, ISBN-13: 978-0-323-31162-5**

Editor: Joanne Husovski
Developmental Editor: Susan Showalter

*Dermatologic Clinics* (ISSN 0733-8635) is published quarterly by Elsevier Inc., 360 Park Avenue South, New York, NY 10010-1710. Months of publication are January, April, July, and October. Business and editorial offices: 1600 John F. Kennedy Blvd., Suite 1800, Philadelphia, PA 19103-2899. Customer service office: 11830 Westline Drive, St. Louis, MO 63146. Periodicals postage paid at New York, NY, and additional mailing offices. Subscription prices are USD 365.00 per year for US individuals, USD 559.00 per year for US institutions, USD 425.00 per year for Canadian individuals, USD 681.00 per year for Canadian institutions, USD 495.00 per year for international individuals, USD 681.00 per year for international institutions, USD 165.00 per year for US students/residents, and USD 240.00 per year for Canadian and international students/residents. International air speed delivery is included in all *Clinics* subscription prices. All prices are subject to change without notice. **POSTMASTER:** Send address changes to *Dermatologic Clinics*, Elsevier Health Sciences Division, Subscription Customer Service, 3251 Riverport Lane, Maryland Heights, MO 63043. **Customer Service: 1-800-654-2452 (U.S. and Canada); 314-447-8871 (outside U.S. and Canada). Fax: 314-447-8029. E-mail: journalscustomerservice-usa@elsevier.com (for print support); journalsonlinesupport-usa@elsevier.com (for online support).**

*Reprints.* For copies of 100 or more, of articles in this publication, please contact the Commercial Reprints Department, Elsevier Inc., 360 Park Avenue South, New York, New York 10010-1710. Tel.: 212-633-3874; Fax: 212-633-3820; Email: reprints@elsevier.com.

The *Dermatologic Clinics* is covered in *MEDLINE/PubMed (Index Medicus)*, *Current Contents/Clinical Medicine*, *Excerpta Medica*, *Chemical Abstracts*, and *ISI/BIOMED*.

# Contributors

## CONSULTING EDITOR

**BRUCE H. THIERS, MD**
Professor and Chairman, Department of
Dermatology and Dermatologic Surgery,
Medical University of South Carolina,
Charleston, South Carolina

## EDITOR

**HENRY W. LIM, MD**
Chairman and C.S. Livingood Chair,
Department of Dermatology, Henry Ford
Hospital; Senior Vice President for Academic
Affairs, Henry Ford Health System, Detroit,
Michigan

## ASSISTANT EDITOR

**SO YEON PAEK, MD**
Resident Physician, Department of
Dermatology, Henry Ford Hospital, Detroit,
Michigan

## AUTHORS

**FAHAD ALMUTAWA, MD**
Department of Medicine, Kuwait University,
Al-Jabriya, Safat, Kuwait

**ALEXANDER V. ANSTEY, MD, FRCP**
Professor, Department of Dermatology,
Royal Gwent Hospital, Newport; Institute of
Medical Education, Cardiff University, Cardiff,
United Kingdom

**MICHAEL N. BADMINTON, BSc, MBChB,
PhD, FRCPath**
Department of Medical Biochemistry
and Immunology, University Hospital
of Wales; Institute of Molecular and
Experimental Medicine, School of
Medicine, Cardiff University, Cardiff,
United Kingdom

**ELMA D. BARON, MD**
Associate Professor, Department of
Dermatology, University Hospitals Case
Medical Center, Louis Stokes Cleveland
Veterans Affairs Medical Center, Case Western
Reserve University, Cleveland, Ohio

**HANAN BUABBAS, PhD**
Medical Photophysics Laboratory, Asaad al
Hamad Dermatology Center, Khaldeyah,
Kuwait City, Kuwait

**SCOTT N. BYRNE, PhD**
Senior Lecturer in Immunology and Head;
Cellular Photoimmunology Group, Infectious
Diseases and Immunology, Department of
Dermatology, Sydney Medical School, Royal
Prince Alfred Hospital, The University of
Sydney, Darlington, New South Wales,
Australia

**CATHER M. CALA, BA**
Department of Dermatology, University of
Alabama at Birmingham, Birmingham,
Alabama

**ANNA L. CHIEN, MD**
Assistant Professor and Director of
Clinical Trials Research Program,
Department of Dermatology, Johns Hopkins
Medical Institutions, Baltimore,
Maryland

**MELVIN W. CHIU, MD, MPH**
Division of Dermatology, Department of
Medicine, David Geffen School of Medicine at
UCLA, Los Angeles, California

**DAVID CHOI, BS**
Department of Dermatology, Yale School of
Medicine, New Haven, Connecticut

**ROBERT S. DAWE, MBChB, MD, FRCPE**
Consultant Dermatologist and Honorary
Clinical Reader in Dermatology; Photobiology
Unit, Department of Dermatology, Ninewells
Hospital and Medical School, University of
Dundee, Dundee, Scotland, United Kingdom

**MELODY J. EIDE, MD, MPH**
Departments of Dermatology and Public
Health Sciences, Henry Ford Hospital, Detroit,
Michigan

**CRAIG A. ELMETS, MD**
Professor and Chairman, Department of
Dermatology, UAB Skin Diseases Research
Center, UAB Comprehensive Cancer Center,
Birmingham VA Medical Center, University of
Alabama at Birmingham, Birmingham,
Alabama

**ALEXANDRA GRUBER-WACKERNAGEL,
MD**
Senior Lecturer in Dermatology and Staff
Specialist; Research Unit for
Photodermatology, Department of
Dermatology, Medical University of Graz, Graz,
Austria

**ANNE HAN, MD**
Department of Dermatology, Johns Hopkins
Medical Institutions, Baltimore, Maryland

**JUDY Y. HU, MD**
Global Health Research LLC, Chatham,
New Jersey

**SALLY H. IBBOTSON, MBChB, MD, FRCPE**
Clinical Senior Lecturer in Dermatology and
Honorary Consultant Dermatologist;
Photobiology Unit, Department of
Dermatology, Ninewells Hospital and Medical
School, University of Dundee, Dundee,
Scotland, United Kingdom

**SEWON KANG, MD**
Noxell Professor and Chair, Department of
Dermatology, Johns Hopkins Medical
Institutions, Baltimore, Maryland

**SWATI KANNAN, MD**
Department of Dermatology, Henry Ford
Health System, Henry Ford Hospital,
Detroit, Michigan

**RUWANI KATUGAMPOLA, BM, MRCP, MD**
Department of Dermatology,
University Hospital of Wales, Cardiff,
United Kingdom

**BONITA KOZMA, MD**
Department of Dermatology, Henry Ford
Hospital, Detroit, Michigan

**HENRY W. LIM, MD**
Chairman and C.S. Livingood Chair,
Department of Dermatology, Henry Ford
Hospital; Senior Vice President for Academic
Affairs, Henry Ford Health System, Detroit,
Michigan

**SILVIA E. MANCEBO, BS**
Dermatology Service, Memorial Sloan
Kettering Cancer Center, New York,
New York

**GILLIAN M. MURPHY, MB BCh**
Dermatology Department, Beaumont Hospital;
National Photodermatology Unit, Dermatology
Department, Mater Misericordiae University
Hospital, Dublin, Ireland

**SANDRA MUVDI, MD, MSc**
Research and Education Department,
Research and Education Office, Centro
Dermatológico Federico Lleras Acosta,
Bogotá, Colombi

**RATTANAVALAI NITIYAROM, MD**
Assistant Professor, Department of
Pediatrics, Faculty of Medicine, Siriraj Hospital,
Mahidol University, Bangkoknoi, Bangkok,
Thailand

**SUSAN M. O'GORMAN, MB BCh**
Dermatology Department, Beaumont Hospital, Dublin, Ireland

**DAVID M. OZOG, MD**
Vice Chairman, Department of Dermatology, Henry Ford Hospital, Detroit, Michigan

**SO YEON PAEK, MD**
Resident Physician, Department of Dermatology, Henry Ford Hospital, Detroit, Michigan

**ALI M. RKEIN, MD**
Department of Dermatology, Henry Ford Hospital, Detroit, Michigan

**DANJA SCHULENBURG-BRAND, MBChB, MMed (Chem Path)**
Department of Medical Biochemistry and Immunology, University Hospital of Wales, Cardiff, United Kingdom

**AMANDA K. SUGGS, MD**
Photomedicine Research Fellow, Department of Dermatology, University Hospitals Case Medical Center, Case Western Reserve University, Cleveland, Ohio

**MARIAM B. TOTONCHY, MD**
Department of Dermatology, Yale School of Medicine, New Haven, Connecticut

**MARTHA C. VALBUENA, MD**
Photodermatology Unit, Centro Dermatológico Federico Lleras Acosta, Bogotá, Colombia

**STEVEN Q. WANG, MD**
Dermatology Service, Memorial Sloan Kettering Cancer Center, New York, New York

**PETER WOLF, MD**
Professor of Dermatology and Bioimmunotherapy and Head; Research Unit for Photodermatology, Department of Dermatology, Medical University of Graz, Graz, Austria

**CHANISADA WONGPRAPARUT, MD**
Assistant Professor, Department of Dermatology, Faculty of Medicine, Siriraj Hospital, Mahidol University, Bangkoknoi, Bangkok, Thailand

**HUI XU, PhD**
Professor, Department of Dermatology, UAB Skin Diseases Research Center, UAB Comprehensive Cancer Center, Birmingham VA Medical Center, University of Alabama at Birmingham, Birmingham, Alabama

# Contents

**Introduction to Photobiology**                                                 255

Elma D. Baron and Amanda K. Suggs

Photobiology is the study of the local and systemic effects of incident radiation on living organisms. Solar radiation is made up of ultraviolet, visible and infrared radiation. Ultraviolet radiation is made up of UV-C, UV-B, and UV-A. Sun exposure can lead to sunburn, tanning, vitamin D production, photoaging, and carcinogenesis. Phototherapy is the use of nonionizing radiation to treat cutaneous disease. Various types of artificial light sources are used for photo testing and phototherapy.

**Evaluation of Patients with Photodermatoses**                                  267

David Choi, Swati Kannan, and Henry W. Lim

The systematic evaluation of photosensitive patients involves a comprehensive history, physical examination, phototesting, and, if necessary, photopatch testing and laboratory evaluation. Polymorphous light eruption, chronic actinic dermatitis, solar urticaria, and photosensitivity secondary to systemic medications are the most commonly encountered photodermatoses in dermatology clinics worldwide.

**Photoimmunology**                                                              277

Craig A. Elmets, Cather M. Cala, and Hui Xu

The discipline that investigates the biologic effects of ultraviolet radiation on the immune system is called *photoimmunology*. Photoimmunology evolved from an interest in understanding the role of the immune system in skin cancer development and why immunosuppressed organ transplant recipients are at a greatly increased risk for cutaneous neoplasms. In addition to contributing to an understanding of the pathogenesis of nonmelanoma skin cancer, the knowledge acquired about the immunologic effects of ultraviolet radiation exposure has provided an understanding of its role in the pathogenesis of other photodermatologic diseases.

**Photoaging**                                                                   291

Anne Han, Anna L. Chien, and Sewon Kang

This article discusses photoaging or premature skin aging from chronic ultraviolet exposure. This is an important cosmetic concern for many dermatologic patients. Clinical signs include rhytids, lentigines, mottled hyperpigmentation, loss of translucency, and decreased elasticity. These changes are more severe in individuals with fair skin and are further influenced by individual ethnicity and genetics. Photoaging may be prevented and treated with a variety of modalities, including topical retinoids, cosmeceuticals, chemical peels, injectable neuromodulators, soft tissue fillers, and light sources.

> Photocarcinogenesis is the result of a complex interplay between ultraviolet radiation, DNA damage, mutation formation, DNA repair, apoptosis, and the immune system. Recent trends show an increase in incidence of both melanoma and nonmelanoma skin cancers. Some individuals have a genetic predisposition toward increased risk for skin cancer, whereas others experience increased risk through ultraviolet exposure and subsequent mutation formation. The initiation and propagation pathways of melanoma and nonmelanoma skin cancers differ but have some elements in common. The increase in incidence of skin cancer has been discovered to vary among age groups and gender.

> Polymorphous light eruption is an immunologically mediated photodermatosis with high prevalence, particularly among young women in temperate climates, characterized by pruritic skin lesions of variable morphology, occurring in spring or early summer on sun-exposed body sites. A resistance to ultraviolet radiation (UVR)-induced immunosuppression and a subsequent delayed-type hypersensitivity response to a photoantigen have been suggested as key factors in the disease. Molecular and immunologic disturbances associated with disease pathogenesis include a failure of skin infiltration by neutrophils and other regulatory immune cells on UVR exposure linked to a disturbed cytokine microenvironment. Standard management is based on prevention.

> Actinic prurigo is a chronic photodermatosis with onset in childhood or before 20 years of age. It is most prevalent in Amerindians and Latin American mestizos, although it has been reported worldwide. Patients present with photodistributed, erythematous excoriated papules, cheilitis, and conjunctivitis. There is strong association with human leukocyte antigen DR4, especially the DRB1*0407 subtype. Treatment consists of photoprotection and the use of thalidomide.

> Hydroa vacciniforme (HV) and solar urticaria (SU) are uncommon immunologically mediated photodermatoses. HV occurs almost exclusively in children, usually beginning in childhood and remitting spontaneously by adolescence. Association with chronic Epstein-Barr virus infection has been reported in HV, which raises the possibility of lymphoproliferative disorders in these patients. SU is characterized by skin erythema, swelling, and whealing immediately after sun exposure. Although several treatment options are available, the management of both conditions remains a challenge.

> Chronic actinic dermatitis (CAD) is an immunologically mediated photodermatosis characterized by pruritic eczematous and lichenified plaques located predominantly

on sun-exposed areas with notable sparing of eyelids, skin folds, and postauricular skin. CAD is thought to be due to secondary photosensitization of an endogenous antigen in the skin. Management of CAD should include strict photoprotection and topical agents, including corticosteroids and calcineurin inhibitors. Other treatments with noted efficacy include oral prednisone, cyclosporine, azathioprine, and mycophenolate mofetil. Photoprotection and avoidance of allergens, if identified, may lead to spontaneous resolution of CAD in 50% of patients over 15 years.

## Drug-Induced Photosensitivity                                           363

Robert S. Dawe and Sally H. Ibbotson

Drug-induced photosensitivity is common. The principal mechanism of systemic drug photosensitivity is phototoxicity and the principal mechanism of topical drug photosensitivity is photoallergy. Photopatch testing is helpful to determine suspected topical agent photoallergies (eg, from ultraviolet filters in sunscreens) but generally not helpful in detecting systemic drug photosensitivity. Drug-induced photosensitivity is usually best managed by stopping the suspected drug. Other measures, including phototherapy using wavelengths that do not elicit the response, are sometimes necessary.

## The Cutaneous Porphyrias                                                 369

Danja Schulenburg-Brand, Ruwani Katugampola, Alexander V. Anstey, and Michael N. Badminton

The porphyrias are a group of mainly inherited disorders of heme biosynthesis where accumulation of porphyrins and/or porphyrin precursors gives rise to 2 types of clinical presentation: cutaneous photosensitivity and/or acute neurovisceral attacks. The cutaneous porphyrias present with either bullous skin fragility or nonbullous acute photosensitivity. This review discusses the epidemiology, pathogenesis, clinical presentation, laboratory diagnosis, complications, and current approach to porphyria management. Although focusing mainly on their dermatological aspects, the article also covers the management of acute porphyria, which by virtue of its association with variegate porphyria and hereditary coproporphyria, may become the responsibility of the clinical dermatologist.

## Photoaggravated Disorders                                               385

Susan M. O'Gorman and Gillian M. Murphy

Photoaggravated skin disorders are diseases that occur without UV radiation but are sometimes or frequently exacerbated by UV radiation. In conditions, such as lupus erythematosus, photoaggravation occurs in a majority of patients, whereas in conditions, such as psoriasis and atopic dermatitis, only a subset of patients demonstrate photoaggravation. Polymorphous light eruption is a common photodermatosis in all skin types, making it important to differentiate photoaggravation of an underlying disorder, such as lupus erythematosus, from superimposed polymorphous light eruption. Disease-specific treatments should be instituted where possible. A key component of management of photoaggravated conditions is photoprotection with behavioral change, UV-protective clothing, and broad-spectrum sunscreen.

## UV-Based Therapy                                                        399

Mariam B. Totonchy and Melvin W. Chiu

UV phototherapy has a long history of use for the treatment of select diseases in dermatology. Its use has evolved into more effective and targeted modalities, including psoralen + UV-A photochemotherapy, narrowband UV-B, excimer laser, and UV-A1 phototherapy. With its proven record of efficacy and safety, UV phototherapy is an excellent option in the treatment of an ever-growing number of skin conditions.

Photodynamic therapy (PDT) relies on the interaction between a photosensitizer, the appropriate wavelength, and oxygen to cause cell death. First introduced about 100 years ago, PDT has continued to evolve in dermatology into a safe and effective treatment option for several dermatologic conditions. PDT is also used by pulmonologists, urologists, and ophthalmologists. This article focuses on the history of PDT, mechanism of action, photosensitizers and light sources used, therapeutic applications and expected dermatologic outcomes, as well as management of adverse events.

Ultraviolet radiation plays a major role in the development of nonmelanoma and melanoma skin cancers. Photoprotection by sunscreens has been shown to prevent the development of actinic keratosis, squamous cell carcinoma, melanoma, and photoaging. However, these benefits are only derived if the users apply sunscreen appropriately and practice other sun protection measures. This review discusses the health benefits provided by sunscreen use, updates the latest regulatory landscape on sunscreen, and addresses the controversies and limitations associated with sunscreen use.

Ultraviolet (UV) radiation (UVR) has well-known adverse effects on the skin and eyes. Little attention is given to physical means of photoprotection, namely glass, window films, sunglasses, and clothing. In general, all types of glass block UV-B. For UV-A, the degree of transmission depends on the type, thickness, and color of the glass. Adding window films to glass can greatly decrease the transmission of UV-A. Factors that can affect the transmission of UVR through cloth include tightness of weave, thickness, weight, type of fabrics, laundering, hydration, stretch, fabric processing, UV absorbers, color, and fabric-to-skin distance.

# DERMATOLOGIC CLINICS

# Preface
# Photodermatology

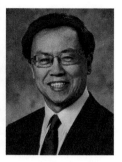

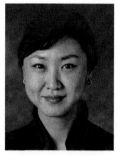

Henry W. Lim, MD
Editor

So Yeon Paek, MD
Assistant Editor

Photodermatology is an integral part of our specialty. On a daily basis, we address issues of photodamage and photoprotection with our patients, deliver phototherapy for various dermatoses, and take care of patients with photosensitivity disorders, ranging from drug-induced photosensitivity to polymorphous light eruption to the porphyrias. Training in photodermatology is an important component of residency education. A good understanding of photodermatology is one area that sets us as dermatologists apart from our colleagues in medicine.

It is a privilege for us to be invited to prepare this special issue on photodermatology. We are pleased that we have been able to recruit superb authors to cover all aspects of this subspecialty, from basic principles of photobiology and photodermatoses to phototherapy and photoprotection. The authors are all prominent clinician-investigators who have made important contributions and have special expertise on the topic. Their participation is an important aspect of the success of this project. To all the authors, we would like to express our sincere thanks!

We trust that you will find this issue to be informative and useful for your daily practice. We hope that you will enjoy reading this as much as we have enjoyed preparing it.

Editor
Henry W. Lim, MD
Department of Dermatology
Henry Ford Hospital
3031 West Grand Boulevard
Suite 800, Detroit, MI 48202, USA

Assistant Editor
So Yeon Paek, MD
Department of Dermatology
Henry Ford Hospital
3031 West Grand Boulevard
Suite 800, Detroit, MI 48202, USA

E-mail addresses:
hlim1@hfhs.org (H.W. Lim)
spaek1@hfhs.org (S.Y. Paek)

Dermatol Clin 32 (2014) xiii
http://dx.doi.org/10.1016/j.det.2014.05.001
0733-8635/14/$ – see front matter © 2014 Published by Elsevier Inc.

# Introduction to Photobiology

Elma D. Baron, MD[a],*, Amanda K. Suggs, MD[b]

## KEYWORDS

- Ultraviolet radiation • Ultraviolet light • Phototherapy • Photobiology • Sunburn • Melanogenesis
- Vitamin D production • Photoaging

## KEY POINTS

- Solar radiation is made up of ultraviolet, visible, and infrared radiation.
- Ultraviolet radiation is made up of UV-C, UV-B, and UV-A.
- Most ultraviolet radiation that reaches the earth is UV-A.
- Sun exposure has a wide range of biological effects, including sunburn, tanning, vitamin D production, photoaging, and carcinogenesis.
- Phototherapy uses properties of ultraviolet light that are useful in the treatment of certain dermatologic conditions.

## INTRODUCTION

Photobiology deals with the local and systemic effects of incident radiation on living organisms. This introductory article on cutaneous photobiology focuses on the effects of ultraviolet (UV) radiation (UVR), both from its natural source (ie, the sun) and artificial sources (ie, those used in phototherapy), on skin function and diseases. Although visible light and infrared radiation also have effects on skin cells, there is more information on UVR.

Phototherapy is the use of nonionizing radiation to treat cutaneous disease. For more than a century, phototherapy has played a pivotal role in the treatment of dermatologic diseases. In 1903, Niels Finsen received the Nobel Prize in Medicine for using light to treat a cutaneous mycobacterial disease. In the middle of the 20th century, advancements in UV-B light therapy expanded treatment options for patients with psoriasis. In the 1970s, photochemotherapy (ie, using psoralen as a photosensitizer in combination with UV-A radiation [PUVA]) made its debut. PUVA became an established player in the treatment of skin diseases in the last quarter of the 20th century. More recent advances in the last few decades (ie, narrowband UV-B therapy, laser therapy, targeted phototherapy, photodynamic therapy [PDT], UV-A1) have also revolutionized photodermatology.[1,2]

## UVR

### Solar Radiation

The rays of the sun hit the earth in the form of UVR, visible, and infrared radiation. These 3 entities are components of the electromagnetic spectrum, which also includes radiowaves, microwaves, radiographs, and $\gamma$ radiation (**Fig. 1**). Solar radiation is made up of approximately 50% visible light, 40% infrared, and 9% UVR.[3] Visible radiation is that which is perceived by the human eye.[4] Each color of visible light represents a different wavelength range (see **Fig. 1**). UVR is the area of the electromagnetic spectrum that is considered most biologically active and therefore of greatest impact on health and disease.

[a] Department of Dermatology, University Hospitals Case Medical Center, Louis Stokes Cleveland Veterans Affairs Medical Center, Case Western Reserve University, 11100 Euclid Avenue, Lakeside 3500, Mailstop 5028, Cleveland, OH 44106-5028, USA; [b] Department of Dermatology, University Hospitals Case Medical Center, Case Western Reserve University, 11100 Euclid Avenue, Cleveland, OH 44106, USA
* Corresponding author.
E-mail address: elma.baron@uhhospitals.org

Dermatol Clin 32 (2014) 255–266
http://dx.doi.org/10.1016/j.det.2014.03.002
0733-8635/14/$ – see front matter © 2014 Elsevier Inc. All rights reserved.

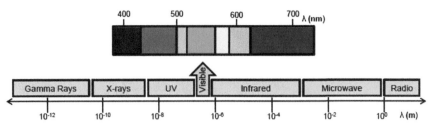

**Fig. 1.** Electromagnetic spectrum.

## UVR

UVR spans the wavelengths 100 to 400 nm and is subdivided into UV-C, UV-B, and UV-A. There are subtle differences in the subdivisions described in the literature. In this article, the subdivision most commonly chosen in photobiology is used (ie, UV-C, 200–290 nm; UV-B, 290–320 nm; and UV-A, 320–400 nm).[4] Other ranges referenced in the literature include: UV-C at 200 to 280 nm, UV-B at 280 to 320 nm, UV-A at 320 to 400 nm, UV-C at 200 to 280 nm, UV-B at 280 to 315 nm, and UV-A at 315 to 400 nm.[5] The stratospheric ozone prevents wavelengths shorter than approximately 290 nm from hitting the earth. Most UV radiation that reaches the earth is UV-A. Only a small percentage (approximately 5%) of UV-B is present in terrestrial sunlight. UV-C is typically filtered by the ozone layer.[6] The amount of solar energy at a specific wavelength that can affect the earth varies with season, region, altitude, pollution, and the path that the solar radiation traverses through the ozone.[7] The amount of UV in sunlight also varies throughout the day. Being of a longer wavelength, UV-A is present consistently from sunrise to sunset, whereas UV-B peaks around noon. Approximately 50% of UV-A exposure occurs in the shade as a result of surface reflection and its penetration to cloud cover. Windows and automotive glass do not shield against UV-A but do shield against UV-B.[8]

For the purposes of phototherapy, UV-B has been further subdivided into broadband UV-B (290–320 nm) and narrrowband UV-B (311 nm–313 nm). UV-A radiation has been subdivided into UV-A1 (340–400 nm) and UV-A2 (320–340 nm), primarily because the biological effect of UV-A2 is closer to that of UV-B. The specific applications of these modalities are discussed in more detail in the article by Rkein and Ozog elsewhere in this issue.

## Light-Skin Interactions

Light has both the properties of waves and particles known as photons. In cutaneous photobiology, it is important to understand what happens to photons when they encounter the skin surface. They can undergo reflection, scattering, or absorption. According to the Grothus-Draper law, light can have a biological effect only if it is absorbed. Once radiation is absorbed by molecules in the skin (termed chromophores), energy is transferred to produce heat or drive photochemical reactions. This process results in detectable responses at the cellular and molecular levels that could lead to a clinical outcome (**Fig. 2**).[9,10]

### Reflection, scattering, and absorption

Reflection happens at the skin surface. Light reflected from the skin can be used for diagnostic

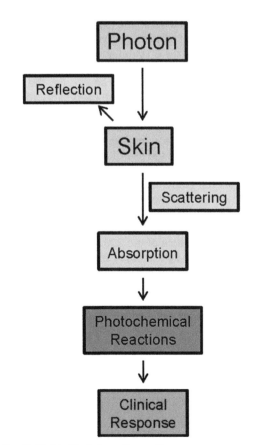

**Fig. 2.** Light-skin interaction pathway.

purposes but does not have much of a therapeutic role. Scattering alters the direction of the light transmission through the skin. How deep a photon can go is influenced by how much it is scattered by structures in the skin. Most scattering takes place in the dermis as a result of the presence of collagen. Scattering of radiation is also wavelength dependent; shorter wavelengths scatter more, whereas longer wavelengths penetrate deeper.[9,10]

The depth of light penetration is critical for phototherapy. UV-B is generally absorbed in the epidermis and upper dermis, whereas UV-A (because of its longer wavelengths) penetrates well into the dermis (Fig. 3). Shorter wavelength visible light such as blue light can be used in PDT for epidermal growths (such as actinic keratoses). Red light, which is of a longer visible wavelength, can target deeper structures such as sebaceous glands and thicker lesions.[11] Nonetheless, penetration depth is only 1 part of the equation. The light must also be of the appropriate wavelength to be absorbed by the target molecule or chromophore. Only on absorption can a photon exert a clinical effect.

Different wavelength(s) target different chromophores, which results in a variety of cutaneous effects.[11] Chromophores can be cellular/molecular components, such as amino acids, nucleotides, lipids, and 7-dehydrocholesterol (a vitamin D precursor). They can also be porphyrins (exogenous or endogenous), tattoo pigments, or photosensitizing drugs (eg, psoralens).[10] DNA directly absorbs UV-B and is therefore a chromophore targeted by UV-B phototherapy. In cosmetic laser treatments, endogenous chromophores targeted are mainly hemoglobin, melanin, and water.[12] Exogenous substances (ie, aminolevulinic acid solution, which converts to protoporphyrin IX) may also be used to act as chromophores, depending on the phototherapeutic modality.

Absorption is wavelength dependent and is influenced by the physicochemical structure of the chromophore.[4,10] Each chromophore has an absorption spectrum, which is the range of wavelengths that are absorbed by that molecule. For example, the absorption spectrum for melanin is 250 to 1200 nm.[13] The absorption maximum (ie, peak) is the wavelength or wavelengths that have the highest probability of being absorbed.[4]

### Photochemical reactions

When the chromophore absorbs the photon, it changes to a transient, excited state. Energy is released as light or heat when the chromophore returns from the excited state to the ground state. This process causes the chromophore to undergo chemical changes or transfer energy to a different molecule.[14] Sufficient amounts of energy (ie, photons) must be present for a cellular response to occur.[11] Only absorbed light can lead to a photochemical reaction, causing cellular changes, which eventually evoke a clinical response.[1] Fig. 4 is an example of a photochemical reaction that takes place when a chromophore, in this case a drug such as psoralen, absorbs UV-A. Action spectrum refers to the wavelengths of the radiation that are most efficient for inducing the desired effect.[9]

### BASIC PRINCIPLES OF PHOTOTHERAPY

To better appreciate the accompanying articles, this introduction briefly discusses the basics of phototherapy. The specifics for different types of phototherapy are discussed in other articles elsewhere in this issue.

As mentioned earlier, phototherapy is the use of nonionizing radiation to treat cutaneous disorders. Phototherapy is typically administered in a physician's office or treatment center. For some types of phototherapy, the patient stands in a booth lined with UV bulbs; more focused light sources, such as those used in targeted phototherapy, may also be used for treatment. The

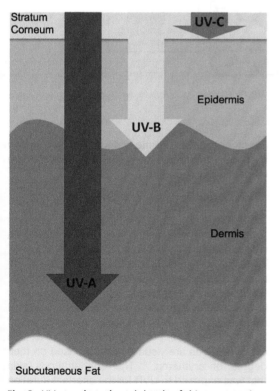

Fig. 3. UV wavelength and depth of skin penetration.

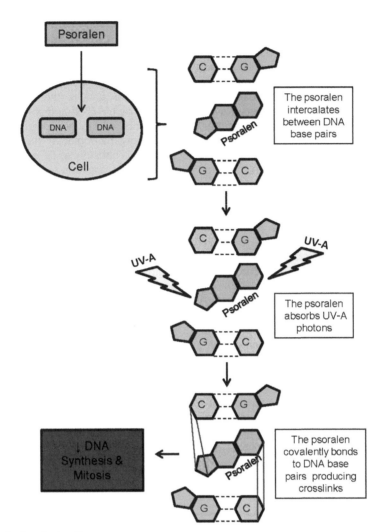

**Fig. 4.** PUVA photochemical pathway.

initial dose is determined empirically by assessing the patient's Fitzpatrick skin phototype (SPT), which is mainly based on history of burning versus tanning responses. The minimal erythema dose (MED) can also be used as the guide to deliver phototherapy.

## MED

To more quantitatively determine the appropriate dosage of UV radiation to administer in phototherapy, the MED is used.[15] A few dosing-related terms used in photodermatology are defined first. Irradiance (usually expressed as $J/s.cm^2$ or $mJ/s.cm^2$) is the intensity of the incident radiation on the patient. The irradiance of a light source or device can be measured by a radiometer. The exposure time (in seconds) is the length of time at which the patient receives UVR. The dose (in $J/cm^2$ or $mJ/cm^2$) is the amount of light energy that the patient receives. These 3 values are related in the equation:

$$\text{Dose } (mJ/cm^2) = \text{irradiance } (mJ/s.cm^2) \times \text{exposure time (s)}$$

MED, also known as the sunburn threshold, is a way to measure an individual's sensitivity to UVR.[2] The MED is the amount of UVR that produces minimal erythema: a faint pink response on the skin, which is best appreciated 16 to 24 hours after UV exposure. To determine the MED, adjacent areas of skin are exposed to increasing doses of UVR.[15] After a specified amount of time, the exposed areas are visually graded based on their degree of erythema.[16] The erythematous skin that was exposed to UVR for the shortest duration is the visual MED.[15] The visual clinical evaluation of these spots is subjective and, thus, varies from 1 observer to another. Nonetheless, a study by Bodekaer and colleagues[16] involving a few individuals did show that objectively measured skin erythema (by a skin reflectance meter) and subjectively measured skin erythema were in good agreement. To objectively calculate the MED, a chromameter can be used to measure the amount of erythema associated with each exposed area. The intensity of UVR (and thus the MED) varies depending on the UV device used, the lamp, and how far the lamp is from the skin.[15] Previous UV exposure or tanning also affects the MED, which is why it is usually performed in relatively sun-protected areas of the skin, such as the lower back or buttock.

The MED allows treatment to safely start at a dose that is usually higher than empirical starting doses based on SPT. This strategy usually results in achieving clinical response at a quicker pace, with fewer treatment sessions. MED is frequently used for UV-B phototherapy. The minimal phototoxic dose (MPD) is used for PUVA.[2] MPD is also defined as the lowest dose to produce erythema. The main difference is that it involves oral ingestion of 8-methoxypsoralen 1 hour before phototesting and is typically evaluated at 72 hours. However, because of the relative complexity of performing MPD, the SPT-based protocol is more commonly used to deliver PUVA therapy.

## Acute and Chronic Effects of UVR

Norman Paul established the association between sun exposure and skin cancer at the start of the 20th century. It was later postulated that UV-B caused sunburn and that UV-B–induced sunburn led to skin cancer. At the time, UV-B was considered the causative wavelength for skin carcinogenesis, and all other wavelengths were regarded as safe, Thus, sun protection products focused on blocking only UV-B rays, and it was believed that it was possible to tan without burning or causing harmful effects on the skin. Products were labeled suntan lotions for this reason. The sun protection factor (SPF) was introduced by Franz Greiter in the 1960s. By the late 1960s, UV-B exposure was noted to cause aging of the skin, and a decade later, UV-A was identified as another spectrum responsible for photoaging. As a result of these findings, in the 1980s, sun protection products changed their labeling from suntan lotions to sunscreens. Later, the concept of broad-spectrum protection was adopted, leading to the development of sunscreens with both UV-A and UV-B filters.

## UV Damage on a Molecular Level

### DNA damage and repair

DNA is a major target of UV-B.[8] Although DNA maximally absorbs from 245 to 290 nm,[14] UV-C (200–290 nm) does not penetrate the atmosphere, and thus, it is UV-B (290–320 nm) that primarily targets DNA. UV-B radiation is capable of traversing the stratum corneum. Epidermal DNA in keratinocytes and Langerhans cells directly absorbs UV-B, which is more cytotoxic and mutagenic than UV-A. UV-B causes most cyclobutane pyrimidine dimers (CPDs) and pyrimidone (6-4) pyrimidone photoproducts. These photoproducts are considered the signature lesions of UVR-induced DNA damage.[17,18] The 5-6 double-bond of pyrimidine (thymine or cytosine) bases is the most efficient area of DNA that absorbs UVR. A photon is absorbed by one of the pyrimidines that form a cyclobutane ring between the 2 adjacent pyrimidines. This ring is formed at the 5 and 6 positions, which results in a CPD. CPD is the most common product when DNA damage from UVR occurs. If a bond is formed at the 6-4 linkage, it is instead referred to as a pyrimidine-pyrimidone photoproduct.[7] Both of these photoproducts are structurally damaging. They distort the DNA helix, which halts RNA polymerase and inhibits gene expression.

UV-A, which comprises about 95% of terrestrial solar radiation, also inflicts damage in cellular DNA, despite DNA having minimal absorption within the wavelength range of UV-A.[18] The mechanisms are believed to be indirect and involve induction of oxidative stress.[17] DNA damage can also be caused by oxidation, most frequently at the 8 position of guanine. Oxidation by UVR results in formation of 8-oxo-guanine (8oG); thymine glycol is another oxidized base from UVR.[2] UV-A results in more oxidative damage than does UV-B. However, UV-A has also been shown to produce more CPD than 8oG.[18] Thus, CPD is still the most common product of DNA damage from UVR. The chromophores responsible for UV-A effects have not been defined and may be nonspecific, but presumably include proteins, lipids, and other cellular components.

DNA damage can influence DNA repair and gene expression. This situation can result in inhibition of antiinflammatory cytokines and, conversely, increased production of immunosuppressive cytokines. It can also lead to the production of collagen-degrading proteins (eg, matrix metalloproteinases).[2] Multiple proteins and enzymes are recruited to facilitate DNA repair. Nucleotide excision repair is used to repair bulky products such as CPD.[6] Base excision repair is used to repair modified bases such as 8oG. Other methods are also in place for DNA repair. If these methods fail, cell apoptosis or DNA mutations are the result.

During DNA repair or replication, errors can occur, and incorrect bases can be inserted. Erroneous additions, deletions, or rearrangements can occur, but most of these mutations are not catastrophic, because the genetic code is redundant and large portions of DNA are not used. However, if mutations occur at oncogenes or tumor suppressor genes, tumorigenesis may be favored. For instance, mutations of the tumor suppressor gene, p53, are found in many UV-induced skin cancers, such as squamous cell carcinomas.[17]

Perhaps the best example that shows the importance of DNA repair after UVR damage is seen in the genetic disorder known as xeroderma pigmentosum (XP). This is an autosomal-recessive condition characterized by deficient repair of UV-induced photoproducts.[17] The capacity to undergo DNA repair in patients with XP is decreased by up to 50%. However, their risk of carcinogenesis from UVR is increased by a factor of 1000. Patients with this disorder develop skin cancers in the first 2 decades of life, in addition to premature photoaging.[17]

### UVR-induced apoptosis

After UVR exposure, sunburn cells, or apoptotic keratinocytes, can be observed histologically.[17] Sunburn cells can be seen as early as half an hour after UVR.[14] This is a protective mechanism of the body to get rid of cells that may be at risk for malignant transformation.[5] Keratinocytes are more vulnerable to UVR than are melanocytes. This vulnerability is because keratinocytes cycle more often than melanocytes. Cells are more vulnerable to undergo apoptosis when they are undergoing DNA synthesis.[17] UV-B can lead to G1 and G2 phase cell cycle arrest. Hence, the cell cycle can be stopped before DNA replication (G1/S checkpoint) or chromosome segregation (G2/M checkpoint).[19] If the keratinocyte is severely damaged, it is likely to be destroyed by apoptosis, whereas a melanocyte may be able to survive.[17]

Apoptosis is a finely regulated process, with numerous checks and balances. There are antiapoptotic and proapoptotic pathways.[5] At least 3 mechanisms are known to activate the pathways leading to apoptosis: DNA damage, membrane receptor clustering, and formation of reactive oxygen species (ROS). Apoptosis causes morphologic changes in the cell, such as cell shrinkage and membrane blebbing, with chromatin condensation and DNA fragmentation.[5] This process leads to a cell with a pycnotic nucleus (the so-called sunburn cell) and to apoptotic bodies of membrane enclosed fragmented DNA.[5,19] These apoptotic bodies undergo phagocytosis by macrophages. This process is believed to occur in specific keratinocytes, sparing the surrounding tissues.

### Role of lipids

The combination of molecular oxygen plus UVR results in ROS, which can damage stratum corneum free lipids and the membranes of living cells.[7] ROS can oxidize lipids in 1 of 2 ways: directly, by oxidizing the double bonds of the lipid, or indirectly, via a chain reaction of oxidized lipids. The processing of the damaged lipid membranes in living cells is by enzymatic and nonenzymatic reactions, which can result in the expression of stress response genes or the production of prostaglandins, which mediate inflammatory reactions.[19]

### Role of proteins

UV effects on proteins are not as severe as those on DNA and lipids. This situation may be because the skin has several proteins, which are destroyed and remanufactured constantly. Nonetheless, protein components of the skin can be oxidized by ROS. ROS breakdown collagen and elastin fibers, leading to reduced dermal structural support and volume, a major factor in the wrinkling of the epidermis.[13] UVR can also cross-link collagen, elastin, and other proteins in the dermis, resulting in destruction of these proteins, which leads to the clinical effect of photoaging.[7]

Some proteins are cell surface receptors, and absorption of UVR may result in receptor clustering and other changes. This situation leads to the production of extracellular signals, resulting in cell activation.

## UV Damage on a Clinical Level

### Sun exposure: acute and chronic effects

**Sunburn and tanning** A sunburn is an acute inflammatory response to UV exposure, which causes vasodilation of dermal blood vessels. UV-B is the main culprit, and UV-B photons are about 1000-fold more efficient than longer wavelength UV-A at inducing erythema.[8]

An individual's inherent tendency to either burn or tan when exposed to UVR underlies the concept of SPT, or Fitzpatrick skin type, which is divided into 6 categories. Individuals with darker skin and higher Fitzpatrick SPT usually burn less and tan more, whereas Fitzpatrick SPT I individuals always burn and never tan (**Table 1**).[7]

Melanocytes are epidermal dendritic cells, which make up 5% to 10% of the basal cell layer. Melanin is packaged in melanosomes, which are

**Table 1
Fitzpatrick SPT**

| SPT | Reaction to Sun Exposure |
|-----|--------------------------|
| I | Always burns, never tans |
| II | Always burns, sometimes tans |
| III | Sometimes burns, gradually tans |
| IV | Sometimes burns, tans well |
| V | Rarely burns, always tans. Brown skin |
| VI | Never burns, always tans. Dark brown/ black skin |

transferred into keratinocytes via a dendritic process. This process causes the skin to be more pigmented (ie, tanner).[3,7] Melanin is a complex polymer of tyrosine derivatives. Melanosomes have eumelanin (brown/black pigment) and pheomelanin (yellow/red pigment).[3,19] Differences in skin color are not caused by the number of melanocytes in the skin but by variations in melanogenesis, differences in the amount of these pigments within melanosomes, and the size and density of melanosomes.[3] There is a mix of carotenoids and hemoglobin in the skin, which also contribute to skin color. The density of melanocytes is different throughout the body. The head and forearms have more melanocytes, whereas the palms and soles have fewer. In general, all skin types contain more eumelanin than pheomelanin. However, red hair can contain high levels of pheomelanin.[3]

Tanning is the darkening of skin that happens within hours to a few days after UVR.[17] There are 3 main steps, which may have overlapping mechanisms and features: (1) immediate pigment darkening; (2) persistent pigment darkening; and (3) delayed tanning. The first step, immediate pigment darkening, occurs within minutes of UVR exposure. It is caused by the redistribution of melanosomes (the packagers of melanin) and photo-oxidation of melanin (ie, the pigment), which is already present in the skin. The skin becomes initially gray and fades to brown within minutes. The second step, persistent pigment darkening, occurs within 1 hour after UVR and lasts 3 to 5 days, during which the skin is tan to brown. It is postulated that this step is a result of further oxidation of melanin. True melanogenesis (ie, the synthesis of new melanin) is primarily represented by the third step (delayed tanning), which typically starts 2 to 3 days after exposure. The tan is usually at its maximum from 10 days to 3 to 4 weeks and fades over several weeks to months as the melanin within the keratinocytes is sloughed off. The length

of the tan is dependent on the amount of UVR received and the individual's skin type.[3]

The purpose of melanogenesis goes beyond the cosmetic appearance of a tan. The increased pigmentation is helpful against future UV damage. A critical player in this process is the melanocortin 1 receptor (MC1R), which genetically influences variations in skin and hair color. The MC1R protein (a G-coupled receptor) sits on the melanocyte surface and regulates melanogenesis. When keratinocytes and melanocytes are exposed to UVR, α-melanocyte stimulating hormone and adrenocorticotropic hormone are secreted. This process leads to the upregulation of MC1R expression, which, after a series of molecular events, leads to melanogenesis.[7]

Melanin is important for photoprotection and functions as a broadband UV absorber, which decreases the penetration of UV through the epidermis. However, melanin does not provide total protection. It absorbs only 50% to 75% of UVR, and its SPF is only about 1.5 to 2 (maximum, 4).[3,19] Melanin also serves as a physical barrier to scatter UVR and functions as an antioxidant and scavenger for free oxygen radicals.[3]

**Vitamin D production** For most people, the major source of vitamin D is exposure to UV-B in sunlight, aside from dietary intake. Vitamin D, an antioxidant, has numerous health benefits, such as calcium absorption and bone maintenance. Synthesis of vitamin D starts in the epidermis (**Fig. 5**), with photolysis of 7-dehydrocholesterol (7-DHC), which is located within the cell membranes of keratinocytes, by UV-B. This process creates previtamin D, which is converted to a more stable form, vitamin $D_3$ (cholecalciferol) by thermal isomerization. Vitamin $D_3$ then goes into circulation and is picked up by vitamin D binding protein. Vitamin $D_3$ is taken to the liver to be hydroxylated to 25-hydroxyvitamin $D_3$ before it is transferred to the kidney to be converted into 1α25-dihydroxyvitamin $D_3$ (calcitriol), the biologically active form.[3,7,19,20] Skin pigmentation does have an effect on vitamin D production, because melanin competes with 7-DHC for UV-B photons.[20]

**Photoaging** Intrinsic (ie, chronologic) aging depends on natural chronologic senescence of cells. However, extrinsic factors such as UVR exposure can induce premature skin aging or photoaging. Phenotypically, photoaged skin is leathery in appearance and shows more wrinkles, telangiectasias, laxity, and uneven skin pigment. Histologically, the epidermis is thicker in photoaged skin.[14] However, the dermis shows most of the chronic

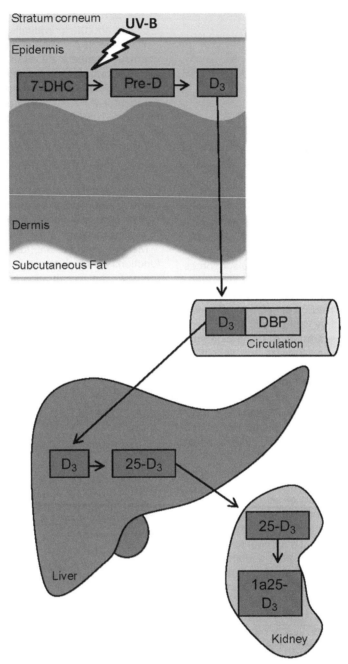

**Fig. 5.** Vitamin D synthesis. $D_3$, vitamin $D_3$ (cholecalciferol); DBP, vitamin D binding protein; Pre-D, previtamin D; 1a25-$D_3$, 1α25 dihydroxyvitamin $D_3$ (calcitriol); 7-DHC, 7-dehydrocholesterol; 25-$D_3$, 25-hydroxyvitamin $D_3$.

damage, especially secondary to the more deeply penetrating UV-A. UV-A leads to ROS production, which damages DNA, proteins, and lipids, as mentioned earlier. ROS also trigger cytokine cascades, leading to photoaging and alteration of the structural components of the skin.[21] Type I collagen, the most abundant protein in the dermis, and type III collagen give the skin its strength and elasticity. UVR-induced matrix metalloproteins cause direct degradation of the collagen. The products of collagen degradation also indirectly inhibit collagen synthesis.[22] In photoaged skin, there is disorganization and degradation of collagen fibrils, as well as reduced synthesis of type I and type III procollagen. Immediately after UVR, there is a decrease in type I procollagen synthesis. In very photodamaged skin, ongoing procollagen synthesis is diminished. Photoprotection with sunscreen and UV protective clothing can help prevent photoaging and slow its progression. Studies have shown that regular use of broad-spectrum sunscreen can prevent sunburn and photoaging effects such as rhytides (ie, wrinkles) and uneven pigmentation.[21]

**Carcinogenesis** Both melanoma and nonmelanoma cancers are influenced by UVR. Since 2004, there has been a 3% increase in the incidence of melanoma among Caucasians each year.[23] UVR from excess sun exposure is the most important modifiable risk factor for melanoma.[23]

Cutaneous melanomas arise from epidermal melanocytes. Melanoma formation is associated with intense, intermittent UVR exposure. It is frequently seen on areas of the body that are exposed to the sun only intermittently (ie, the lower legs in women and the back in men).[23] It is more common in people with indoor occupations, who receive intermittent UVR exposure on vacations and weekends. A history of 5 or more severe sunburns in adolescence more than doubles a person's risk of developing melanoma.[17] Similarly, artificial UV exposure via tanning beds is believed to be a potential contributor to the increase in incidence of melanoma in young women.[23] Unlike the severely UV-damaged keratinocyte, which undergoes apoptosis, the severely damaged melanocyte may not. Thus, intermittent, intense UVR exposure leads to less capacity to repair DNA and greater retention of damaged melanocytes.[17]

Basal and squamous cell carcinomas develop from epidermal keratinocytes and hair follicles. Unlike melanoma, which is associated with intense, intermittent UVR exposure, basal and squamous cell carcinomas are linked to cumulative exposure to UVR. They occur most often on chronically sun exposed areas of the body (ie, face, forearms, back of the hands), particularly in those with daily increased UVR exposure over their lifetime (eg, farmers, sailors, fishermen).[17]

*Phototherapy*

The biological effects of UV light and even visible light spectra may be used clinically in the treatment of certain skin diseases, such as psoriasis, atopic dermatitis, cutaneous T-cell lymphoma, and other photoresponsive dermatoses.

UV-B is used for the treatment of inflammatory cutaneous disorders, such as psoriasis. An acute phototoxic reaction manifesting as erythema is the most common acute side effect from overexposure to UV-B. This process occurs about 24 hours after treatment. Its equivalent for PUVA

may occur as late as 72 hours after exposure. Conjunctivitis and keratitis can occur if adequate eye protection is not used during treatment.[2]

UV therapy can provoke a photodermatosis (eg, polymorphous light eruption) or drug-induced photosensitivity. If a culprit phototoxic medication is being used, drug-induced photosensitivity can lead to an exaggerated sunburn effect.

PDT, in which a photosensitizer is applied to the skin before controlled exposure to visible light, is used for treatment of neoplasms such as actinic keratoses, squamous cell carcinomas, and basal cell carcinomas. It also has benefit in some inflammatory conditions, such as acne. The acute side effects of PDT are typically phototoxic reactions and pain. The phototoxic reactions are characterized by erythema, edema, or hyperpigmentation.[12] Pain depends on the type of photosensitizer being used. This pain, often referred to as a smarting reaction, is the most common side effect of PDT at the time of treatment; analgesia may be needed for pain control.[1]

Chronic side effects of UV phototherapy include lentigines, photoaging, actinic keratoses, and skin cancer formation. There has yet to be confirmation that UV-B phototherapy increases the risk of basal or squamous cell carcinomas.[2] A meta-analysis of 11 studies evaluating skin cancer risk after UV-B phototherapy[24] found no significant increased risk of nonmelanoma or melanoma skin cancer. However, there is a dose-related increased risk for cutaneous malignancy, particularly squamous cell carcinoma, after cumulative high-dose systemic PUVA therapy.[1,2] Male genitalia, in particular, have greater risk for squamous cell carcinoma after PUVA exposure.[1] Lower-dose UV-A is used to minimize this risk. The risk for malignancy after PUVA is heightened with concomitant use of immunosuppressive medications such as cyclosporine and azathioprine. Although less established, there is also concern for increased melanoma risk in patients with PUVA.[1,25,26] PUVA exposure does not significantly increase the risk of cataracts in patients who use eye protection.[27]

*Phototesting with Artificial Light Sources*

Phototesting is the process of evaluating a patient's sensitivity to specific wavelengths of UV and visible radiation, sometimes performed in the research setting, or at times, conducted in the clinic for the purpose of narrowing down the etiologic spectrum behind a photoaggravated skin rash. At times, these artificial light sources are also used for phototherapy. Artificial sources of radiation can imitate solar radiation or isolate certain areas of the optical radiation spectrum. All artificial sources of radiation can generate light, modify light to the appropriate spectral output, and deliver the light to the source (ie, skin). Most medical light devices generate radiation by converting electrical energy to light energy. Optical filters and specific chromophores are used to isolate certain wavelengths. Mirrors, lenses, and fibers are then used to direct the light to the specified target.[9]

Many lamps produce an assortment of wavelengths and are characterized by the wavelengths that they produce (ie, UV-A vs UV-B). The quality and quantity of light that reaches the skin (ie, the emission spectrum) is the most important property of the lamp. The manufacturer usually determines the emission spectra of a device. The emission spectrum is a plot of the irradiance of a lamp as a function of wavelength.[9] The irradiance, which can be measured by a radiometer, is the intensity of the incident radiation on the skin of the patient. The irradiance is used to calculate the MED (as mentioned earlier) by dose = irradiance × exposure time.

Solar simulators are light sources that mimic natural sunlight. They are used to test sunscreens[28] and for the diagnostic workup of photosensitivity.[29] The following sections describe some of the more common artificial light sources available.

### Arc lamps

The arc lamp was the first effective artificial light source. In arc lamps, 2 electrodes are sealed in a transparent envelope with gas (eg, mercury or xenon). A high voltage is applied across this apparatus. The electric current leads to an excitation of electrons within the gas. Light is emitted when the gas returns to its ground state, and hence, it is also known as a gas discharge lamp. The plasma between the electrodes is the arc.[9] Different gases and pressures lead to different spectral output. Xenon arc lamps are used as solar simulators.

### Excimer

The excimer is a relatively new technology for delivering targeted UV therapy. Monochromatic excimer light uses a xenon-chloride gas combination. It emits wavelengths at 308 nm. The excimer (or excited dimer) is an excited complex of noble gas plus reactive gas (a halogen), which forms an excited complex. When this complex decomposes, it gives off excess energy as UVR. There are 2 devices that use this gas combination. One is the excimer laser, which is characterized by intermittent (pulsing), monochromatic (1 wavelength), and coherent (targeted) light. The excimer laser is approved by the US Food and Drug Administration for treatment of psoriasis, atopic

dermatitis, and vitiligo. The other device is the excimer lamp, which gives off polychromatic, incoherent (nontargeted) light, with a range of wavelengths from 306 to 310 nm and a peak around 308 nm. The lamp can treat a range of body surface areas.[30]

### Fluorescent lamps

Fluorescence is the re-emission of absorbed light. A photon is absorbed by a fluorophore (ie, a chromophore for fluorescence), then re-emitted. The emitted photon is of lower energy than the initial photon that was absorbed. In a fluorescent lamp, mercury is sealed in cylindrical glass tubes. Current is applied to the ends of the tubes. The mercury is vaporized to a higher energy state. Radiation is released when mercury falls back to its ground state. In fluorescent lamps, the primary radiation is absorbed by phosphors, which are the fluorophores that coat the tube. The phosphors then re-emit light at longer wavelengths.[9]

Fluorescent lamps are the most frequently used sources of therapeutic UVR in dermatology. Depending on the size, some UV lamps can deliver full body treatments, whereas others are more suitable for target areas (ie, palms and soles). Different phosphors lead to UV-A, UV-B, or visible light. Fluorescent lamps can also be used for diagnosis. The Wood lamp is commonly used in the office setting for diagnosing dermatologic conditions, such as vitiligo, fungal infections, and erythrasma. The Wood lamp emits UV-A radiation at 365 nm. Fluorophores in the form of collagen, elastin, and porphyrins absorb the UV-A. They then re-emit fluorescent light at a longer wavelength, which is visible.

### Light-emitting diodes

Light-emitting diodes (LEDs) are semiconductors that change electrical current to light.[11] They emit low-intensity, narrowband light.[31] Emitted light can be in the range of UV to near infrared (247–1300 nm), depending on what the device is being used for.[11] LEDs can deliver the same wavelengths of light as lasers but at a lower energy output. For instance, laser power output is often measured in watts, whereas LED power output is often measures in milliwatts. An LED device can be made up of panels, which allow treatment of large areas[31] with acceptably short treatment times (seconds to minutes).[11]

LEDs have been used safely in PDT of neoplasms, acne, wound healing, cosmetic photorejuvenation, and other indications.

### Lasers

Laser is an acronym for light amplification by stimulated emission of radiation. In stimulated emission, the photon that strikes an excited molecule has energy that is equivalent to the energy transition between the excited to ground state of that molecule. Hence, the incident and emitted photons are of the same wavelength, phase, and direction. This characteristic gives lasers their monochromatic (ie, single wavelength) and coherent spectral output.[9]

The vital components of a laser are its lasing medium, longitudinal optical cavity, and external energy source. The lasing medium can be solid, liquid, or gas. The laser cavity holds the laser medium. An external energy source causes the excitation of the molecules in the medium. Stimulated emission occurs in the laser medium. The laser pumping source (ie, external energy source) is usually a radiofrequency generator or an intense light source (eg, flashlamp). Depending on the pumping source used, lasers can produce light in either continuous or pulsed modes. Lasers are classified by their lasing medium, wavelength, or mode of operation (ie, continuous or pulsed).[9]

Lasers are used in dermatology to generate heat within the skin via selective photothermolysis (ie, selective thermal damage). Depending on the wavelength, lasers can select a given chromophore and destroy it, with minimal damage to the surrounding tissue.[14] Hemoglobin, melanin, artificial pigment (tattoos), and collagen are some of the skin structures that can be targeted by lasers.[1] The wavelength and pulse duration can be chosen depending on the target. The laser wavelength is determined by the depth and absorption characteristics of the target chromophore. The pulse duration is chosen based on the size of the target; smaller targets require shorter pulse.[9] Laser output is reproducible (ie, the same wavelength is emitted during each pulse) and offers the user good control to navigate where the treatment is going.

## SUMMARY

The sun is our natural source of light. It emits energy essential to life and allows the skin cells to biochemically synthesize vitamin D, which helps prevent bone disorders and other diseases. However, excessive sun exposure can lead to sunburn, photoaging, and skin cancer; hence, appropriate and adequate photoprotection is necessary. Susceptibility to harmful effects of UV light is influenced by inherent factors, such as an individual's skin type, genetics, and photosensitivities, as well as external and societal factors. Artificial sources of UV and visible light may be optimized for phototherapy for certain skin diseases.

Phototherapy also has its side effects, and risk-benefit ratios must be discussed and carefully considered.

## REFERENCES

1. Zanolli M. The modern paradigm of phototherapy. Clin Dermatol 2003;21(5):398–406.
2. Iordanou E, Berneburg M. Phototherapy and photochemotherapy. J Dtsch Dermatol Ges 2010;8(7): 533–41.
3. Brenner M, Hearing VJ. The protective role of melanin against UV damage in human skin. Photochem Photobiol 2008;84(3):539–49.
4. Diffey B, Kochevar I. Basic principles of photobiology. In: Lim H, Honigsmann H, Hawk JL, editors. Photodermatology. New York: Informa Healthcare; 2007. p. 15–27.
5. Murphy G, Young AR, Wulf HC, et al. The molecular determinants of sunburn formation. Exp Dermatol 2001;10(3):155–60.
6. Dupont E, Gomez J, Bilodeau D. Beyond UV radiation: a skin under challenge. Int J Cosmet Sci 2013;35(3):224–32.
7. Longo D, Fauci AS, Kasper DL, et al. Photosensitivity and other reactions to light. Harrison's principles of internal medicine. 18th edition. New York: McGraw-Hill; 2011.
8. Schaefer H, Moyal D, Fourtanier A. Recent advances in sun protection. Semin Cutan Med Surg 1998;17(4):266–75.
9. Lui H, Anderson RR. Radiation sources and interaction with the skin. In: Lim H, Honigsmann H, Hawk JL, editors. Photodermatology. New York: Informa Healthcare; 2007. p. 29–40.
10. Hamzavi I, Lui H. Using light in dermatology: an update on lasers, ultraviolet phototherapy and photodynamic therapy. Dermatol Clin 2005;23(2): 199–207.
11. Barolet D. Light-emitting diodes (LEDs) in dermatology. Semin Cutan Med Surg 2008;27(4):227–38.
12. Babilas P, Schreml S, Szeimies RM, et al. Intense pulsed light (IPL): a review. Lasers Surg Med 2010;42(2):93–104.
13. Ciocon D, Boker A, Goldberg DJ. Intense pulsed light: what works, what's new, what's next. Facial Plast Surg 2009;25(5):290–300.
14. Rabe J, Mamelak AJ, McElgunn PJ, et al. Photoaging: mechanisms and repair. J Am Acad Dermatol 2006;55(1):1–19.
15. Heckman C, Chandler R, Kloss JD, et al. Minimal erythema dose (MED) testing. J Vis Exp 2013;75:e50175.
16. Bodekaer M, Philipsen PA, Karlsmark T, et al. Good agreement between minimal erythema dose test reactions and objective measurements: an in vivo study of human skin. Photodermatol Photoimmunol Photomed 2013;29(4):190–5.

17. Gilchrest B, Eller MS, Geller AC, et al. The pathogenesis of melanoma induced by ultraviolet radiation. N Engl J Med 1999;340(17):1341–8.

18. Courdavault S, Baudouin C, Charveron M, et al. Larger yield of cyclobutane dimer than 8-oxo-7, 8-dihydroguanine in the DNA of UVA-irradiated human skin cells. Mutat Res 2004;556(1–2):135–42.

19. Garmyn M, Yarosh DB. The molecular and genetic effects of ultraviolet radiation exposure on skin cells. In: Lim H, Honigsmann H, Hawk JL, editors. Photodermatology. New York: Informa Healthcare; 2007. p. 41–54.

20. Kift R, Berry JL, Vail A, et al. Lifestyle factors including less cutaneous sun exposure contribute to starkly lower vitamin D levels in UK South Asians compared with the white population. Br J Dermatol 2013;169(6):1272–8.

21. McCullough J, Kelly KM. Prevention and treatment of skin aging. Ann N Y Acad Sci 2006;1067:323–31.

22. Fisher G, Kang S, Varani J, et al. Mechanisms of photoaging and chronological skin aging. Arch Dermatol 2002;138(11):1462–70.

23. Chen S, Geller AC, Tsao H. Update on the epidemiology of melanoma. Curr Dermatol Rep 2013;2(1):24–34.

24. Lee E, Koo J, Berger T. UVB phototherapy and skin cancer risk: a review of the literature. Int J Dermatol 2005;44(5):355–60.

25. Stern R, Nichols KT, Vakeva L. Malignant melanoma in patients treated for psoriasis with methoxsalen (psoralen) and ultraviolet A radiation (PUVA). N Engl J Med 1997;336(15):1041–5.

26. Stern R. The risk of melanoma in association with long-term exposure to PUVA. J Am Acad Dermatol 2001;44(5):755–61.

27. Malanos D, Stern RS. Psoralen plus ultraviolet A does not increase the risk of cataracts: a 25-year prospective study. J Am Acad Dermatol 2007; 57(2):231–7.

28. Food and Drug Administration, HHS. Sunscreen products for over-the-counter human use. Final monograph FR. Fed Regist 1999;64(98):27666–93.

29. Roelandts R. The diagnosis of photosensitivity. Arch Dermatol 2000;136:1152–7.

30. Park K, Liao W, Murase JE. A review of monochromatic excimer light in vitiligo. Br J Dermatol 2012; 167(3):468–78.

31. Dierickx C, Anderson RR. Visible light treatment of photoaging. Dermatol Ther 2005;18(3):191–208.

# Evaluation of Patients with Photodermatoses

David Choi, BS[a], Swati Kannan, MD[b], Henry W. Lim, MD[b],*

## KEYWORDS

- Photodermatoses • Polymorphous light eruption • Chronic actinic dermatitis • Solar urticaria
- Actinic prurigo • Phototoxic dermatitis • Evaluation of photodermatoses

## KEY POINTS

- There are 4 general categories of photodermatoses: (1) immunologically mediated photodermatoses, (2) drug-induced and chemical-induced photosensitivity, (3) defective DNA repair disorders, and (4) photoaggravated conditions.
- Significant components of the history include age of onset, exposure to photosensitizers, interval between sun exposure and development of eruptions, season and duration of eruption, effect of window glass, and family history.
- Careful evaluation of the distribution of lesions on sun-exposed, relatively sun-exposed, and sun-protected areas should be done during the physical examination.
- Phototesting can be used to confirm the presence of a photosensitivity disorder, and photopatch testing is used to evaluate patients with photoallergic contact dermatitis.
- For most photodermatoses, strict photoprotection is first-line therapy.

## OVERVIEW

Only a limited portion of the solar spectrum reaches the Earth's surface, and this includes 2% of ultraviolet radiation (UVR), 32% of visible light, and 66% of infrared light. UVR is divided into ultraviolet B (UVB; 290–320 nm, the sunburn spectrum) and ultraviolet A (UVA; 320–400 nm). UVA is further subdivided into UVA-1 (340–400 nm) and UVA-2 (320–340 nm). UVB, and to a lesser extent UVA-2, is mainly responsible for erythema, whereas UVA is predominantly responsible for tanning, photoaging, and drug-induced photosensitivity.[1]

Cutaneous photosensitivity is due to the existence of molecules called chromophores that absorb UVR during exposure to the sun. DNA is the most abundant chromophore, triggering UVR-related changes such as tanning, sun burning, hyperplasia, aging, and carcinogenesis.[2] Only certain individuals, however, develop aberrant reactions to UVR, also known as photodermatoses.

Photodermatoses are disorders that are caused or exacerbated by exposure to UVR or visible light, and can be classified into 4 broad categories: (1) immunologically mediated photodermatoses, previously referred to as idiopathic; (2) drug-induced and chemical-induced photosensitivity (either exogenous from ingested or externally applied drugs or chemicals, or endogenous, as in cutaneous porphyrias); (3) photoaggravated dermatoses, including autoimmune diseases, infectious conditions, and nutritional deficiencies; and (4) defective DNA repair disorders.[3] **Box 1** lists the photodermatoses by these categories. Furthermore, photodermatoses can range from extremely rare disorders such as hydroa vacciniforme (prevalence of 0.34 per 100,000) to common disorders such as polymorphous light eruption (PMLE; prevalence 10%–20% of the general population).

Patients with photodermatoses can present with diverse clinical features, and diagnosis can often

Disclosures: None.
[a] Department of Dermatology, Yale School of Medicine, 333 Cedar Street, New Haven, CT 06510, USA;
[b] Department of Dermatology, Henry Ford Health System, Henry Ford Hospital, 3031 West Grand Boulevard, Suite 800, Detroit, MI 48202, USA
* Corresponding author.
E-mail address: hlim1@hfhs.org

Dermatol Clin 32 (2014) 267–275
http://dx.doi.org/10.1016/j.det.2014.03.006
0733-8635/14/$ – see front matter © 2014 Elsevier Inc. All rights reserved.

is performed. In those patients requiring photopatch testing, 2 sets of photoallergens are applied, usually on the back. The sites are then covered with opaque dressings. During the third visit, the results of the phototest are read, and the minimal erythema dose (MED) for UVB (MED-B) and UVA (MED-A) is determined. MED is defined as the lowest dose of UVA or UVB that will produce perceptible erythema over the entire exposed site. At the same visit, one set of photoallergens are exposed to UVA. On the fourth visit, both irradiated and nonirradiated photopatch test sites are read; the patient may be asked to return on the eighth to tenth day for assessment of delayed positive response. **Table 1** summarizes the key steps in evaluating a patient with photodermatoses.[4]

## HISTORY

A thorough evaluation of the patient's history is an important step in establishing the correct diagnosis.

### Age of Onset

The age of onset is helpful in directing the differential diagnosis, as some photodermatoses more commonly manifest in certain age groups (**Box 2**). For example, the average age of onset for PMLE is 23 years. Juvenile spring eruption, a PMLE variant, often presents in childhood or during early adolescence.[7,8] Other photodermatoses characterized by childhood onset include actinic prurigo,

**Table 1**
**Evaluation of a photosensitive patient**

| | |
|---|---|
| First visit | Thorough history and physical examination |
| Second visit | Phototesting with UVA, UVB, and/or visible light<br>First reading of the phototest reactions<br>Application of duplicate sets of photoallergens if photopatch testing is required |
| Third visit | Second reading of phototest results and determination of MED for UVA and UVB<br>Exposure of one set of photoallergens to UVA |
| Fourth visit | Reading of all irradiated and nonirradiated photopatch test sites |
| Fifth visit | Assessment of delayed positive responses at the photopatch test sites |

*Abbreviations:* MED, minimal erythema dose; UVA, ultraviolet A; UVB, ultraviolet B.
*Data from* Refs.[1,3–6]

be difficult, especially if patients present during disease-free intervals. Therefore, proper evaluation of the patient is critical. The evaluation begins with a detailed history, thorough physical examination, phototesting, and, if necessary, photopatch testing. Laboratory investigations such as skin biopsy, antinuclear antibody (ANA) panel, plasma, urine, and stool porphyrins can be helpful in the appropriate setting.

A thorough evaluation of photosensitivity requires several clinic visits, described in subsequent paragraphs. On the first visit the patient should be evaluated with a comprehensive history and physical examination. On the second visit, phototesting with UVA, UVB, and/or visible light

*When the Patient is a Child:*

- Juvenile spring eruption
- Childhood porphyrias (ie, erythropoietic protoporphyria, congenital erythropoietic protoporphyria)
- Actinic prurigo
- Hydroa vacciniforme
- Genodermatoses

*When the Patient is an Adult:*

- Polymorphous light eruption
- Drug-induced photosensitivity
- Solar urticaria
- Lupus erythematosus
- Porphyria cutanea tarda

*When the Patient is Elderly:*

- Chronic actinic dermatitis
- Drug-induced photosensitivity
- Dermatomyositis

*Data from* Refs.[1,4–10]

erythropoietic protoporphyria, and congenital erythropoietic porphyria. Chronic actinic dermatitis occurs most commonly in men older than 50 years.[9,10]

## Seasonal Variation, Interval Before Onset, Duration of the Eruption

Subtle differences in seasonal variation, interval between sun exposure and onset of cutaneous lesions, and duration of eruption help to differentiate among the various types of photodermatoses. PMLE appears in spring or early summer, and the likelihood of recurrence typically decreases as summer progresses, suggesting a "hardening" or immunologic tolerance. PMLE also tends to be chronic and recurrent, and can worsen with each season. The interval between sun exposure and the development of lesions in PMLE ranges from 30 minutes to several hours; the lesions resolve within a few days if further sun exposure is avoided.[11,12]

Patients with chronic actinic dermatitis (CAD) suffer with a persistent eczematous eruption throughout the year, which typically becomes exacerbated in the summertime. Symptoms of CAD

can persist for several years, with approximately 20% of patients entering remission within 10 years of disease onset.[9,13]

In solar urticaria, lesions appear within 5 to 10 minutes of exposure and resolve within 1 to 3 hours.[14,15] Similarly to PMLE, solar urticaria may demonstrate hardening as the season progresses. Following cutaneous or systemic exposure to a phototoxic agent and appropriate UVR, phototoxicity develops within hours.

## Family History

It is crucial to obtain the family history when evaluating the porphyrias, such as congenital erythropoietic porphyria (autosomal recessive), familial form of porphyria cutanea tarda (autosomal dominant), hereditary coproporphyria (autosomal dominant), variegate porphyria (autosomal dominant), and erythropoietic protoporphyria (autosomal dominant, rarely autosomal recessive). Positive family history has been reported in 5% to 75% of patients with actinic prurigo, depending on the patient population studied.[16,17] A family history of autoimmune or connective tissue disease should also be obtained, as these conditions are associated with photoaggravated dermatoses.[18]

## Systemic Abnormalities

Visceral and neurologic manifestations such as abdominal pain, vomiting, and motor neuropathy, along with blistering skin lesions or skin fragility, can indicate that the patient may have one of the porphyrias: hereditary coproporphyria or variegate porphyria.[19,20] Polyarthritis, Raynaud phenomenon, or pulmonary disease, such as interstitial lung disease, along with photosensitivity suggest a possible diagnosis of systemic lupus erythematosus or dermatomyositis.

Rare genodermatoses involving DNA repair defects or chromosomal instability, such as xeroderma pigmentosum or Bloom syndrome, can manifest with photosensitivity, along with systemic signs such as skin cancer or craniofacial defects.

## Window Glass

Whereas basic window glass filters out UVB and transmits UVA and visible light, automobile glass provides different properties of UV protection depending on the type of glass. Windshields are made from laminated glass, which can block a large amount of UVA (up to 380 nm). However, most side and rear windows are tinted and not laminated glass. Thus, a significant amount of UVA-1 can still reach vehicle passengers through side and rear windows and induce a cutaneous eruption in photosensitive patients.[21]

## Exposure to Photosensitizers

Detailed inquiry into possible exposure to photosensitizing agents is important for certain photodermatoses. Exposure to photosensitizers can result in 2 types of reactions: phototoxicity and photoallergy. An exaggerated sunburn-like reaction is characteristic of a phototoxic reaction, which results from simultaneous exposure to exogenous agents (via ingestion, injection, or topical application) and to UVR or visible light. There are 2 types of phototoxic reactions: (1) systemic dermatitis in individuals systemically exposed to a photosensitizing agent and subsequent UVR; and (2) local phototoxic dermatitis, occurring in individuals topically exposed to a photosensitizing agent and subsequent UVR. Common phototoxic sensitizers include antiarrhythmics, diuretics (furosemides), and psoralens. A photoallergic reaction, which is a delayed type of hypersensitivity, presents with pruritic, eczematous dermatitis; however, morphologically differentiating this type of reaction from a phototoxic reaction can be difficult. Common photoallergens include sunscreen agents such as oxybenzone, nonsteroidal anti-inflammatory drugs, antimicrobials such as chlorhexidine, and fragrances.[2] Common phototoxic and photoallergic agents are listed in **Table 2**.

## EPIDEMIOLOGY AND PREVALENCE

PMLE is the most common photodermatosis, with a prevalence of 10% in Boston, 14% in London, and 21% in Sweden. Actinic prurigo is most commonly seen in Mestizos and in populations living in higher altitudes in the Americas; it has also been well reported in patients residing in the United Kingdom.[16] Drug-induced or chemical-induced photosensitivity occurs most commonly in adults.

**Table 2**
**The most common phototoxic and photoallergic agents**

| Common Phototoxic Agents | Common Photoallergic Agents |
|---|---|
| Antiarrhythmics | Topical Agents |
| Amiodarone | Sunscreen agents |
| Quinidine | UVA absorbers: benzophenones |
| Diuretics | Fragrances |
| Furosemide | 6-Methylcoumarin |
| Thiazides (chlorothiazide, dyazide) | Musk ambrette |
| Nonsteroidal anti-inflammatory drugs | Sandalwood oil |
| Nabumetone | Antibacterial agents |
| Naproxen | Dibromosalicylanilide |
| Piroxicam | Tetrachlorosalicylanilide |
| Phenothiazines | Bithionol |
| Chlorpromazine | Sulfonamides |
| Prochlorperazine | Chlorhexidine |
| Furocoumarins | Fenticlor |
| Psoralens (5-methoxypsoralen, 8-methoxypsoralen, 4,5′,8-trimethylpsoralen) | Hexachlorophene |
| Antibacterial | Antifungals |
| Quinolones (ciprofloxacin, lomefloxacin, nalidixic acid, sparfloxacin) | Thiobischlorophenol |
| Tetracyclines (demeclocycline, doxycycline) | Buclosamide |
| Sulfonamides | Bromochlorosalicylanilide |
| Antifungals | Systemic Agents |
| Voriconazole | Antiarrhythmics |
| Griseofulvin | Quinidine |
| Antipsychotic drugs | Antifungal |
| Phenothiazines (chlorpromazine, prochlorperazine) | Griseofulvin |
| St. John's wort | Antimalarial |
| Hypericin | Quinine |
| Tar (topical) | Antimicrobials |
| Photodynamic therapy agents | Quinolones |
| Porfimer | Sulfonamides |
| Verteporfin | Nonsteroidal anti-inflammatory drugs |
| | Diclofenac |
| | Ketoprofen |
| | Piroxicam |

Data from Refs.[1,2,5,22,23]

## PATHOPHYSIOLOGY

In brief, the skin contains chromophores, such as DNA, that absorb UV photons during exposure. The absorbed energy is then re-emitted as harmless and longer wavelengths of radiation (ie, fluorescence) or harmful thermochemical reactions that can lead to molecular, cellular, tissue, and clinical changes. Reactive oxygen species can also be generated during this exposure. This abnormal response can be produced by an endogenous cause, as occurs in the porphyrias, or an exogenous cause following ingestion or application of a photosensitizing drug. In photoallergic dermatitis, the chemical agent on the skin absorbs photons and forms a new, modified photoproduct that subsequently binds to surrounding proteins to form a new antigen, eliciting a type-IV delayed hypersensitivity reaction.

The porphyrias, notably, are caused by a deficiency in enzymes required to form heme molecules. This enzyme defect leads to a pathologic accumulation of porphyrins, which absorb light in the Soret band (major peak absorption at 400–410 nm). The photoexcited porphyrins initiate a cascade of events, eventually resulting in a clinical presentation of photosensitivity.[17]

## CLINICAL FINDINGS

The physical examination should pay close attention to the distribution of lesions on sun-exposed, relatively sun-protected, or completely sun-protected areas. Photodermatoses manifest in sun-exposed regions including the forehead, the cheeks, the V-region or nape of the neck, the dorsum of the hands, and the extensor aspects of bilateral forearms. It is also important to examine the relatively sun-protected areas, such as the nasolabial folds, the posterior auricular areas, the upper eyelids, the periorbital areas in patients who wear glasses, the superior aspects of the pinna (which may be covered by hair), and the submental area. Relatively sun-protected sites are spared in photodermatoses, although these areas may be involved in airborne contact dermatitis.

Photodermatoses are characterized by diverse morphologies, and a comprehensive perusal of the skin can assist the physician in arriving at the correct diagnosis. Urticarial lesions are seen in solar urticaria and erythropoietic protoporphyria.[14,24] Porphyria cutanea tarda is characterized by increased photosensitivity, skin fragility, blisters, milia, crusts, and scars at mainly sun-exposed sites (Fig. 1).[24] Papular lesions commonly characterize PMLE and acute exacerbations of CAD.[11] In

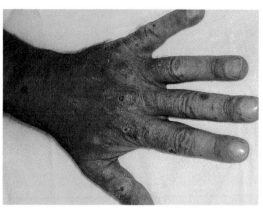

**Fig. 1.** Dorsal hand of a man showing skin fragility resulting in crusted erosions of porphyria cutanea tarda.

PMLE, lesions consist of mildly pruritic, grouped, erythematous, or skin-colored papules of varying sizes. However, darkly pigmented individuals typically present with grouped, pinhead-sized papules (Fig. 2).[25] Juvenile spring eruption, which normally affects young boys, is characterized by vesicles affecting the helices of the ears.

Actinic prurigo distinctively presents as a pruritic and crusted papular eruption. The most severe form of actinic prurigo classically afflicts Native Americans, especially Mestizos (individuals with a mixed ancestry of Native American and Caucasian backgrounds), and frequently occurs in conjunction with cheilitis and conjunctivitis (Fig. 3).[26] CAD appears as a chronic eczematous eruption that is frequently associated with lichenification, owing to the pruritic and chronic nature of the lesions (Fig. 4).

Photoallergy resembles allergic contact dermatitis and presents with pruritic, eczematous lesions, whereas phototoxic reactions demonstrate an exaggerated sunburn-like reaction.

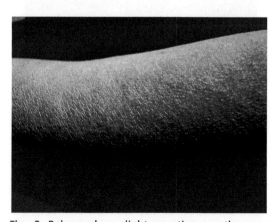

**Fig. 2.** Polymorphous light eruption on the arm, showing pinhead papules coalescing into plaques, occurring a day after sun exposure.

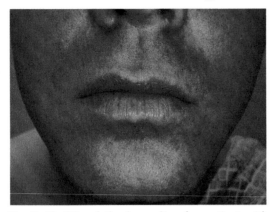

**Fig. 3.** Cheilitis of the lower lip of a patient with actinic prurigo.

Phytophotodermatitis represents a localized phototoxic reaction that displays linear streaks of erythema, arising a day after skin exposure to plants containing furocoumarins and sunlight.[2] **Table 3** lists the differential diagnoses based on lesion morphology.

### Histology

The histology for many photodermatoses can be nonspecific; however, there are certain characteristic findings that can help distinguish one over the other. Actinic prurigo characteristically displays

| Table 3 |
|---|
| **The differential diagnosis of photodermatoses most commonly associated with lesion morphology** |

| Morphology | Possible Diagnosis |
|---|---|
| Urticaria or urticarial | Solar urticaria<br>Erythropoietic protoporphyria |
| Papule | Polymorphous light eruption<br>Actinic prurigo<br>Chronic actinic dermatitis |
| Vesicle | Polymorphous light eruption<br>Juvenile spring eruption<br>Porphyria cutanea tarda<br>Variegate porphyria<br>Coproporphyria<br>Phototoxicity<br>Photoallergy<br>Hydroa vacciniforme |
| Erosion, crust | Actinic prurigo<br>Hydroa vacciniforme<br>Porphyrias (PCT, VP, CEP, HC) |
| Eczema and/or lichenification | Chronic actinic dermatitis |
| Erythema | Phototoxicity |
| Scars | Hydroa vacciniforme<br>PCT<br>VP<br>CEP |

*Abbreviations:* CEP, congenital erythropoietic porphyria; HC, hereditary coproporphyria; PCT, porphyria cutanea tarda; VP, variegate porphyria.
*Data from* Refs.[1,2,5,14,26,27]

lymphoid follicles on tissue biopsied from the lips.[28] CAD may contain atypical mononuclear cells in the epidermis and dermis.[29] The cutaneous porphyrias are distinguished by immunoglobulin, and complement deposition along the dermoepidermal junction and in perivascular regions.

Furthermore, biopsies of phototoxicity reveal scattered necrotic keratinocytes ("sunburn cells") and a dermal infiltrate composed of primarily lymphocytes and neutrophils; alternatively, photoallergy is characterized by epidermal spongiosis and a dermal lymphohistiocytic infiltrate.

### Laboratory and Photobiology Tests

#### Blood tests
Certain blood tests such as ANA, anti-SSA (Ro), anti-SSB (La), and plasma porphyrin levels can narrow the differential diagnosis when PMLE, lupus, or porphyrias are suspected. If plasma

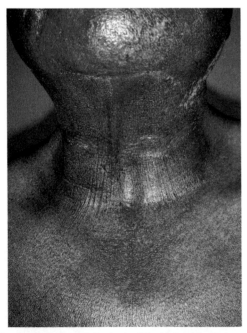

**Fig. 4.** Chronic actinic dermatitis. Lichenification and hyperpigmentation on sun-exposed sites, with sparing of skin folds on the neck and photoprotected areas on the upper chest.

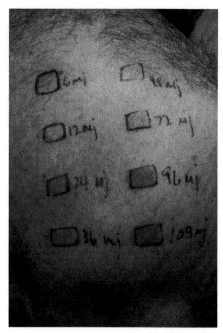

**Fig. 5.** Phototesting results at 24 hours after exposure. The lowest dose of broadband ultraviolet B (UVB) that resulted in erythema covering the entire irradiated site is at 24 mJ/cm², which is the minimal erythema dose for UVB in this patient.

porphyrin levels are elevated, a complete porphyrin profile, which includes erythrocyte, urine, and stool porphyrin levels, is indicated to further specify the type of cutaneous porphyria.[24]

### Phototesting

Phototesting can confirm the presence of a photosensitivity disorder and is most helpful for the diagnosis of immunologically mediated photodermatoses (**Fig. 5**).[30] Using an opaque template with several windows, the uninvolved skin of the back or the abdomen is exposed to varying doses of UVA, UVB, and/or visible monochromatic or broad-spectrum radiation. Following light exposure, the first reading is performed in 20 minutes to detect urticarial lesions as seen in solar urticaria.[31] The MED is determined 24 hours after exposure. MED is defined as the lowest dose of UVA or UVB (ie, MED-A or MED-B) that will produce perceptible erythema over the entire exposed site (see **Fig. 5**). **Table 4** outlines the expected phototesting results for the most common photodermatoses.

Provocative light testing is used to reproduce an eruption so that the morphology of the lesion can be examined in greater detail. This test involves exposing the same site for up to 3 to 4 consecutive days.[27,33] Usually, 80% of the MED is used as the starting dose, and an increase of 10% to 20% is performed on consecutive days. This test is primarily useful in confirming the diagnosis of PMLE. Though not commonly performed, the provocative skin test can also be used to confirm the photosensitive form of lupus erythematosus. In lupus erythematosus, the reading is delayed because the formation of lesions often occurs 1 to 2 weeks after phototesting or provocative light testing.[34] For photoaggravated dermatoses, with the exception of lupus erythematosus the patient presents with characteristic clinical features of the primary disorder and a negative phototest.

### Photopatch testing

Photopatch testing evaluates patients with photoallergic contact dermatitis. In a study involving 100 patients, positive photopatch tests resulted in the diagnosis of photoallergic contact dermatitis in about 10% of cases.[32] Photopatch testing is similar to a standard patch test used for evaluation of allergic contact dermatitis; a notable difference includes irradiation of the patch sites with UVA in the photopatch testing. Duplicate sets of photoallergen panels are placed on the back, and the sites are then covered with an opaque material to protect them from exposure to light. After 24 hours, one of the panels is irradiated with a dose of 10 J/cm² of UVA, or 50% of MED-A if the MED-A

**Table 4**
**Expected phototest and photopatch test results**

| Disorder | MED for UVA | MED for UVB | Visible Light | Photopatch Test |
|---|---|---|---|---|
| Polymorphous light eruption | NL/↓ | NL/↓ | NL | Negative |
| Chronic actinic dermatitis | ↓ | ↓ | NL/↓ | Negative/Positive |
| Solar urticaria | Urticaria | Urticaria | Urticaria | Negative |
| Phototoxicity | ↓ | NL | NL | Negative |
| Photoallergy | ↓ | NL | NL | Positive |

*Abbreviation:* NL, normal.
*Data from* Refs.[1,4,5,23,32]

is significantly reduced. The other panel acts as the control. **Table 5** shows the photopatch test results that can be expected for photoallergy, contact allergy, and both.[32,35]

## TREATMENT

In almost all photodermatoses, strict photoprotection, which includes seeking shade during peak daylight hours (10–2 PM for UVB, throughout the day for UVA), wearing sun-protective clothing and a wide-brimmed hat, and applying broad-spectrum sunscreens with sun-protection factor of at least 30, is the first line of therapy. However, depending on the specific photodermatosis and its severity, additional therapies may be needed. In the more severe forms of PMLE, prophylactic narrow-band UVB phototherapy or psoralen-UVA (PUVA) can be administered 2 to 3 times weekly for a total of 15 treatments in early spring to induce tolerance.[36] Gradual exposure to UVA or PUVA has also been helpful in building tolerance to UVR in patients with solar urticaria.[37] In addition, high-dose oral nonsedating antihistamines, taken 1 hour before expected sun exposure, can prevent or decrease the severity of solar urticaria.

In phototoxicity and photoallergy, identifying and avoiding the offending agent is clearly the most important factor in treating patients. Similarly, the treatment of photoaggravated dermatoses should focus on identifying and treating the underlying systemic or cutaneous disorder. Most phototoxic reactions can be treated in a manner similar to that for sunburn, which includes symptomatic relief with cool compresses, emollients, oral analgesics, and topical corticosteroids. Photoallergic reactions are treated in the same way as for contact allergies, with the application of topical corticosteroids. In very severe or refractory cases of PMLE or CAD, oral prednisone, azathioprine, or cyclosporine has been beneficial in relieving the severity and duration of the lesions.[38–40]

## SUMMARY

A systematic approach to the evaluation of the photosensitive patient includes history, physical examination, phototesting, photopatch testing, and laboratory evaluation. Polymorphous light eruption, CAD, solar urticaria, and photosensitivity secondary to systemic medications are the most frequently encountered photodermatoses in dermatologic clinics.

## REFERENCES

1. Bylaite M, Grigaitiene J, Lapinskaite GS. Photodermatoses: classification, evaluation and management. Br J Dermatol 2009;161(Suppl 3):61–8.
2. Lim HW, Hawk JL. Photodermatoses. In: Bolognia JL, Jorizzo JL, Schaffer JV, editors. Dermatology. 2nd edition. London: Mosby; 2007. p. 1467–86.
3. Meola T, Lim HW, Soter NA. Evaluation of the photosensitive patient. In: Lim HW, Solter NA, editors. Clinical photomedicine. New York: Marcel Dekker; 1993. p. 153–66.
4. Yashar SS, Lim HW. Classification and evaluation of photodermatoses. Dermatol Ther 2003;16(1):1–7.
5. Lim HW, Hawk JL. Evaluation of the photosensitive patient. In: Lim HW, Honigsmann H, Hawk JL, editors. Photodermatology. New York: Informa Healthcare; 2007. p. 139–48.
6. Roelandts R. The diagnosis of photosensitivity. Arch Dermatol 2000;136(9):1152–7.
7. Stratigos AJ, Antonious C, Papadakis P, et al. Juvenile spring eruption: clinicopathologic features and phototesting results in 4 cases. J Am Acad Dermatol 2004;50(Suppl 2):S57–60.
8. Lava SA, Simonetti GD, Ragazzi M, et al. Juvenile spring eruption: an outbreak report and systematic review of the literature. Br J Dermatol 2013;168(5):1066–72.
9. Dawe RS, Crombie IK, Ferguson J. The natural history of chronic actinic dermatitis. Arch Dermatol 2000;136(10):1215–20.
10. Que SK, Brauer JA, Soter NA, et al. Chronic actinic dermatitis: an analysis at a single institution over 25 years. Dermatitis 2011;22(3):147–54.
11. Boonstra HE, van Weelden H, Toonstra J, et al. Polymorphous light eruption: a clinical, photobiologic, and follow-up study of 110 patients. J Am Acad Dermatol 2000;42(2 Pt 1):199–207.
12. Epstein JH. Polymorphous light eruption. Photodermatol Photoimmunol Photomed 1997;13(3):89–90.
13. Lim HW, Morison WL, Kamide R, et al. Chronic actinic dermatitis. An analysis of 51 patients evaluated in the United States and Japan. Arch Dermatol 1994;130(10):1284–9.
14. Farr PM. Solar urticaria. Br J Dermatol 2000;142(1):4–5.

**Table 5**
**Expected photopatch test results**

| Diagnosis | Unirradiated | Irradiated (UVA) |
|---|---|---|
| Photoallergy | NL | + |
| Contact allergy | + | + |
| Both contact allergy and photoallergy | + | ++ |

*Abbreviation:* NL, normal.
*Data from* Refs.[1,2,4,5,23,32]

15. Watanabe M, Matsunaga Y, Katayama I. Solar urticaria: a consideration of the mechanism of inhibition spectra. Dermatology 1999;198(3):252–5.

16. McGregor JM, Grabcznska S, Vaughan R, et al. Genetic modeling of abnormal photosensitivity in families with polymorphic light eruption and actinic prurigo. J Invest Dermatol 2000;115(3):471–6.

17. Frank J, Poblete-Gutierrez PA. Porphyrias. In: Bolognia JL, Jorizzo JL, Schaffer JV, editors. Dermatology. 3rd edition. London: Mosby; 2012. p. 717–27.

18. Callen JP. Photosensitivity in collagen vascular diseases. Semin Cutan Med Surg 1999;18(4):293–6.

19. Barohn RJ, Sanchez JA, Anderson KE. Acute peripheral neuropathy due to hereditary coproporphyria. Muscle Nerve 1994;17(7):793–9.

20. Brodie MJ, Thompson GG, Moore MR, et al. Hereditary coproporphyria. Demonstration of the abnormalities in haem biosynthesis in peripheral blood. Q J Med 1977;46(182):229–41.

21. Almutawa F, Vandal R, Wang SQ, et al. Current status of photoprotection by window glass, automobile glass, window films, and sunglasses. Photodermatol Photoimmunol Photomed 2013;29(2):65–72.

22. Lim HW. Abnormal responses to ultraviolet radiation: photosensitivity induced by exogenous agents. In: Goldsmith L, Katz S, Gilchrest B, et al, editors. Fitzpatrick's dermatology in general medicine. 8th edition. New York: McGraw-Hill; 2012. Chapter 92.

23. DeLeo VA, Suarez SM, Maso MJ. Photoallergic contact dermatitis. Results of photopatch testing in New York, 1985 to 1990. Arch Dermatol 1992;128(11):1513–8.

24. Lim HW, Cohen JL. The cutaneous porphyrias. Semin Cutan Med Surg 1999;18(4):285–92.

25. Kerr HA, Lim HW. Photodermatoses in African Americans: a retrospective analysis of 135 patients over a 7-year period. J Am Acad Dermatol 2007;57(4):638–43.

26. Ross G, Foley P, Baker C. Actinic prurigo. Photodermatol Photoimmunol Photomed 2008;24(5):272–5.

27. Holzle E, Plewig G, Hofmann C, et al. Polymorphous light eruption. Experimental reproduction of skin lesions. J Am Acad Dermatol 1982;7(1):111–25.

28. Fotiades J, Soter NA, Lim HW. Results of evaluation of 203 patients for photosensitivity in a 7.3-year period. J Am Acad Dermatol 1995;33(4):597–602.

29. Heller P, Wieczorek R, Waldo E, et al. Chronic actinic dermatitis. An immunohistochemical study of its T-cell antigenic profile, with comparison to cutaneous T-cell lymphoma. Am J Dermatopathol 1994;16(5):510–6.

30. Fazel N, Lim HW. Evaluation and management of the patient with photosensitivity. Dermatol Nurs 2002;14(1):23–4, 27–30.

31. Kapoor R. Phototesting in solar urticaria. J Am Acad Dermatol 2009;60(5):877.

32. Neumann NJ, Holzle E, Lehmann P, et al. Pattern analysis of photopatch test reactions. Photodermatol Photoimmunol Photomed 1994;10(2):65–73.

33. Holzle E, Plewig G, Lehmann P. Photodermatoses—diagnostic procedures and their interpretation. Photodermatol 1987;4(2):109–14.

34. Kuhn A, Sonntag M, Richter-Hintz D, et al. Phototesting in lupus erythematosus tumidus—review of 60 patients. Photochem Photobiol 2001;73(5):532–6.

35. Bell HK, Rhodes LE. Photopatch testing in photosensitive patients. Br J Dermatol 2000;142(3):589–90.

36. Man I, Dawe RS, Ferguson J. Artificial hardening for polymorphic light eruption: practical points from ten years' experience. Photodermatol Photoimmunol Photomed 1999;15(3–4):96–9.

37. Kullavanijaya P, Lim HW. Photoprotection. J Am Acad Dermatol 2005;52(6):937–58 [quiz: 959–62].

38. Hawk JL, Lim HW. Chronic actinic dermatitis. In: Lim HW, Honigsmann H, Hawk JL, editors. Photodermatology. New York: Informa Healthcare; 2007. p. 169–83.

39. Patel DC, Bellaney GJ, Seed PT, et al. Efficacy of short-course oral prednisolone in polymorphic light eruption: a randomized controlled trial. Br J Dermatol 2000;143(4):828–31.

40. Murphy GM, Maurice PD, Norris PG, et al. Azathioprine treatment in chronic actinic dermatitis: a double-blind controlled trial with monitoring of exposure to ultraviolet radiation. Br J Dermatol 1989;121(5):639–46.

# Photoimmunology

Craig A. Elmets, MD[a],*, Cather M. Cala, BA[b], Hui Xu, PhD[a]

## KEYWORDS

- Photoimmunology • Nonmelanoma skin cancer • Ultraviolet radiation • Polymorphous light eruption
- Chronic actinic dermatitis • Cutaneous lupus erythematosus • Phototherapy • Photosensitivity

## KEY POINTS

- Photoimmunology investigates the immunologic effects of UV radiation exposure.
- Photoimmunology originated from observations about the biologic behavior of nonmelanoma skin cancers and the recognition that immunosuppressed organ transplant recipients were at an increased risk for sunlight-induced skin cancers.
- Experiments in animal models showed that alterations in the host cell–mediated immune response are necessary for skin cancers to develop.
- UV mediates its effects by causing a disproportionate increase in regulatory T cells, altering the function of antigen-presenting cutaneous dendritic cells, and stimulating the production of soluble immunosuppressive mediators.
- Knowledge generated about the UV effects on the immune system has contributed to a broader understanding of the pathogenesis of several photosensitivity diseases and to the generation of more effective and safer forms of phototherapy.

The area of photodermatology that investigates the complex interrelationship between UV radiation and the body's immune system is referred to as *photoimmunology*. Its foundation derives from clinical observations in patients with UV-induced skin cancers, but the acquisition of knowledge about the interactions of UV radiation with the immune system has implications beyond skin cancer. It has helped us to understand the mechanisms by which phototherapy is effective in psoriasis and other dermatologic diseases and, in so doing, has expanded the spectrum of illnesses amenable to UV radiation treatments. Furthermore, photoimmunology has enhanced our understanding of the role of the immune system in several different photodermatologic disorders.

## EVIDENCE OF PHOTOIMMUNOLOGIC EFFECTS OF UV RADIATION IN HUMANS

The possibility that UV radiation, especially within the UVB range (290–320 nm), might modulate immunologic function was suspected long before there was supportive experimental evidence and was based on careful observations in individuals who developed solar UV radiation–induced skin cancers. In contrast to many of the cancers that arise in other organs, cutaneous squamous cell carcinomas (SCCs) develop gradually, rarely metastasize, and are associated with a chronic inflammatory infiltrate. SCCs develop from actinic keratoses, more than 25% of which undergo spontaneous regression, presumably by activation of cell-mediated immune defenses directed at antigens expressed by the preneoplastic cells.[1]

Funded by NIH grants and contracts: P30 AR050948, P30 CA013148, N01 CN05014-69 and by VA Merit Review 18-103-02.

Conflicts of Interest: None.

[a] Department of Dermatology, UAB Skin Diseases Research Center, UAB Comprehensive Cancer Center, Birmingham VA Medical Center, University of Alabama at Birmingham, EFH 414, 1720 2nd Avenue South, Birmingham, AL 35294-0009, USA; [b] Department of Dermatology, University of Alabama at Birmingham, EFH 414, 1720 2nd Avenue South, Birmingham, AL 35294-0009, USA

* Corresponding author.

E-mail address: celmets@uab.edu

It has also been observed that cutaneous SCC are more frequent in immunosuppressed individuals. More than 50% of renal transplant recipients on long-term immunosuppressive therapy have developed at least one nonmelanoma skin cancer.[2–5] Although there is a 10-fold increased risk of basal cell carcinomas (BCCs) in organ transplant recipients, the likelihood of developing SCCs is even greater by 65 to 250 times,[6] resulting in an inverted SCC/BCC ratio. The predisposition to skin cancer is not restricted to transplant patients. Patients with lymphoma and chronic lymphocytic leukemia, who also have subtle defects in cellular immune function, also have an increased incidence of BCCs and SCCs.[7,8]

Immunologic abnormalities have been detected in patients with skin cancer who are otherwise immune competent. These patients demonstrate suppressed reactions to skin test antigens and decreased sensitization rates to the contact allergen dinitrochlorobenzene (DNCB), which are immune responses mediated by T lymphocytes.[9,10] In addition, when BCCs are examined histologically, a disproportionate number of regulatory T cells are present in the inflammatory infiltrate.[11] Finally, people who have received large numbers of psoralen plus UVA photochemotherapy (PUVA) treatments are known to have an increased incidence of skin cancer.[12,13] These patients have been reported to have decreased immunization rates to contact allergens[14] and reduced numbers of circulating peripheral blood CD4$^+$ T cells.[15,16]

## EXPERIMENTAL EVIDENCE FOR THE PHOTOIMMUNOLOGIC EFFECTS OF UV RADIATION

More direct evidence of the ability of UV radiation to impair immune responses is derived from a classic series of experiments in animal models.[17] Mice that are chronically exposed to UV radiation, like humans, develop UV-induced tumors (Fig. 1A). When these tumors are removed and are transplanted to the skin of genetically identical recipient mice, the tumors initially engraft but do not enlarge and ultimately regress because a host immune response develops against the tumors (see Fig. 1B). On the other hand, when the same tumors are transplanted to genetically identical recipients that have received subcarcinogenic doses of UV radiation, the tumors grow progressively, are not immunologically eradicated, and ultimately kill their host (see Fig. 1C). The conclusions that can be derived from these experiments are as follows: (1) UV radiation, in addition to causing mutations in keratinocytes, also

prevents activation of host immune responses that have evolved to destroy mutant keratinocytes before they can develop into clinically apparent tumors. (2) Only when there are both mutant keratinocytes and UV-induced immunologic alterations is it possible for skin tumors to occur (see Fig. 1D).

## MECHANISMS OF UV-INDUCED IMMUNE SUPPRESSION

There has been great interest in determining the mechanisms by which UV radiation mediates its effects on the immune system. Those studies have focused on 5 features: (1) the role of regulatory T cells, (2) the contribution to alterations in antigen-presenting cell (APC) function, (3) the effect of UV-induced cytokines and soluble mediators, (4) the molecular target that initiates UV-induced immune suppression, and (5) the participation of toll-like receptors (TLRs) and innate immunity.

### Regulatory T Cells

Studies have shown that UV radiation alters T cell–mediated immunity and, in so doing, causes immune suppression. Under normal circumstances, cutaneous exposure to antigens, such as contact allergens or tumor antigens expressed on skin cancers, results in the generation of both effector and regulatory T-lymphocytes, which are specific for the exposed antigen (Fig. 2A). Effector cells promote an immune response directed against the inciting antigen, whereas regulatory T cells dampen the reaction. The overall magnitude of the response depends on the ratio of effector to regulatory T cells that develop (see Fig. 2C). When large numbers of effector T cells develop and small numbers of regulatory T cells are present, a vigorous immune response occurs, whereas in situations in which smaller numbers of effector T cells and proportionally larger numbers of regulatory T cells are generated, there is a modest immune response. Following UV exposure, the generation of regulatory T cells is unaffected, whereas the number of effector T cells is diminished (see Fig. 2B).[18] The disproportionate number of regulatory T cells relative to effector T cells leads to a suppressed immune response (see Fig. 2C). The regulatory T cells that occur following UV exposure carry the phenotypic markers CD4$^+$, CD25$^+$, CTLA4$^+$, and FoxP3$^+$ and secrete the immunosuppressive cytokine interleukin-10 (IL-10).[19,20] In addition, a second population of cells called NKT cells have characteristics of both natural killer (NK) cells and T cells and express the CD4$^+$ and DX5$^+$ (CD49b$^+$) proteins. NKT cells suppress immune responses

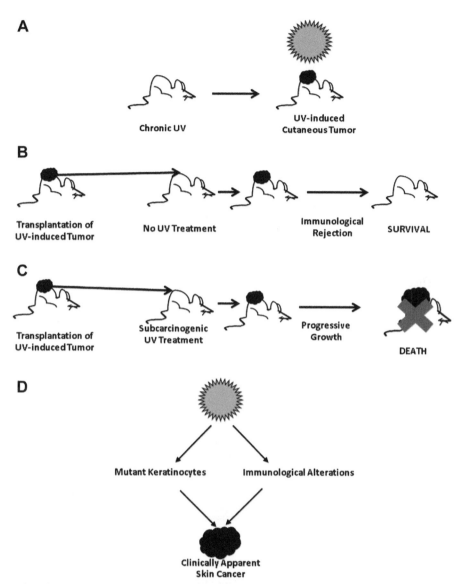

Fig. 1. UV-induced immune suppression and photocarcinogenesis. (*A*) Chronic exposure of mice, as in humans, results in the development of UV-induced nonmelanoma skin cancers. (*B*) UV-induced tumors that are transplanted to genetically identical recipients that have not been exposed to UV radiation results in rejection of the tumor by the host immune response. (*C*) UV-induced tumors that are transplanted to genetically identical recipients that have received subcarcinogenic doses of UV radiation grow progressively and ultimately result in death of the recipient. (*D*) UV-induced tumors only develop when mutations in keratinocytes and UV-induced immunosuppression occurs.

following UV radiation exposure and produce the Th2 cytokine IL-4, which suppresses antitumor immunity.[21]

## APCs

The recognition that regulatory T cells contribute to the suppressed immune response following UV exposure coincided with the discovery that T cells are only activated when antigen is presented to them by APCs. The skin contains several populations of APCs, including epidermal Langerhans cells, different types of dermal dendritic cells, and macrophages/monocytes, some of which migrate into the skin after UVB exposure.[22] Depending on the type and status of the APC, different subpopulations of T cells are activated. UV radiation has been shown to have a deleterious influence on cutaneous dendritic cell function for effector T-cell activation and less of an effect on APC function for regulatory T cells (see Fig. 2).[23,24] Recent evidence from animal models

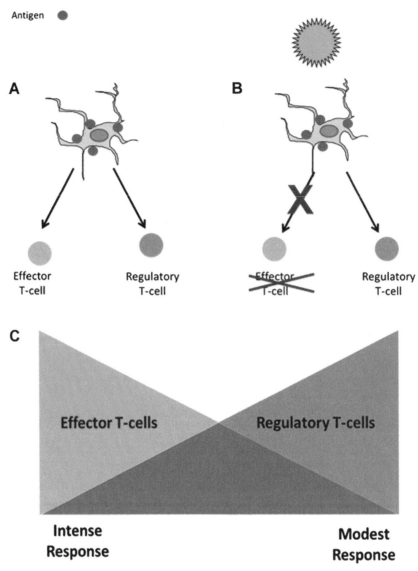

Fig. 2. Cell-mediated immune responses reflect the balance between regulatory and effector T cells. (A) When antigens, including tumor antigens, are present in the skin, they are taken up by cutaneous dendritic cells, which is a necessary precondition for the generation of effector and regulatory T-lymphocytes. (B) When the skin has been UV irradiated and then encounters an antigen, the generation of regulatory T cells proceeds unimpeded; but the generation of effector T cells is diminished. (C) The overall magnitude of the cutaneous cell-mediated immune response represents the balance between the effector and regulatory T cells that are generated. Following UV exposure, there are relatively more regulatory T cells, resulting in a more modest response.

indicates that epidermal Langerhans cells are required for the generation of regulatory T cells following UV exposure.[25] UV radiation produces its effects on cutaneous dendritic cells both through indirect and direct effects on the cells (Fig. 3). The indirect effects include stimulation of keratinocytes to produce immunosuppressive soluble mediators, such as IL-4, IL-10, tumor necrosis factor (TNF)-α, and prostaglandin (PGE2),[26–29] and stimulation of the migration of immunosuppressive macrophages into sites of UV injury.[30,31]

Also, the regulatory T cells that are generated following UV exposure have a negative influence on the presentation of antigen to effector T cells, thereby serving as a positive feedback loop for immunosuppression.

### Initial Molecular Events

DNA is now generally considered to be the molecular structure within cells that initiates the immunosuppressive effects of UV radiation.[32–34] Those wavelengths within the solar spectrum that are

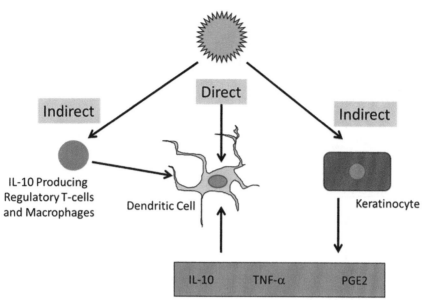

**Fig. 3.** Direct and indirect effects of UV radiation on the antigen-presenting function of cutaneous dendritic cells. Following UV exposure, the antigen-presenting function of cutaneous dendritic cells is altered by direct effects on the APC itself and by indirect effects. The indirect effects are mediated by UV-irradiated keratinocyte production of soluble mediators, such as IL-10, prostaglandin E2 (PGE2), and TNF-α, which then act on cutaneous dendritic cells. In addition, macrophages, which migrate into the skin following UV exposure, and regulatory T cells both secrete the immunosuppressive molecule IL-10, which diminishes the capacity of cutaneous APCs to activate effector T cells.

most effective at causing immunosuppression lie primarily within the UVB range and correspond closely with those that are most damaging to DNA.[35] In fact, patients with xeroderma pigmentosum (XP), a disease in which there is an inherited defect in DNA repair, have an increased propensity to develop actinic keratoses, BCCs, SCCs, and melanomas at an unusually early age. Patients with XP also have impaired delayed-type hypersensitivity (DTH) responses, reduced circulating CD4/CD8 T-cell ratios, defective NK cell function, and impaired production of interferon-γ, further supporting the concept of DNA as the molecular target of UVR-induced immunosuppression.[36–40] In animal models, UV-induced immune suppression can be reversed by topical application of enzymes that repair DNA damage.[32,33,41] When used in patients with XP, topical application of DNA repair enzymes prevents the development of actinic keratoses and BCCs.[42]

Transurocanic acid is present in large amounts in the stratum corneum of the skin and undergoes photoisomerization to its cis-urocanic acid conformation following UV exposure. Cis-urocanic acid has been shown to be a mediator of UV-induced immunosuppression.[43] Recent studies have shown that cis-urocanic acid mediates its immunosuppressive effects by interfering with the repair of UV-induced DNA damage.[34]

### Cytokines and Other Soluble Mediators

UV radiation is known to stimulate epidermal production of a variety of soluble mediators. These mediators include TNF-α[44]; PGE2[45,46]; serotonin[47]; platelet-activating factor[48,49]; and neuropeptides, such as calcitonin gene–related peptide (CGRP) and α-melanocyte-stimulating hormone (α-MSH).[50] UVR is also proficient at generating reactive oxygen intermediates.[51] These molecules have been shown to be important mediators of UV-induced immunosuppression, and interfering with their activity reverses their immunosuppressive effects in experimental animal models (**Fig. 4**).[27,28,46,47,49,52–54] Many of these agents, including cis-urocanic acid, platelet-activating factor, and serotonin, produce their immunosuppressive effects by interfering with repair of DNA damage.[34] CGRP inhibits the Langerhans cell antigen-presenting function,[55] and this may be the mechanism by which it causes UV-induced immune suppression. α-MSH is a stimulus for IL-10 production by keratinocytes and monocytes.[56,57]

Two other cytokines that play a prominent role in UV-induced immunosuppression are IL-10 and IL-12. IL-10 is an immunosuppressive cytokine produced by UV-irradiated keratinocytes, macrophages that migrate into UV-irradiated skin, and

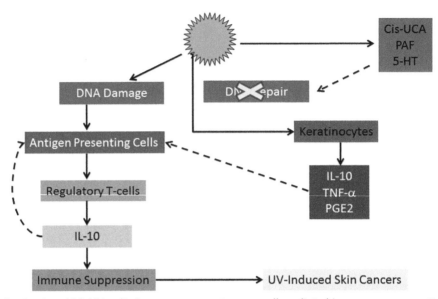

**Fig. 4.** Mechanism by which UV radiation suppresses cutaneous cell-mediated immune responses. Following UV exposure, DNA damage occurs, which, in addition to its other effects, initiates photoimmunosuppression. Furthermore, UV exposure of the skin results in the generation of soluble mediators, including serotonin (5-HT), cis-urocanic acid (Cis-UCA), and platelet-activating factor (PAF), all of which antagonize activation of DNA repair enzymes. In addition, UV exposure prompts keratinocytes to produce immunosuppressive mediators, which alter the antigen-presenting function of cutaneous dendritic cells. Regulatory T cells are generated that produce IL-10, which suppresses host T cell–mediated defense mechanisms and facilitates the growth and development of UV-induced tumors. The solid line indicates stimulatory. The dashed line indicates inhibitory.

regulatory T cells that are generated following UV exposure.[58–60] IL-10 acts on dendritic cells in such a manner as to enhance the generation of UV-induced regulatory T cells. IL-12, on the other hand, promotes T cell–mediated immunity by supporting the production of effector T cells, which produce the proinflammatory cytokine interferon-γ. Studies in animal models have shown that the administration of IL-12 will reverse the immunosuppressive effects of UV radiation.[61,62] IL-12 stimulates the production of enzymes that repair UV-damaged DNA,[63] which may also contribute to its ability to abrogate the immunosuppressive effects of UV. Polyphenols present in green tea and other natural and dietary products have been shown to prevent UV-induced immunosuppression and carcinogenesis, at least in part, by stimulating the production of IL-12.[64–67]

### TLRs and Innate Immunity

TLRs are highly conserved molecules that are present on the surface of immune cells and epithelial cells including epidermal keratinocytes.[68] They are important in the activation of several pathways of the innate immune response. TLRs recognize patterns within antigens that are foreign to the immune system, which include foreign pathogens; pathogen-associated molecular patterns; as well as endogenous antigens that are altered from their normal state, damage-associated molecular patterns. Of the 13 TLRs that have been identified thus far, 2 (TLR3 and TLR4) have been shown to be involved in the recognition of UV radiation–induced damage of RNA and DNA, respectively. These receptors initiate pathways that ultimately enhance UV-induced immunosuppression.

TLR3 is a cell surface receptor, present on keratinocytes. Following UV exposure, damage to keratinocytes occurs, which results in the release of double-stranded, small nuclear RNA (snRNA).[69] Once released, these snRNAs induce the expression of TLR3 on nonirradiated cells and then bind to the same TLR3 receptors, the expression of which they have provoked. TLR3 activation causes keratinocytes to produce proinflammatory cytokines, such as IL-6 and TNF-α. TNF-α is a known mediator of UV-induced immune suppression. Direct evidence of TLR3 in UV-induced immune suppression has come from studies in experimental animal models. UV-irradiated mice expressing TLR3 develop a suppressed T cell–mediated allergic contact hypersensitivity response, whereas the immune response in mice that are genetically deficient in TLR3 is normal.

A receptor involved in the recognition of UV-induced DNA damage is TLR4.[70] As was mentioned, UV-damaged DNA can be repaired by DNA repair enzymes. In the skin, TLR4 is found primarily on dendritic cells. Following UV exposure, dendritic cells in the skin that express the TLR4 molecule have a diminished capacity to synthesize IL-12. As was mentioned (see above), IL-12 stimulates the synthesis of DNA repair enzymes. The decrease in DNA repair in cutaneous dendritic cells renders them unable to effectively activate effector T cells and leads to suppression of the cell-mediated immune response. In contrast, in experimental systems, TLR4-deficient animals repair UV-damaged DNA normally and do not exhibit UV-induced immune suppression.

## PHOTOIMMUNOLOGIC DISEASES

The information derived from animal models about the photoimmunologic effects of UV radiation, coupled with observations made in patients, have been the basis for theories about the immunopathogenesis of several photodermatologic disorders, including polymorphous light eruption (PMLE), chronic actinic dermatitis, and cutaneous lupus erythematosus.

### PMLE

PMLE is the most common photodermatosis, with prevalence rates ranging from 1% to 21%, depending on the geographic location surveyed.[71–73] Wavelengths within the UVA are most commonly reported to prompt the inflammatory reaction, although in some patients, UVB and even UVC[74] have been associated with flares of the disease. PMLE has many features in common with DTH reactions in the skin. Within a few hours of sun exposure, CD4$^+$ T cells can be detected infiltrating the UV-exposed site.[75] The CD4$^+$ T cell infiltrate is followed over the next few days by an influx of CD8$^+$ T cells. In addition, the adhesion molecules E-selectin (CD62), vascular cell adhesion molecule 1 (CD106, also known as VCAM1), and intercellular adhesion molecule-1 (CD54, also known as ICAM1), all of which facilitate the migration and retention of T cells into inflamed skin, can easily be detected in PMLE skin, whereas they are not found in normal skin.[76] Although they are not first-line therapies for the disease, the fact that PMLE can be controlled with immunosuppressive agents, such as azathioprine and cyclosporine, is also consistent with the concept that it is an immunologically mediated disease.

It has been proposed that UV is less effective at suppressing cell-mediated immune responses in patients with PMLE (**Fig. 5**). There is decreased migration of CD11b$^+$ macrophages, which are known to secrete IL-10, into UV-irradiated skin in

patients with PMLE.[77] Moreover, a series of studies in which attempts were made to sensitize PMLE and normal control subjects to the contact allergen DNCB through UV-irradiated skin, demonstrated that UV-induced suppression of the contact allergic reaction was more effective in control subjects than in patients with PMLE.[78] In other words, patients with PMLE are resistant to the immunosuppressive effects of UV radiation.

### Chronic Actinic Dermatitis

Patients with chronic actinic dermatitis (CAD) have an exquisite photosensitivity that results in a subacute to chronic inflammatory process that begins in sun-exposed skin and can generalize to non–sun-exposed cutaneous surfaces.[79–81] Patients with CAD may or may not have a positive photoallergic response; but even in those who do, the dermatitis persists despite the removal of the substance causing the problem. Many of these patients initially have a photosensitivity to UVB, but this frequently extends to the UVA and even visible light.

The photopathogenesis of CAD is incompletely understood but is thought to be immunologic in nature.[81] Biopsies of involved skin demonstrate leukocyte epidermotropism, dermal infiltrates comprised primarily of T cells, and keratinocytes that express major histocompatibility class II molecules, features which are also present in DTH reactions in the skin.[81–83] Another characteristic suggesting that CAD is immunologically mediated is that the disease responds to immunosuppressive agents.[79,81]

There are 2 theories about the immunopathogenesis of CAD.[81] The first theory postulates that these patients have an exaggerated immune reaction to a photoantigen. This type of reaction is suppressed in normal individuals but, for some reason, is activated in those with CAD. The second theory proposes that there is cross-reactivity between a photoallergen and endogenous antigens. In this scenario, a photoallergen initiates the immune response. Because of cross-reactivity, the endogenous antigen allows the response to persist even though the photoallergen is no longer present.

### Cutaneous Lupus Erythematosus

Patients with cutaneous lupus erythematosus are frequently photosensitive, as sun sensitivity is one of the defining characteristics of the disease.[84,85] Rates vary depending on the type of lupus.[86,87] Wavelengths within the UVA and/or UVB are responsible for production of cutaneous lesions.[88,89]

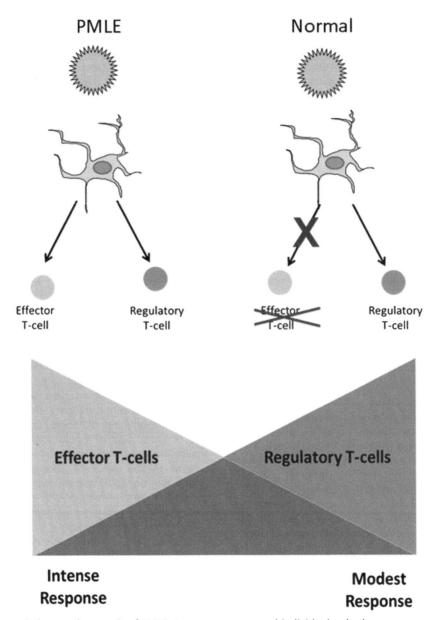

**Fig. 5.** Proposed photopathogenesis of PMLE. In contrast to normal individuals who have a suppressed immune response following UV exposure, the immune response in patients with PMLE is not suppressed.

UV exposure can prompt the development of lupus, aggravate the activity in existing skin lesions, and provoke systemic manifestations of the disease. With the exception of tumid lupus, cutaneous lupus is associated with vacuolar destructive changes in the basal cell layer of the epidermis. All forms of cutaneous lupus are associated with a dermal mononuclear infiltrate.

Antibodies to the Ro antigen are commonly present in subacute and neonatal lupus erythematosus (**Fig. 6**A). The Ro antigen is normally present within the nucleus of cells; but when keratinocytes

are exposed to UV radiation, it translocates to the cell surface membrane.[90] In that location, anti-Ro antibodies can bind to the molecule. It is hypothesized that cells that express Fc receptors for immunoglobulin G (IgG) are able to attach to the Fc portion of the anti-Ro antibody and exert a cytotoxic effect, resulting in keratinocyte lysis.

Cell destruction in cutaneous lupus may also occur via apoptotic keratinocytes and activation of a proinflammatory pathway (see **Fig. 6**B).[91,92] Following UV exposure, keratinocytes undergo apoptosis, which can be observed histologically

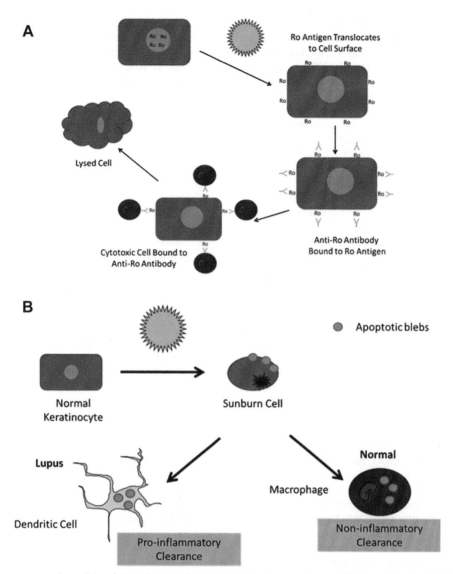

**Fig. 6.** Two proposed models of the photopathogenesis of cutaneous lupus. (*A*) In patients with Ro-positive lupus, UV exposure of the skin results in translocation of the Ro protein to the surface of the keratinocyte, which enables anti-Ro antibodies to bind. Cytotoxic cells that express Fc receptors for the immunoglobulin G molecule bind to the Fc portion of the anti-Ro antibody, which is attached to UV-irradiated keratinocytes expressing the Ro antigen on their surface. Thus, cytotoxicity occurs, leading to keratinocyte lysis. (*B*) Following UV exposure, apoptotic keratinocytes (sunburn cells) result. Apoptotic blebs are released from the dying keratinocytes. In unaffected individuals, these apoptotic blebs are removed by macrophages via noninflammatory mechanisms. In patients with lupus, the apoptotic bodies are taken up by dendritic cells and enter a proinflammatory pathway.

as a sunburn cell. Under normal conditions, the apoptotic blebs that are released from degenerating keratinocytes are taken up by macrophages and are cleared by noninflammatory pathways. In patients with lupus, however, these apoptotic blebs may be taken up by dendritic cells, which then can activate cell-mediated immune processes that eventuate in formation of cutaneous lupus lesions.

## PHOTOIMMUNOLOGIC EFFECTS OF PHOTOTHERAPY

Our ability to develop new phototherapeutic modalities is caused by the recognition that different types of UV radiation have unique molecular and biologic effects.[93,94] Most of the radiation within the UVB (290–320 nm) range penetrates only to the superficial dermis. Its primary effects on DNA are to cause cyclobutane pyrimidine dimers, although it is known to also cause photochemical changes. In the stratum corneum, UV exposure converts transurocanic acid to its cis-urocanic acid. Direct cellular targets of UVB are primarily Langerhans cells and keratinocytes in the epidermis; UVB depletes the epidermis Langerhans cells and stimulates keratinocytes both to produce immunosuppressive cytokines and to alter the expression of adhesion molecules that are required for adherence of T cells to keratinocytes. These immunologic effects help to explain why UVB radiation and, more recently, narrowband UVB have been effective in treating psoriasis,[95,96] atopic dermatitis,[97–99] and early forms of cutaneous T-cell lymphoma.[100,101]

In contrast, longer wavelength UVA1 radiation (340–400 nm) penetrates more deeply into the skin and has its major effects in the mid to lower dermis.[94] The major molecular consequence of UVA1 exposure is the production of reactive oxygen intermediates. UVA1 depletes the dermis of mast cells and dendritic cells, causes apoptosis of dermal CD4$^+$ T cells, and stimulates the production of matrix metalloproteinases by fibroblasts. These distinguishing characteristics of UVA1 have been exploited for therapeutic benefit for acute flares of atopic dermatitis and dyshidrosis, the pruritus associated with mastocytosis, as well as morphea,[102] scleroderma,[102] and other sclerodermoid inflammatory syndromes.[103] In atopic dermatitis, UVA1 has been shown to be more successful than combined UVA/UVB phototherapy.[104,105] It has also been shown to be effective in cutaneous T-cell lymphoma,[106] in which UVA1 acts directly on CD4$^+$ T cells and causes apoptosis.[107] Its efficacy in morphea and other sclerodermoid conditions is caused by its ability to augment matrix metalloproteinase-1, which degrades collagen.[108,109] In mastocytosis, UVA1 has been effective because of its ability to deplete the skin of mast cells.[102]

The primary molecular defect in PUVA photochemotherapy differs from that of both UVB and UVA1.[94] The addition of psoralen results in the production of bifunctional adducts with DNA. Like UVA1, UVA used in PUVA photochemotherapy penetrates into the mid to lower dermis, thereby altering dermal dendritic cells, stimulating fibroblast production of IL-1, and damaging dermal CD4$^+$ T cells. These effects help to explain its efficacy in psoriasis[110] and cutaneous T-cell lymphoma.[111,112]

## SUMMARY

UV radiation has been shown to alter immunologic function, both in the skin and systemically. In so doing, it contributes to the pathogenesis of non-melanoma skin cancer and participates in the development of lupus and other photosensitivity diseases in which immune mechanisms play a role. On the other hand, the immunologic effects of UV radiation have been exploited as a therapeutic modality to treat diseases, such as psoriasis, atopic dermatitis, cutaneous T-cell lymphoma, morphea, and mastocytosis.

## REFERENCES

1. Marks R, Rennie G, Selwood TS. Spontaneous remission of solar keratoses: the case for conservative management. Br J Dermatol 1986;115:649–55.
2. Hartevelt MM, Bouwes Bavinck JN, Kootte AM, et al. Incidence of skin cancer after renal transplantation in the Netherlands. Transplantation 1990;49:506–9.
3. Bouwes-Bavinck JN, Vermeer BJ, van-der-Woude FJ, et al. Relation between skin cancer and HLA antigens in renal-transplant patients. N Engl J Med 1991;325:843–8.
4. Webb MC, Compton F, Andrews PA, et al. Skin tumours posttransplantation: a retrospective analysis of 28 years' experience at a single centre. Transplant Proc 1997;29:828–30.
5. Jensen P, Moller B, Hansen S. Skin cancer in kidney and heart transplant recipients and different long-term immunosuppressive therapy regimens. J Am Acad Dermatol 2000;42:307.
6. Euvrard S, Kanitakis J, Claudy A. Skin cancers after organ transplantation. N Engl J Med 2003;348:1681–91.
7. Mellemgaard A, Geisler CH, Storm HH. Risk of kidney cancer and other second solid malignancies in patients with chronic lymphocytic leukemia. Eur J Haematol 1994;53:218–22.
8. Maule M, Scelo G, Pastore G, et al. Risk of second malignant neoplasms after childhood leukemia and lymphoma: an international study. J Natl Cancer Inst 2007;99:790–800.
9. Weimar VM, Ceilley RI, Goeken JA. Cell-mediated immunity in patients with basal and squamous cell skin cancer. J Am Acad Dermatol 1980;2:143–7.
10. Yoshikawa T, Rae V, Bruins-Slot W, et al. Susceptibility to effects of UVB radiation on induction of contact hypersensitivity as a risk factor for skin cancer in man. J Invest Dermatol 1990;95:530–6.
11. Kaporis HG, Guttman-Yassky E, Lowes MA, et al. Human basal cell carcinoma is associated with Foxp3+ T cells in a Th2 dominant microenvironment. J Invest Dermatol 2007;127:2391–8.
12. Stern RS, Liebman EJ, Vakeva L. Oral psoralen and ultraviolet-A light (PUVA) treatment of psoriasis and persistent risk of nonmelanoma skin cancer.

PUVA follow-up study. J Natl Cancer Inst 1998;90: 1278–84.

13. Stern RS. Carcinogenic risk of psoralen plus ultraviolet radiation therapy: evidence in humans. Natl Cancer Inst Monogr 1984;66:211–6.

14. Volden G, Molin L, Thomsen K. PUVA-induced suppression of contact sensitivity to mustine hydrochloride in mycosis fungoides. Br Med J 1978;2:865–6.

15. Moscicki RA, Morison WL, Parrish JA, et al. Reduction of the fraction of circulating helper-inducer T cells identified by monoclonal antibodies in psoriatic patients treated with long-term psoralen/ultraviolet-A radiation (PUVA). J Invest Dermatol 1982; 79:205–8.

16. Morison WL, Wimberly J, Parrish JA, et al. Abnormal lymphocyte function following long-term PUVA therapy for psoriasis. Br J Dermatol 1983; 108:445–50.

17. Kripke ML. Antigenicity of murine skin tumors induced by ultraviolet light. J Natl Cancer Inst 1974;53:1333–6.

18. Elmets CA, Bergstresser PR, Tigelaar RE, et al. Analysis of mechanism of unresponsiveness produced by haptens painted on skin exposed to low dose ultraviolet radiation. J Exp Med 1983; 158:781–94.

19. Schwarz A, Maeda A, Wild MK, et al. Ultraviolet radiation-induced regulatory T cells not only inhibit the induction but can suppress the effector phase of contact hypersensitivity. J Immunol 2004;172: 1036–43.

20. Schwarz A, Navid F, Sparwasser T, et al. In vivo reprogramming of UV radiation-induced regulatory T-cell migration to inhibit the elicitation of contact hypersensitivity. J Allergy Clin Immunol 2011;128: 826–33.

21. Moodycliffe AM, Nghiem D, Clydesdale G, et al. Immune suppression and skin cancer development: regulation by NKT cells. Nat Immunol 2000; 1:521–5.

22. Xu H, Timares L, Elmets CA. Host defenses in the skin. In: Rich RR, Fleisher TA, Shearer WT, et al, editors. Clinical immunology: principles and practice. 4th edition. St. Louis, MO: Elsevier Saunders; 2013. p. 228–38.

23. Ullrich SE, Byrne SN. The immunologic revolution: photoimmunology. J Invest Dermatol 2012;132: 896–905.

24. Schwarz T. 25 years of UV-induced immunosuppression mediated by T cells-from disregarded T suppressor cells to highly respected regulatory T cells. Photochem Photobiol 2008;84:10–8.

25. Schwarz A, Noordegraaf M, Maeda A, et al. Langerhans cells are required for UVR-induced immunosuppression. J Invest Dermatol 2010;130:1419–27.

26. Shreedhar V, Giese T, Sung VW, et al. A cytokine cascade including prostaglandin E2, IL-4, and IL-10 is responsible for UV-induced systemic immune suppression. J Immunol 1998;160:3783–9.

27. Kurimoto I, Streilein JW. Tumor necrosis factor-alpha impairs contact hypersensitivity induction after ultraviolet B radiation via TNF-receptor 2 (p75). Exp Dermatol 1999;8:495–500.

28. Streilein JW. Sunlight and skin-associated lymphoid tissues (SALT): if UVB is the trigger and TNF alpha is its mediator, what is the message? J Invest Dermatol 1993;100:47S–52S.

29. Yoshikawa T, Streilein JW. Genetic basis of the effects of ultraviolet light B on cutaneous immunity. Evidence that polymorphism at the TNFa and Lps loci governs susceptibility. Immunogenetics 1990; 32:398–405.

30. Meunier L, Bata-Csorgo Z, Cooper KD. In human dermis, ultraviolet radiation induces expansion of a CD36+ CD11b+ CD1- macrophage subset by infiltration and proliferation; CD1+ Langerhans-like dendritic antigen-presenting cells are concomitantly depleted. J Invest Dermatol 1995;105:782–8.

31. Cooper KD, Oberhelman L, Hamilton TA, et al. UV exposure reduces immunization rates and promotes tolerance to epicutaneous antigens in humans: relationship to dose, CD1a-DR+ epidermal macrophage induction, and Langerhans cell depletion. Proc Natl Acad Sci U S A 1992;89: 8497–501.

32. Applegate LA, Ley RD, Alcalay J, et al. Identification of the molecular target for the suppression of contact hypersensitivity by ultraviolet radiation. J Exp Med 1989;170:1117–31.

33. Kripke ML, Cox PA, Alas LG, et al. Pyrimidine dimers in DNA initiate systemic immunosuppression in UV-irradiated mice. Proc Natl Acad Sci U S A 1992;89:7516–20.

34. Sreevidya CS, Fukunaga A, Khaskhely NM, et al. Agents that reverse UV-Induced immune suppression and photocarcinogenesis affect DNA repair. J Invest Dermatol 2010;130:1428–37.

35. Elmets CA, LeVine MJ, Bickers DR. Action spectrum studies for induction of immunologic unresponsiveness to dinitrofluorobenzene following in vivo low dose ultraviolet radiation. Photochem Photobiol 1985;42:391–7.

36. Norris PG, Limb GA, Hamblin AS, et al. Immune function, mutant frequency and cancer risk in the DNA repair defective genodermatoses xeroderma pigmentosum, Cockayne's syndrome and trichothiodystrophy. J Invest Dermatol 1990;94:94–100.

37. Gaspari AA, Fleisher TA, Kraemer KH. Impaired interferon production and natural killer cell activation in patients with the skin cancer-prone disorder, xeroderma pigmentosum. J Clin Invest 1993;92:1135–42.

38. Wysenbeek AJ, Weiss H, Duczyminer-Kahana M, et al. Immunologic alterations in xeroderma pigmentosum patients. Cancer 1986;58:219–21.

39. Morison WL, Bucana C, Hashem N, et al. Impaired immune function in patients with xeroderma pigmentosum. Cancer Res 1985;45:3929–31.

40. Dupuy JM, Lafforet D. A defect of cellular immunity in Xeroderma pigmentosum. Clin Immunol Immunopathol 1974;3:52–8.

41. Cafardi JA, Elmets CA. T4 endonuclease V: review and application to dermatology. Expert Opin Biol Ther 2008;8:829–38.

42. Yarosh D, Klein J, O'Connor A, et al. Effect of topically applied T4 endonuclease V in liposomes on skin cancer in xeroderma pigmentosum: a randomised study. Lancet 2001;357:926–9.

43. Noonan FP, DeFabo EC, Morrison H. Cis-urocanic acid, a product formed by ultraviolet B irradiation of the skin, initiates an antigen presentation defect in splenic dendritic cells in vivo. J Invest Dermatol 1988;90:92–9.

44. Kock A, Schwarz T, Kirnbauer R, et al. Human keratinocytes are a source for tumor necrosis factor a: evidence for synthesis and release upon stimulation with endotoxin or ultraviolet light. J Exp Med 1990;172:1609–14.

45. Pentland AP, Mahoney M, Jacobs SC, et al. Enhanced prostaglandin synthesis after ultraviolet injury is mediated by endogenous histamine stimulation. J Clin Invest 1990;86:566–74.

46. Chung HT, Burnham DK, Robertson B, et al. Involvement of prostaglandins in the immune alterations caused by the exposure of mice to ultraviolet radiation. J Immunol 1986;137:2478–84.

47. Walterscheid JP, Nghiem DX, Kazimi N, et al. Cis-urocanic acid, a sunlight-induced immunosuppressive factor, activates immune suppression via the 5-HT2A receptor. Proc Natl Acad Sci U S A 2006; 103:17420–5.

48. Dy LC, Pei Y, Travers JB. Augmentation of ultraviolet B radiation-induced tumor necrosis factor production by the epidermal platelet-activating factor receptor. J Biol Chem 1999;274:26917–21.

49. Zhang Q, Yao Y, Konger RL, et al. UVB radiation-mediated inhibition of contact hypersensitivity reactions is dependent on the platelet-activating factor system. J Invest Dermatol 2008;128:1780–7.

50. Seiffert K, Granstein RD. Neuropeptides and neuroendocrine hormones in ultraviolet radiation-induced immunosuppression. Methods 2002;28: 97–103.

51. Black HS. Potential involvement of free radical reactions in ultraviolet light-mediated cutaneous damage. Photochem Photobiol 1987;46:213–21.

52. Garssen J, Buckley TL, Van Loveren H. A role for neuropeptides in UVB-induced systemic immunosuppression. Photochem Photobiol 1998;68: 205–10.

53. Legat FJ, Jaiani LT, Wolf P, et al. The role of calcitonin gene-related peptide in cutaneous immunosuppression induced by repeated subinflammatory ultraviolet irradiation exposure. Exp Dermatol 2004;13:242–50.

54. Grabbe S, Bhardwaj RS, Mahnke K, et al. alpha-melanocyte-stimulating hormone induces hapten-specific tolerance in mice. J Immunol 1996;156: 473–8.

55. Hosoi J, Murphy GF, Egan CL, et al. Regulation of Langerhans cell function by nerves containing calcitonin gene-related peptide. Nature 1993;363: 159–63.

56. Bhardwaj RS, Schwarz A, Becher E, et al. Pro-opiomelanocortin-derived peptides induce IL-10 production in human monocytes. J Immunol 1996; 156:2517–21.

57. Redondo P, Garcia-Foncillas J, Okroujnov I, et al. Alpha-MSH regulates interleukin-10 expression by human keratinocytes. Arch Dermatol Res 1998; 290:425–8.

58. Rivas JM, Ullrich SE. The role of IL-4, IL-10, and TNF-alpha in the immune suppression induced by ultraviolet radiation. J Leukoc Biol 1994;56:769–75.

59. Rivas JM, Ullrich SE. Systemic suppression of delayed-type hypersensitivity by supernatants from UV-irradiated keratinocytes. An essential role for keratinocyte-derived IL-10. J Immunol 1992; 149:3865–71.

60. Toichi E, Lu KQ, Swick AR, et al. Skin-infiltrating monocytes/macrophages migrate to draining lymph nodes and produce IL-10 after contact sensitizer exposure to UV-irradiated skin. J Invest Dermatol 2008;128:2705–15.

61. Schwarz A, Maeda A, Kernebeck K, et al. Prevention of UV radiation-induced immunosuppression by IL-12 is dependent on DNA repair. J Exp Med 2005;201:173–9.

62. Schmitt DA, Walterscheid JP, Ullrich SE. Reversal of ultraviolet radiation-induced immune suppression by recombinant interleukin-12: suppression of cytokine production. Immunology 2000;101: 90–6.

63. Schwarz A, Stander S, Berneburg M, et al. Interleukin-12 suppresses ultraviolet radiation-induced apoptosis by inducing DNA repair. Nat Cell Biol 2002;4:26–31.

64. Sharma SD, Katiyar SK. Dietary grape-seed proanthocyanidin inhibition of ultraviolet B-induced immune suppression is associated with induction of IL-12. Carcinogenesis 2006;27:95–102.

65. Vaid M, Singh T, Li A, et al. Proanthocyanidins inhibit UV-induced immunosuppression through IL-12-dependent stimulation of CD8+ effector T cells and inactivation of CD4+ T cells. Cancer Prev Res (Phila) 2011;4:238–47.

66. Katiyar S, Elmets CA, Katiyar SK. Green tea and skin cancer: photoimmunology, angiogenesis and DNA repair. J Nutr Biochem 2007;18:287–96.

67. Meeran SM, Katiyar S, Elmets CA, et al. Silymarin inhibits UV radiation-induced immunosuppression through augmentation of interleukin-12 in mice. Mol Cancer Ther 2006;5:1660–8.

68. Takeda K, Kaisho T, Akira S. Toll-like receptors. Annu Rev Immunol 2003;21:335–76.

69. Bernard JJ, Cowing-Zitron C, Nakatsuji T, et al. Ultraviolet radiation damages self-noncoding RNA and is detected by TLR3. Nat Med 2012;18: 1286–90.

70. Ahmad I, Simanyi E, Guroji P, et al. Toll-like receptor-4 deficiency enhances repair of ultraviolet radiation induced cutaneous DNA damage by nucleotide excision repair mechanism. J Invest Dermatol 2013. [Epub ahead of print].

71. Ros AM, Wennersten G. Current aspects of polymorphous light eruptions in Sweden. Photodermatol 1986;3:298–302.

72. Honigsmann H. Polymorphous light eruption. Photodermatol Photoimmunol Photomed 2008;24: 155–61.

73. Khoo SW, Tay YK, Tham SN. Photodermatoses in a Singapore skin referral centre. Clin Exp Dermatol 1996;21:263–8.

74. Majoie IM, van Weelden H, Sybesma IM, et al. Polymorphous light eruption-like skin lesions in welders caused by ultraviolet C light. J Am Acad Dermatol 2010;62:150–1.

75. Norris PG, Morris J, McGibbon DM, et al. Polymorphic light eruption: an immunopathological study of evolving lesions. Br J Dermatol 1989;120:173–83.

76. Norris PG, Barker JN, Allen MH, et al. Adhesion molecule expression in polymorphic light eruption. J Invest Dermatol 1992;99:504–8.

77. Kolgen W, Van Weelden H, Den Hengst S, et al. CD11b+ cells and ultraviolet-B-resistant CD1a+ cells in skin of patients with polymorphous light eruption. J Invest Dermatol 1999;113:4–10.

78. Palmer RA, Friedmann PS. Ultraviolet radiation causes less immunosuppression in patients with polymorphic light eruption than in controls. J Invest Dermatol 2004;122:291–4.

79. Roelandts R. Chronic actinic dermatitis. J Am Acad Dermatol 1993;28:240–9.

80. Que SK, Brauer JA, Soter NA, et al. Chronic actinic dermatitis: an analysis at a single institution over 25 years. Dermatitis 2011;22:147–54.

81. Hawk JL, Lim HW. Chronic actinic dermatitis. In: Lim HW, Honigsmann H, Hawk JL, editors. Photodermatology. New York: Informa Health; 2007. p. 169–83.

82. Menage Hdu P, Sattar NK, Haskard DO, et al. A study of the kinetics and pattern of E-selectin, VCAM-1 and ICAM-1 expression in chronic actinic dermatitis. Br J Dermatol 1996;134:262–8.

83. Fujita M, Miyachi Y, Horio T, et al. Immunohistochemical comparison of actinic reticuloid with allergic contact dermatitis. J Dermatol Sci 1990;1: 289–96.

84. Foering K, Chang AY, Piette EW, et al. Characterization of clinical photosensitivity in cutaneous lupus erythematosus. J Am Acad Dermatol 2013; 69:205–13.

85. Foering K, Goreshi R, Klein R, et al. Prevalence of self-report photosensitivity in cutaneous lupus erythematosus. J Am Acad Dermatol 2012;66: 220–8.

86. Kim A, Chong BF. Photosensitivity in cutaneous lupus erythematosus. Photodermatol Photoimmunol Photomed 2013;29:4–11.

87. Scheinfeld N, Deleo VA. Photosensitivity in lupus erythematosus. Photodermatol Photoimmunol Photomed 2004;20:272–9.

88. Kuhn A, Wozniacka A, Szepietowski JC, et al. Photoprovocation in cutaneous lupus erythematosus: a multicenter study evaluating a standardized protocol. J Invest Dermatol 2011;131:1622–30.

89. Lehmann P, Holzle E, Kind P, et al. Experimental reproduction of skin lesions in lupus erythematosus by UVA and UVB radiation. J Am Acad Dermatol 1990;22:181–7.

90. LeFeber WP, Norris DA, Ryan SR, et al. Ultraviolet light induces binding of antibodies to selected nuclear antigens on cultured human keratinocytes. J Clin Invest 1984;74:1545–51.

91. Orteu CH, Sontheimer RD, Dutz JP. The pathophysiology of photosensitivity in lupus erythematosus. Photodermatol Photoimmunol Photomed 2001;17: 95–113.

92. Lin JH, Dutz JP, Sontheimer RD, et al. Pathophysiology of cutaneous lupus erythematosus. Clin Rev Allergy Immunol 2007;33:85–106.

93. Cafardi JA, Pollack BP, Elmets CA. Phototherapy. In: Goldsmith LA, editor. Fitzpatrick's dermatology in general medicine. 8th edition. New York: McGraw Hill; 2012. p. 2841–50.

94. Krutmann J, Morita A, Elmets CA. Mechanisms of Photo(chemo)therapy. In: Krutmann J, Hönigsmann H, Elmets CA, editors. Dermatological phototherapy and photodiagnostic methods. 2nd edition. Berlin: Springer-Verlag; 2009. p. 63–77.

95. van Weelden H, De La Faille HB, Young E, et al. A new development in UVB phototherapy of psoriasis. Br J Dermatol 1988;119:11–9.

96. Parrish JA, Jaenicke KF. Action spectrum for phototherapy of psoriasis. J Invest Dermatol 1981;76: 359–62.

97. Clayton TH, Clark SM, Turner D, et al. The treatment of severe atopic dermatitis in childhood with narrowband ultraviolet B phototherapy. Clin Exp Dermatol 2007;32:28–33.

98. Ersoy-Evans S, Altaykan A, Sahin S, et al. Phototherapy in childhood. Pediatr Dermatol 2008;25: 599–605.

99. Jury CS, McHenry P, Burden AD, et al. Narrowband ultraviolet B (UVB) phototherapy in children. Clin Exp Dermatol 2006;31:196–9.

100. Gathers RC, Scherschun L, Malick F, et al. Narrowband UVB phototherapy for early-stage mycosis fungoides. J Am Acad Dermatol 2002;47:191–7.

101. Boztepe G, Sahin S, Ayhan M, et al. Narrowband ultraviolet B phototherapy to clear and maintain clearance in patients with mycosis fungoides. J Am Acad Dermatol 2005;53:242–6.

102. Stege H, Schopf E, Ruzicka T, et al. High-dose UVA1 for urticaria pigmentosa. Lancet 1996;347:64.

103. Tuchinda C, Kerr HA, Taylor CR, et al. UVA1 phototherapy for cutaneous diseases: an experience of 92 cases in the United States. Photodermatol Photoimmunol Photomed 2006;22:247–53.

104. Krutmann J, Czech W, Diepgen T, et al. High-dose UVA1 therapy in the treatment of patients with atopic dermatitis. J Am Acad Dermatol 1992;26:225–30.

105. Krutmann J, Diepgen TL, Luger TA, et al. High-dose UVA1 therapy for atopic dermatitis: results of a multi-center trial. J Am Acad Dermatol 1998;38:589–93.

106. Plettenberg H, Stege H, Megahed M, et al. Ultraviolet A1 (340-400 nm) phototherapy for cutaneous T-cell lymphoma. J Am Acad Dermatol 1999;41:47–50.

107. Morita A, Werfel T, Stege H, et al. Evidence that singlet oxygen-induced human T helper cell apoptosis is the basic mechanism of ultraviolet-A radiation phototherapy. J Exp Med 1997;186:1763–8.

108. Yin L, Yamauchi R, Tsuji T, et al. The expression of matrix metalloproteinase-1 mRNA induced by ultraviolet A1 (340-400 nm) is phototherapy relevant to the glutathione (GSH) content in skin fibroblasts of systemic sclerosis. J Dermatol 2003;30:173–80.

109. Wlaschek M, Briviba K, Stricklin GP, et al. Singlet oxygen may mediate the ultraviolet A-induced synthesis of interstitial collagenase. J Invest Dermatol 1995;104:194–8.

110. Parrish JA, Fitzpatrick TB, Tanenbaum L, et al. Photochemotherapy of psoriasis with oral methoxsalen and longwave ultraviolet light. N Engl J Med 1974;291:1207–11.

111. Rupoli S, Goteri G, Pulini S, et al. Long-term experience with low-dose interferon-alpha and PUVA in the management of early mycosis fungoides. Eur J Haematol 2005;75:136–45.

112. Herrmann JJ, Roenigk HH Jr, Honigsmann H. Ultraviolet radiation for treatment of cutaneous T-cell lymphoma. Hematol Oncol Clin North Am 1995;9:1077–88.

# Photoaging

Anne Han, MD[a], Anna L. Chien, MD[a], Sewon Kang, MD[b],*

## KEYWORDS

- Photoaging • Dermatoheliosis • Photodamage • Rhytids • Skin rejuvenation

## KEY POINTS

- Photoaging is caused by chronic ultraviolet exposure leading to a complex process of skin changes that occur predominately on the sun-exposed cutaneous surfaces.
- Photoaging is more pronounced in fair-skin individuals and is characterized by subtle differences across ethnicities.
- Clinical manifestations of photoaging include rhytids, lentigines, telangiectasias, mottled pigmentation, coarse texture, laxity, and loss of translucency.
- Patients are concerned about their appearance related to photoaging and are influenced by society, culture, and personal values.
- A variety of modalities exist to prevent and treat photodamage, including sun protection, topical retinoids, cosmeceuticals, chemical peels, neuromodulators, soft tissue fillers, and light sources such as lasers.

## INTRODUCTION

Photoaging is characterized by a complex process of skin changes induced over time by ultraviolet light exposure. It results in premature aging of the skin and is superimposed on the changes caused by chronologic aging. Not all photoaging is equal. The process is influenced by skin type and ethnicity. The degree of photoaging also depends on geographic location (ie, latitude and altitude), extent of sun exposure in relation to occupation and lifestyle, and photoprotective practices, including using sunscreens and photoprotective clothing, and seeking shade. Many patients use antiaging products or have corrective procedures.

Generally, patients are concerned about appearance and are influenced by society, culture, and personal values. Aesthetic ideals of beauty vary, yet the appearance of youthfulness remains a constant benchmark. Photoaging plays an important role in the degree to which youthfulness is retained despite advancing age.[1]

This article discusses the clinical features, epidemiology, histopathology, pathogenesis, and management of photoaging.

## HISTORY

The term photoaging was first coined in 1986 and has been used interchangeably with the term dermatoheliosis.[2] However, the latter is a faulty neologism that implies a pathologic condition (osis) of the sun (helio).[3] Thus, photoaging is more accurate and is used exclusively throughout this article.

## EPIDEMIOLOGY

Photoaging is more prevalent among populations with fair skin. Fitzpatrick skin types I, II, and III are more prone to photoaging than skin types IV, V, and VI. Ethnic origin, in particular Northern European descent, also plays an important role. In an Australian study of participants younger than the age of 30, moderate to severe photoaging was

Disclosures: None.
[a] Department of Dermatology, Johns Hopkins Medical Institutions, 601 North Caroline Street, 6th Floor, Baltimore, MD 21287, USA; [b] Department of Dermatology, Johns Hopkins Medical Institutions, 1550 Orleans Street, 2nd Floor, Baltimore, MD 21287, USA
* Corresponding author.
E-mail address: swk@jhmi.edu

Dermatol Clin 32 (2014) 291–299
http://dx.doi.org/10.1016/j.det.2014.03.015
0733-8635/14/$ – see front matter © 2014 Elsevier Inc. All rights reserved.

observed in 72% of men and 47% of women.[4] In populations with darker skin, wrinkling is not readily apparent until the age of 50 and the severity is not as marked as in fairer skinned populations of similar age.[5] One study found that the onset of wrinkles in Chinese women occurred on average 10 years later than in French women.[6]

Photoaging is directly associated with cumulative sun exposure and, by extension, increasing age. Other factors include geographic location, such as high altitude and proximity to the equator where the harmful effects of ultraviolet light from the sun are most severe. Lifestyle practices, including outdoor occupations and outdoor recreational activities, increase cumulative sun exposure. For example, farmers, sailors, construction workers, and truck drivers frequently show severe effects of sun exposure over a lifetime. Indoor tanning is a practice that is also responsible for accelerated photoaging.[7]

Factors that diminish the features of photoaging include rigorous sun-protection practices. In Asian culture, in particular, women fastidiously avoid exposing their face to the sun.[8] They may wear large brimmed hats, carry parasols, and avoid the beach or other outdoor activities. These practices are highly influenced by societal ideals of beauty and attractiveness.

## PATHOGENESIS

Both UV-A (320–400 nm) and UV-B (290–320 nm) seem to be implicated in the photoaging process, although UV-A is emerging as the major contributor because it penetrates deeper into the dermis and reaches the earth at least 10-fold more abundantly than UV-B.[9] UV-B radiation is mainly absorbed in the epidermis by cellular DNA, inducing damage with formation of cyclobutane pyrimidine dimers. UV-B is responsible for sunburn, photocarcinogenesis, and immunosuppression.[10]

Cumulative UV-A radiation causes damage to the dermal extracellular matrix and blood vessels. UV-A also indirectly damages DNA, as well as lipids and proteins, through the generation of reactive oxygen species (ROS). ROS cause oxidative damage to cellular components such as cell membranes, mitochondria, and DNA. Mitochondria are the main endogenous source of ROS and are produced during the conversion of ADP to ATP. Endogenous ROS, including superoxide anion, hydrogen peroxide, and singlet oxygen, activate cytokine and growth factor receptors, which in turn induce transcription factor activator protein 1 (AP-1) and NF-κB.

**Fig. 1** demonstrates the pathogenesis of photoaging. UV radiation activates growth factor and

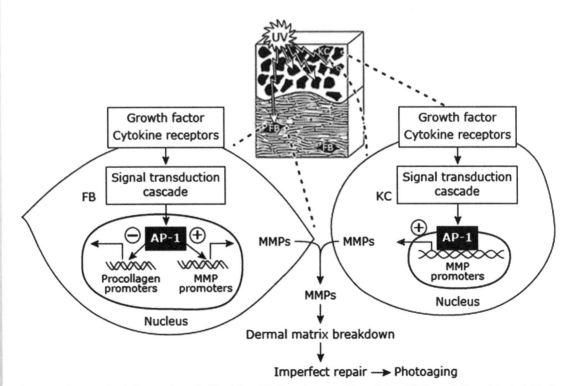

**Fig. 1.** Pathogenesis of photoaging. FB, fibroblast; KC, keratinocyte. (*From* Fisher GJ, Kang S, Varani J, et al. Mechanisms of photoaging and chronologic skin aging. Arch Dermatol 2002;138:1462; with permission.)

cytokine receptors, which induce transcription factor AP-1. The induction of AP-1 promotes collagen breakdown by upregulating matrix metalloproteinases (MMP), including interstitial collagenase (MMP-1), stromelysin-1 (MMP-3), and 92 kDa gelatinase (MMP-9).[11] The combined actions of MMP-1, MMP-3, and MMP-9 degrade most of type I and III dermal collagen.[12] Furthermore, AP-1 inhibits collagen production by decreasing gene expression of types I and III procollagen in the dermis. AP-1 binds to the transcriptional complex responsible for procollagen transcription or blocks the activity of transforming growth factor beta (TGF-β), a cytokine that promotes procollagen formation. With repeated sun exposure, degraded collagen accumulates over time and attenuation of collagen production results in the clinical and histologic features of photoaging.[13]

The activation of NF-κB by ROS regulates the expression of proinflammatory cytokines, such as interleukin (IL)-1β, TNF-α, IL-6, IL-8, and various adhesion molecules. These cytokines, in turn, can amplify AP-1 and NF-κB pathways, further enhancing the response to UV radiation.[14,15]

## CLINICAL MANIFESTATIONS

Photoaging can manifest as rhytids, lentigines, telangiectasias, mottled pigmentation, coarse texture, loss of translucency, sallow color, laxity, and decreased elasticity and turgor. More severe photoaging may result in accentuated ridging, deep furrows, leathery appearance, severe atrophy, open comedones, milia, cobblestone effect from elastosis, actinic purpura, and epidermal and dermal thickening.[16] Chronologic aging is dominated by fine lines and increased skin laxity. The latter is primarily due to soft tissue volume loss from fat atrophy, gravity-induced soft tissue redistribution, and reduction of facial skeletal support related to bone resorption.

Photoaging is significantly affected by an individual's skin type and ethnicity. Darker skin is more photoprotected than fair skin because of the increased melanin content. A cadaveric study comparing black and white skin found the photoprotective effect of melanin against UV radiation has an average sun protective factor (SPF) of 13.4.[17] Thus, individuals with higher Fitzpatrick skin types are inherently more protected because they generally experience the effects of photoaging 10 to 20 years later and with less severity.

Ethnicity plays a strong factor in determining the specific clinical features of photoaging. Wrinkle patterns and pigmentary changes differ between white and Asian skin.[18] A population study evaluating the effects of ethnicity and genetics on photoaging was conducted in the Pokhara valley of Nepal, which is cohabited by two distinct ethnic groups of Aryan-origin and Mongolian-origin.[19] It was found that Aryan-origin participants showed deeper wrinkles, particularly around the eye area and forehead, even though they had darker skin on average. Thus, ethnic origin and genetics are independent factors in determining the effects of photoaging. Another epidemiologic study investigating the role of genetics compared Japanese women from Japan and white women from Germany. The Japanese women had less facial wrinkling and more pigment spots than their German counterparts. Plausible explanations for the underlying differences include higher antioxidant levels in fasting blood (for less wrinkling) and greater frequency of the SLC45A2 gene allele involved in melanin synthesis (for more pigmented lesions) in Japanese women.[20] These metabolic and genetic differences may further illuminate the role of ethnicity and genetics in the complex process of photoaging.

## HISTOLOGY

Microscopic changes in photodamaged skin affect the epidermis and dermis. **Fig. 2** compares the histology of normal, sun-protected skin and damaged, photoaged skin. In photoaging, epidermal changes include either atrophy with thinning of the spinous layer and flattening of the dermoepidermal junction (loss of rete ridges), or epidermal thickening and acanthosis.[21] In the dermis, there is decreased extracellular matrix and breakdown of collagen fibers, which clinically manifest as rhytids.[22] The most pronounced histologic feature of photoaging is disintegration of elastic fibers, also called solar elastosis, which results in deposition of amorphous masses of abnormally thickened, curled, and fragmented elastic fibers.[23] Increased numbers of atypical melanocytes and keratinocytes may be seen. By contrast, histologic changes of chronologically aged skin are less complex and characterized by epidermal atrophy with decreased amounts of fibroblasts and collagen content.

## PHOTOBIOLOGIC EVALUATION

Photoaging can be characterized on a scale from minimal to severe involvement. Multiple photoaging scales have been developed by experts in the field. In one of the earliest efforts, Griffiths and colleagues[24] used five photographic standards with assigned grades of 0, 2, 4, 6, and 8 (**Fig. 3**) to develop a photonumeric nine-point scale illustrating the severity of photodamage

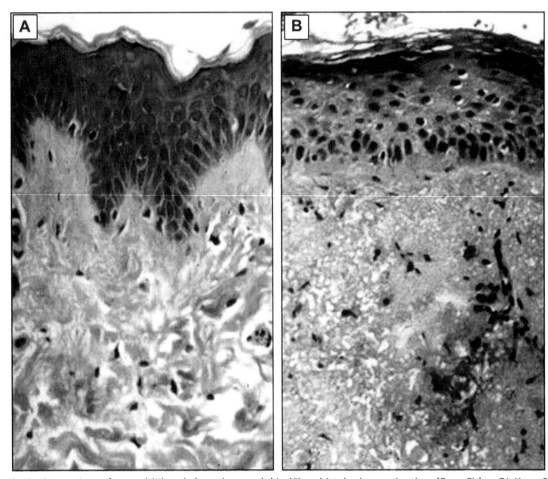

**Fig. 2.** Comparison of normal (*A*) and photodamaged skin (*B*) on histologic examination. (*From* Fisher GJ, Kang S, Varani J, et al. Mechanisms of photoaging and chronologic skin aging. Arch Dermatol 2002;138:1462; with permission. *From* Kang S, Bergfeld W, Gottlieb AB, et al. Long-term efficacy and safety of tretinoin emollient cream 0.05% in the treatment of photodamaged facial skin. Am J Clin Dermatol 2005;6:245; with permission.)

(0 = no photodamage, 8 = severe). Helfrich and colleagues[25] studied photoprotected skin of the upper inner arm and developed a similar photonumeric nine-point scale to assess chronologic aging. Chung and colleagues[26] designed two photonumeric scales, one for wrinkling and the other for dyspigmentation, to grade the severity of photoaging in Asian skin. The Glogau classification divides the degree of photoaging into four groups: mild, moderate, advanced, and severe. It predominately measures the severity of rhytids.[27] The Wrinkle Severity Rating Scale and Global Aesthetic Improvement Scale is a five-point photonumeric scale designed to quantify facial folds (1 = absent, 5 = severe). It has been used in clinical research studies to provide objective quantification of improvement after skin rejuvenation interventions such as soft tissue fillers.[28] Carruthers and Carruthers[29] also developed a set of validated grading scales (0 = none, 4 = severe)

to rate brow positioning, forehead lines, melomental folds, and crow's feet for clinical and research purposes.

## TREATMENT

The extent to which photoaging develops may be dramatically affected by preventive measures and even reversed to a certain degree by various cosmetic treatments. Primary prevention is geared toward protection from the sun. Photoprotection, including seeking shade when outdoors and using sunscreens and protective clothing, is the first line of defense against photoaging. These strategies are discussed in detail in the article by Mancebo and colleagues and in the article by Almutawa and Buabbas elsewhere in this issue. Primary prevention also includes avoidance of artificial sources of UV exposure, including tanning beds, and judicious use of therapeutic light boxes for medical

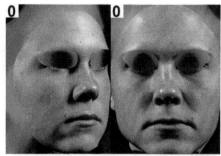

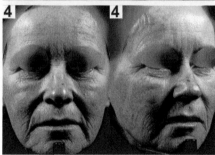

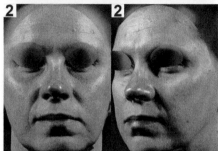

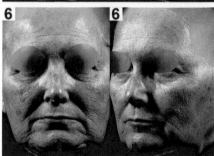

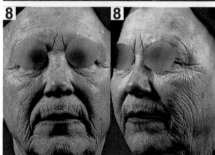

**Fig. 3.** Photonumeric scale for cutaneous photodamage. (*Courtesy of* Regents of the University of Michigan, East Lansing, MI; with permission.)

treatment of dermatoses. Treatment of photoaging includes a variety of topical and procedural interventions, including topical retinoids, cosmeceuticals, chemical peels, injectable neuromodulators, injectable soft-tissue fillers, and light sources.

## Topical Retinoids

Topical retinoids are the mainstay of treatment of patients with mild to moderate photoaging. Retinoids are a class of naturally occurring or synthetic compounds related to vitamin A, also known as retinol. Retinol is naturally converted in the body to its most biologically active form, retinoic acid, as well as to its other derivatives, retinaldehyde and retinyl ester. Various natural and synthetic retinoids increase collagen production, induce epidermal hyperplasia, and decrease keratinocyte and melanocyte atypia.[30–34] Clinically, they reduce the appearance of fine lines, improve skin texture, correct tone and elasticity, and slow the progression of photoaging. **Fig. 4** demonstrates the efficacy of topical tretinoin in the treatment of photoaging.

Tretinoin, or all-trans-retinoic acid, is the most widely investigated photoaging therapy. Tretinoin 0.05% emollient cream (Renova) and tazarotene 0.1% cream (Tazorac or Avage) are the only two retinoids approved by the US Food and Drug Administration (FDA) for this indication.[35] Other topical retinoids used off-label for photoaging include adapalene, a synthetic derivative available by prescription, and retinol, which is found in many antiaging cosmeceutical products.[31]

Topical retinoids may cause irritant reactions, such as scaling, redness, burning, and dermatitis, limiting patient compliance. Retinoids should be initiated at the lowest effective dose to minimize adverse effects. A minimum of 4 months use is necessary before benefits are appreciated.[36] Although tazarotene is the only topical retinoid with a category X designation, topical retinoids are not recommended during pregnancy or lactation.

## Cosmeceuticals

Cosmeceuticals encompass a heterogeneous category of nonprescription topical products, including antioxidants, vitamins, hydroxy acids, and plant extracts.[37] Cosmeceuticals are marketed to the consumer based on claims of their antiaging effects. They are touted to lighten and brighten, reduce wrinkles, correct blemishes, and lead to overall skin rejuvenation. Although some products may have scientific rationale and produce visible results in the treatment of photoaging, they are not classified as drugs. As a result, these products are not subject to the rigorous testing or

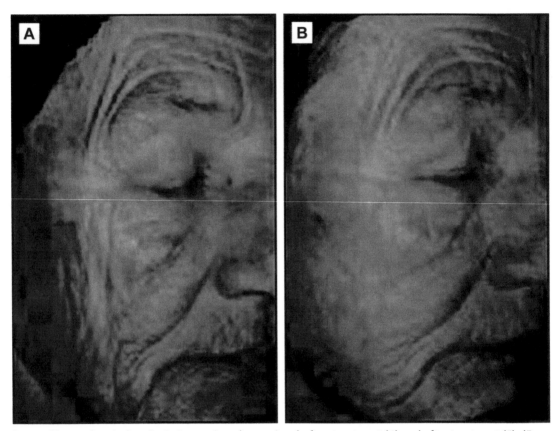

**Fig. 4.** Efficacy of topical tretinoin in treating photoaging: before treatment (*A*) and after treatment (*B*). (*From* Kang S, Bergfeld W, Gottlieb AB, et al. Long-term efficacy and safety of tretinoin emollient cream 0.05% in the treatment of photodamaged facial skin. Am J Clin Dermatol 2005;6:245; with permission.)

regulation by agencies such as the FDA. However, most cosmeceuticals do serve a role in keeping the skin moisturized and many are combined with topical retinol to enhance their antiaging benefits. For instance, in a small randomized study, nonprescription 1% topical retinol was as effective as 0.02% tretinoin in improving photoaging.[38]

## Chemical Peels

Chemical peels used in the treatment of photoaging involve controlled wounding of the skin by applying a caustic substance.[39] Subsequent regeneration of the skin produces a tightening effect and evens the skin tone. Peels may result in a more compact stratum corneum, thicker epidermis, and uniform distribution of melanin.[40] Chemical peels are classified by their intended depth of injury: superficial, medium, or deep. Superficial peels are well-tolerated and require minimal downtime. They cause injury to the epidermis down to the papillary dermis. These peels include alpha-hydroxy acids such as glycolic, lactic, salicylic, and low concentrations of trichloroacetic acid (TCA). Jessner solution is a combination of lactic acid, salicylic acid, and resorcinol in ethanol. Medium-depth peels cause injury down to the upper reticular dermis with increased efficacy as well as risk of side effects. The classic medium-depth peel is TCA 50%, which may lead to unpredictable results due to depth of penetration. Deep peels are rarely performed now. The Baker-Gordon formula, containing phenol and croton oil, is the traditional deep peel. Cardiac monitoring is required because phenol can cause arrhythmias.[41] Adverse effects such as hyperpigmentation, infection, and scarring are more common with medium-depth and deep peels.

## Neuromodulators

Botulinum toxin is an injectable neuromodulator used to reduce fine lines and wrinkles. It is one of the most sought after cosmetic procedures and is remarkably safe when used appropriately. Botulinum toxin is derived from neurotoxins produced by *Clostridium botulinum*, the bacterium responsible for botulism. It weakens and paralyzes skeletal muscle and improves rhytids caused by facial muscle contraction. Common facial areas of treatment include glabellar rhytids, horizontal forehead lines, and lateral canthal lines (crow's feet), in addition to other areas in the midface and lower face.[42] Neuromodulator injections are rapid in-office procedures with minimal to no downtime. The clinical effects are transient, beginning in the first week and generally lasting 3 to 4 months.[43] Currently, three formulations of botulinum toxin serotype A are approved by the FDA for cosmetic applications and are marketed under the trade names Botox, Dysport, and Xeomin.

Absolute contraindications to neuromodulator treatment include infection at the site of injection or known hypersensitivity to any component of the product. Dysport should not be given to patients with allergies to cow milk protein. Relative contraindications include disorders of the neuromuscular junction, such as myasthenia gravis, which may amplify the effect of the toxin. Caution should be exercised with patients who are taking drugs that can interfere with neuromuscular transmission, such as quinine, aminoglycosides, and calcium channel blockers.[44] Common adverse effects are usually minimal, transient, and related to the injection itself, such as local bruising, swelling, and headache. Other, more severe, complications are usually due to improper placement or diffusion, causing temporary disfigurement or functional impairments such as brow ptosis and eyelid ptosis.[45] Some of these complications can be improved with further interventions until the effect of the toxin dissipates.

## Soft Tissue Fillers

Soft tissue filler injections are used for facial rejuvenation to improve coarse wrinkles and gradual loss of tissue volume. A wide variety of injectable fillers are available for cosmetic use, including biodegradable products, permanent fillers, and autologous fat transfer. Careful selection and placement of the appropriate filler is important because properties of fillers vary widely. In addition, specific contraindications for the selected filler should be reviewed before treatment. Biodegradable products, such as hyaluronic acid, and semipermanent fillers, such as calcium hydroxyapatite, are eventually resorbed by the body. They may last from 6 months to 2 years. They offer the advantage of reversibility in the case of undesirable placement but require repeated treatments to maintain the desired effect.

Common side effects immediately following soft tissue augmentation are related to injection site bruising, swelling, and redness. Rarely, more serious complications may arise due to vascular compromise leading to tissue necrosis. This may result from compression or obstruction of blood vessels in the glabella or nasolabial folds. Signs of impending necrosis include blanching, violaceous reticulation, or significant pain.[46,47] Blindness due to retinal embolism following intravascular injection of the supratrochlear artery, a branch of the ophthalmic artery, has also been reported.[48] Late adverse effects of filler injection relate to the formation of subcutaneous nodules, which may be due to filler aggregation, granulomatous inflammatory reactions, or a chronic subclinical infection.[49]

## Light Sources

Laser resurfacing is a skin rejuvenation technology developed to target the cutaneous signs of photodamage. Lasers and other light source procedures are divided into ablative and nonablative resurfacing. Laser procedures are based on the theory of selective photothermolysis.[50] Ablative lasers were first used in the 1980s and markedly improved rhytids, dyspigmentation, skin laxity, and other signs of photoaging by inducing dermal collagen remodeling. The traditional ablative lasers consisted of the 10,600-nm $CO_2$ and 2940-nm erbium:YAG lasers. However, due to a relatively high risk of adverse effects and long recovery period, fractional ablative, as well as other nonablative, lasers have since been developed. The latter technologies are associated with a lower incidence of scarring, infection, dyspigmentation, and prolonged erythema. Nonablative modalities include vascular lasers, pigment lasers, intense pulsed light (IPL), infrared lasers and light sources, and radiofrequency devices.

In managing photoaging, treatments should be tailored to target the specific clinical features in different skin types and ethnic origin, as well as to take into account the variation in potential treatment complications. In a recent review of the literature, procedures that are more invasive, such as chemical peels and laser resurfacing in contrast to botulinum toxin and dermal fillers, pose a greater risk for skin of color.[1] These complications include dyspigmentation, keloid, or hypertrophic scarring. Individuals with darker skin should avoid medium to deep peels. Photorejuvenation with lasers in darker skinned patients is challenging and may be successfully achieved when appropriate settings are used, such as limiting the fluence. Epidermal cooling is essential to avoid unwanted thermal injury and postinflammatory hyperpigmentation.[51] Safer choices of lasers and light sources include IPL, light-emitting diode, 1064-nm laser, fractional nonablative laser, and radiofrequency technology.[52]

## SUMMARY

Photoaging results in premature skin aging from chronic ultraviolet exposure. Individuals with fair skin are predisposed to more severe changes. Clinical signs include rhytids, lentigines, mottled hyperpigmentation, loss of translucency, and decreased elasticity. These features are further influenced by individual ethnicity and genetics. Photoaging may be prevented and treated with a variety of modalities, including topical retinoids, cosmeceuticals, chemical peels, injectable neuromodulators, soft tissue fillers, and light sources. Photoaging remains an important cosmetic concern for many dermatologic patients. Further investigation into the differences between ethnicities, as well as even more effective strategies to prevent and treat photoaging, is warranted.

## REFERENCES

1. Davis EC, Callender VD. Aesthetic dermatology for aging ethnic skin. Dermatol Surg 2011;37(7): 901–17.
2. Kligman LH. Photoaging. Manifestations, prevention, and treatment. Dermatol Clin 1986;4(3): 517–28.
3. Bart RS. Dermatoheliosis? J Am Acad Dermatol 1996;35(4):649–50.
4. Green AC. Premature ageing of the skin in a Queensland population. Med J Aust 1991;155(7): 473–4, 477–8.
5. Goh SH. The treatment of visible signs of senescence: the Asian experience. Br J Dermatol 1990; 122(Suppl 35):105–9.
6. Nouveau-Richard S, Yang Z, Mac-Mary S, et al. Skin ageing: a comparison between Chinese and European populations. A pilot study. J Dermatol Sci 2005;40(3):187–93.
7. Urbach F, Forbes PD, Davies RE, et al. Cutaneous photobiology: past, present and future. J Invest Dermatol 1976;67(1):209–24.
8. Chung JH. Photoaging in Asians. Photodermatol Photoimmunol Photomed 2003;19(3):109–21.
9. Yaar M, Gilchrest BA. Photoageing: mechanism, prevention and therapy. Br J Dermatol 2007; 157(5):874–87.
10. Benjamin CL, Ullrich SE, Kripke ML, et al. p53 tumor suppressor gene: a critical molecular target for UV induction and prevention of skin cancer. Photochem Photobiol 2008;84(1):55–62.
11. Fisher GJ, Kang S, Varani J, et al. Mechanisms of photoaging and chronological skin aging. Arch Dermatol 2002;138(11):1462–70.
12. Sternlicht MD, Werb Z. How matrix metalloproteinases regulate cell behavior. Annu Rev Cell Dev Biol 2001;17:463–516.
13. Fisher GJ, Voorhees JJ. Molecular mechanisms of photoaging and its prevention by retinoic acid: ultraviolet irradiation induces MAP kinase signal transduction cascades that induce Ap-1-regulated matrix metalloproteinases that degrade human skin in vivo. J Investig Dermatol Symp Proc 1998;3(1):61–8.
14. Senftleben U, Karin M. The IKK/NF-kappaB pathway. Crit Care Med 2002;30(Suppl 1):S18–26.
15. Yamamoto Y, Gaynor RB. Therapeutic potential of inhibition of the NF-kappaB pathway in the treatment of inflammation and cancer. J Clin Invest 2001;107(2):135–42.
16. Gordon JR, Brieva JC. Images in clinical medicine. Unilateral dermatoheliosis. N Engl J Med 2012; 366(16):e25.
17. Kaidbey KH, Agin PP, Sayre RM, et al. Photoprotection by melanin–a comparison of black and Caucasian skin. J Am Acad Dermatol 1979;1(3): 249–60.
18. Shirakabe Y, Suzuki Y, Lam SM. A new paradigm for the aging Asian face. Aesthetic Plast Surg 2003;27(5):397–402.
19. Timilshina S, Bhuvan KC, Khanal M, et al. The influence of ethnic origin on the skin photoageing: Nepalese study. Int J Cosmet Sci 2011;33(6):553–9.
20. Vierkotter A, Krutmann J. Environmental influences on skin aging and ethnic-specific manifestations. Dermatoendocrinol 2012;4(3):227–31.
21. Kurban RS, Bhawan J. Histologic changes in skin associated with aging. J Dermatol Surg Oncol 1990;16(10):908–14.
22. Varani J, Warner RL, Gharaee-Kermani M, et al. Vitamin A antagonizes decreased cell growth and elevated collagen-degrading matrix metalloproteinases and stimulates collagen accumulation in naturally aged human skin. J Invest Dermatol 2000;114(3):480–6.
23. Tsuji T. Loss of dermal elastic tissue in solar elastosis. Arch Dermatol 1980;116(4):474–5.
24. Griffiths CE, Wang TS, Hamilton TA, et al. A photonumeric scale for the assessment of cutaneous photodamage. Arch Dermatol 1992;128(3): 347–51.
25. Helfrich YR, Yu L, Ofori A, et al. Effect of smoking on aging of photoprotected skin: evidence gathered using a new photonumeric scale. Arch Dermatol 2007;143(3):397–402.
26. Chung JH, Lee SH, Youn CS, et al. Cutaneous photodamage in Koreans: influence of sex, sun exposure, smoking, and skin color. Arch Dermatol 2001;137(8):1043–51.
27. Glogau RG. Aesthetic and anatomic analysis of the aging skin. Semin Cutan Med Surg 1996;15(3): 134–8.
28. Day DJ, Littler CM, Swift RW, et al. The wrinkle severity rating scale: a validation study. Am J Clin Dermatol 2004;5(1):49–52.

29. Carruthers A, Carruthers J. A validated facial grading scale: the future of facial ageing measurement tools? J Cosmet Laser Ther 2010;12(5):235–41.

30. Cho S, Lowe L, Hamilton TA, et al. Long-term treatment of photoaged human skin with topical retinoic acid improves epidermal cell atypia and thickens the collagen band in papillary dermis. J Am Acad Dermatol 2005;53(5):769–74.

31. Kang S, Duell EA, Fisher GJ, et al. Application of retinol to human skin in vivo induces epidermal hyperplasia and cellular retinoid binding proteins characteristic of retinoic acid but without measurable retinoic acid levels or irritation. J Invest Dermatol 1995;105(4):549–56.

32. Bhawan J, Olsen E, Lufrano L, et al. Histologic evaluation of the long term effects of tretinoin on photodamaged skin. J Dermatol Sci 1996;11(3): 177–82.

33. Fisher GJ, Datta SC, Talwar HS, et al. Molecular basis of sun-induced premature skin ageing and retinoid antagonism. Nature 1996;379(6563):335–9.

34. Griffiths CE, Russman AN, Majmudar G, et al. Restoration of collagen formation in photodamaged human skin by tretinoin (retinoic acid). N Engl J Med 1993;329(8):530–5.

35. CenterWatch. FDA approved drugs in dermatology. [cited 2013 November 17, 2013]. Available at: http://www.centerwatch.com/drug-information/fda-approvals/drug-areas.aspx?AreaID=3. Accessed November 17, 2013.

36. Samuel M, Brooke RC, Hollis S, et al. Interventions for photodamaged skin. Cochrane Database Syst Rev 2005;(1):CD001782.

37. Draelos ZD. The art and science of new advances in cosmeceuticals. Clin Plast Surg 2011;38(3): 397–407, vi.

38. Chien A, Cheng N, Shin J, et al. Topical retinol, a precursor to tretinoin, can deliver comparable efficacy to tretinoin in treatment. J Invest Dermatol 2012;132(S1):S93.

39. Kligman D, Kligman AM. Salicylic acid peels for the treatment of photoaging. Dermatol Surg 1998; 24(3):325–8.

40. Fabbrocini G, De Padova MP, Tosti A. Chemical peels: what's new and what isn't new but still works well. Facial Plast Surg 2009;25(5):329–36.

41. Landau M. Cardiac complications in deep chemical peels. Dermatol Surg 2007;33(2):190–3 [discussion: 193].

42. Carruthers J, Carruthers A. The evolution of botulinum neurotoxin type A for cosmetic applications. J Cosmet Laser Ther 2007;9(3):186–92.

43. Carruthers A. Botulinum toxin type A: history and current cosmetic use in the upper face. Dis Mon 2002;48(5):299–322.

44. Allergan I. Botox Cosmetic (botulinum toxin type A) purified neurotoxin complex (prescribing information). Irvine (CA): Allergan; 2005.

45. Klein AW. Complications, adverse reactions, and insights with the use of botulinum toxin. Dermatol Surg 2003;29(5):549–56 [discussion: 556].

46. Bachmann F, Erdmann R, Hartmann V, et al. The spectrum of adverse reactions after treatment with injectable fillers in the glabellar region: results from the Injectable Filler Safety Study. Dermatol Surg 2009;35(Suppl 2):1629–34.

47. Grunebaum LD, Bogdan Allemann I, Dayan S, et al. The risk of alar necrosis associated with dermal filler injection. Dermatol Surg 2009;35(Suppl 2):1635–40.

48. McCleve DE, Goldstein JC. Blindness secondary to injections in the nose, mouth, and face: cause and prevention. Ear Nose Throat J 1995;74(3): 182–8.

49. Gladstone HB, Cohen JL. Adverse effects when injecting facial fillers. Semin Cutan Med Surg 2007; 26(1):34–9.

50. Anderson RR, Parrish JA. Selective photothermolysis: precise microsurgery by selective absorption of pulsed radiation. Science 1983;220(4596):524–7.

51. Munavalli GS, Weiss RA, Halder RM. Photoaging and nonablative photorejuvenation in ethnic skin. Dermatol Surg 2005;31(9 Pt 2):1250–60 [discussion: 1261].

52. Elsaie ML, Lloyd HW. Latest laser and light-based advances for ethnic skin rejuvenation. Indian J Dermatol 2008;53(2):49–53.

# Photocarcinogenesis
## An Epidemiologic Perspective on Ultraviolet Light and Skin Cancer

Bonita Kozma, MD[a],*, Melody J. Eide, MD, MPH[a,b]

---

**KEYWORDS**

- Melanoma • Nonmelanoma skin cancer • Photocarcinogenesis • Ultraviolet radiation
- Epidemiology

---

**KEY POINTS**

- Ultraviolet (UV) light exposure is a well-known risk factor for developing skin cancer.
- Indoor tanning has been shown to increase cumulative UV exposure and risk of skin cancers, especially in younger fair-skinned populations.
- Cutaneous photocarcinogenesis involves a complex interplay between ultraviolet radiation, cells of the skin, molecular pathways, DNA, and the immune system.

---

## INTRODUCTION

Skin cancer is the most common malignancy worldwide, with increasing incidence seen in many countries, including the United States. In 2013, it is estimated that there will be 3.5 million new cases of nonmelanoma skin cancer (NMSC) and approximately 76,000 new cases of melanoma in the United States alone.[1] It is estimated that around 9000 deaths will occur in the United States because of melanoma in 2013.[1,2]

Ultraviolet (UV) light exposure is a well-known risk factor for the development of skin cancer. Although UV exposure occurs on a daily basis, it is increased through recreational and occupational choices; thus, heightened awareness and understanding of factors and avoidable exposures are key factors to reducing this risk. The International Agency for Research on Cancer (IARC) has classified solar radiation as carcinogenic to humans.[3] This article discusses a brief overview of UV and its biologic effects on cells of the skin

that can lead to mutagenesis and ultimately carcinogenesis. NMSC and melanoma are discussed separately in regards to epidemiology, genetic conditions predisposing patients to each type of skin cancer, and the initiation and propagation of tumors. In addition, public health issues related to UV exposure, such as tanning, workplace exposures, and vitamin D deficiency, are discussed briefly.

## BIOLOGIC EFFECTS OF UV

Solar radiation contains UV, visible light, and infrared radiation. The UV spectrum is divided into UVC (200–290 nm), UVB (290–320 nm), UVA2 (320–340 nm), and UVA1 (340–400 nm). Most all of the UVC wavelength is absorbed by the Earth's ozone, with UVB and UVA reaching the Earth's surface. The wavelength corresponds to level of penetration into the skin, with longer wavelengths penetrating deeper. UVB penetrates to the basal layer of the epidermis and superficial

---

No relationships to disclose.

[a] Department of Dermatology, Henry Ford Hospital, 3031 West Grand Boulevard, Detroit, MI 48202, USA;
[b] Department of Public Health Sciences, Henry Ford Hospital, 3031 West Grand Boulevard, Detroit, MI 48202, USA
* Corresponding author. Department of Dermatology, Henry Ford Health System, 3031 West Grand Boulevard, Suite 800, Detroit, MI 48202.
E-mail address: Bkozma2@hfhs.org

derm.theclinics.com

dermis, with UVA penetrating into the deep dermis.[4] Apart from DNA damage, UVA and UVB also exert different effects on the skin. UVB is more effective than UVA in causing sunburn, whereas UVA leads to immediate (lasting minutes after exposure) and persistent (lasting hours after exposure) pigment darkening. UVA is also responsible for most photoallergic and phototoxic reactions and is capable of penetrating window glass. Both UVA and UVB are involved in photocarcinogenesis.[5] **Fig. 1** overviews photocarcinogenesis.

## DNA Damage

Biologic effects of UV light on the skin occur after the absorption of UV light by chromophores, which are molecules in the skin that absorb photons. The most important chromophore in photocarcinogenesis is DNA. UVB induces the formation of pyrimidine dimers and 4,6 photoproducts. Often there are C to T and CC to TT mutations, which are known as UVB signature mutations. UVA is thought to contribute to carcinogenesis through the formation of free radicals that then cause indirect damage to DNA. Oxidation of guanine to 8-hydroxyguanine is a common mutation from UVA irradiation.[6] However, it is now known that UVA can also form pyrimidine dimers. Single-strand breaks, double-strand breaks, and cross-links between DNA strands can occur as a result of ultraviolet radiation (UVR) exposure.[7] Once a mutation forms, it may be repaired, or the cell may be targeted for apoptosis if the damage is too severe. This is accomplished through *p53*, a tumor suppressor gene that plays a central role in cell repair, apoptosis, and cell-cycle arrest to allow time for repairs. The levels of p53 are increased in normal keratinocytes after UVR exposure.[6] If the *p53* gene is mutated, the cell may not be able to repair itself, leading to permanent damage. The cell may also become resistant to apoptosis.[8] *P53* mutations have been demonstrated in sun-exposed skin, actinic keratoses (AKs), squamous cell carcinoma (SCCs), basal cell carcinoma (BCCs), and melanomas.[6]

It may be more harmful for mutations of *p53* to occur in basal keratinocytes than fully differentiated keratinocytes because basal keratinocytes have the ability to express a stem-cell-like phenotype. Basal keratinocytes with mutated *p53* can give rise to differentiated keratinocytes that also contain mutated *p53*. Clones of cells with mutated *p53* are often found in normal chronically sun-exposed skin, which suggests mutations in *p53* are an early event in photocarcinogenesis.[9,10]

## Cell-Cycle Arrest

For the cell to repair a mutation accurately, it must have time for repair. The cell cycle is divided into G1 (Gap phase), S (DNA synthesis), G2, and M (mitosis) phases. The cell cycle can undergo arrest at various points to allow repair of DNA damage. The G1 checkpoint is important because it prevents a cell from progressing to S phase with a damaged DNA template, which would lead to a mutation formation with DNA replication. Progression to S phase depends on the phosphorylation of retinoblastoma (Rb) by cyclin-dependent kinases (CDK), specifically D-CDK4 (6) kinases. Unphosphorylated Rb is bound by E2F, a transcription factor. Increased levels of *p-53* following UVR

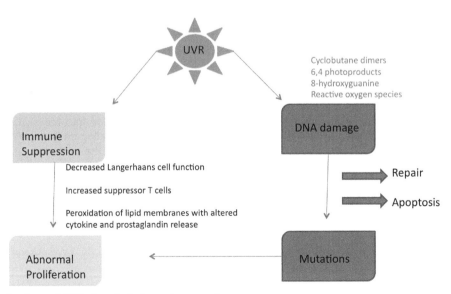

**Fig. 1.** Mechanisms of UV-induced photocarcinogenesis.

exposure leads to induction of p21, a cyclin kinase inhibitor, and to cell-cycle arrest at the G1 checkpoint,[11] which can also occur independent of *p53*.

DNA damage is thought to be sensed by ataxia telangiectasia mutated (ATM) and ATM-Rad3-related protein (ATR), which are protein kinases that signal via other molecules to effectors of cellular repair. ATM and ATR are thought to exhibit some specificity to the type of DNA damage they detect. Because UVA and UVB can produce differing proportions of photoproducts, it is thought that UVA and UVB induce different mechanisms of repair through the transduction paths of ATM and/or ATR. ATM depends on functional *p53*, whereas ATR does not.[12]

Some phases of the cell cycle are more resistant to UV-mediated damage. S phase is the most resistant phase to damage from UVR. ATM phosphorylates Chk2, BRCA1, and NBS1, which are molecules responsible for DNA repair response and the S-phase checkpoint. G2 phase is also comparatively resistant to photodamage. This phase represents the last opportunity to prevent damaged DNA from replicating and being passed on to daughter cells in mitosis. If cells are damaged in G2, they undergo arrest that depends on ATM and BRCA1. If cells are damaged in S phase and passed onto G2, they are arrested in an ATM-independent manner through ATR. Multiple pathways regulating G2 arrest ultimately contribute to regulating CDK1 activity through phosphorylation and subsequent activation or inactivation.[12]

## DNA Repair

Once the cell cycle has been arrested, DNA damage is repaired. Base excision repair (BER) involves the recognition and removal of damaged bases, which may not cause significant distortion of the DNA helix. BER is important in protection from oxidative damage of DNA, which is mainly attributed to UVA. Larger strings of nucleotide damage, such as pyrimidine dimers and 6,4 photoproducts caused commonly by UVB, are repaired by nucleotide excision repair (NER). Two groups of NER are used, depending on if the damage has occurred in a transcriptionally active or transcriptionally silent gene.[12]

Repair speed varies by mechanism. Transcription coupled repair corrects damage quickly in active genes, whereas global genome repair works at a slower pace in inactive genes.[13] There are also differences in repair speed between pyrimidine dimers and 6,4 photoproducts. Young and colleagues[14] demonstrated that bulky dimers were repaired slowly and had a half-life of 33.3 hours

in human skin following irradiation. In contrast, 6,4 photoproducts had a half-life of only 2.3 hours. It is postulated that these differences occur because of the difference in degree of distortion the 2 types of products generated on the DNA helix. Although the 6,4 lesion is smaller, it causes more distortion in the helix than the dimer.[15]

## Apoptosis

If cells have sustained too much damage to be repaired, apoptosis is a mechanism in place to prevent mutation formation. The p53 tumor suppressor protein plays a role in mediating apoptosis, with p53-deficient mice showing decreased apoptotic cells after UVR compared with wild-type mice.[9] p53 increases the transcription of Bax, a pro-apoptotic protein, and bcl-2 can inhibit Bax when the 2 molecules form a heterodimer.[13] Although keratinocytes readily undergo apoptosis through this pathway after exposure to UVR, melanocytes are less likely to undergo apoptosis following UVR exposure. This difference is likely due to the higher concentrations of bcl-2 found in melanocytes compared with keratinocytes.[16] After exposure to UVR, bcl-2 expression is reduced in normal skin cells, which leads to a state favoring apoptosis. High levels of bcl-2 are seen in the tumors of melanoma, SCC, BCC, and AKs, which gives the tumor cells a selective survival advantage over normal cells that undergo apoptosis following UVR damage.[13] Park and Lee[17] demonstrated decreased expression of Bcl-Xl after UVB irradiation, which likely occurs through proteasome-mediated degradation. Pro-apoptotic agents may potentially provide alternative treatment modalities for patients with NMSC.

## UV Effects on the Immune System

In addition to causing DNA damage, UV can also indirectly increase the risk of carcinogenesis through effects on the immune system. UV exposure decreases the detection of damaged cells by the immune system as demonstrated by Kripke.[18] Tumor cells were transplanted onto irradiated and unexposed mice. The tumor cells grew when placed in the radiation-exposed mice, but did not progress in the unexposed mice.

Immune suppression is accomplished through alterations of cytokines, soluble factors, and effects on Langerhans cells and T cells of the skin. Pro-inflammatory cytokines and prostaglandins, such as interleukin (IL)-10, tumor necrosis factor α, and prostaglandin E2 are increased following irradiation of keratinocytes.[19] Simon and colleagues[20] demonstrated that Langerhans cells exposed to UVR could present antigen to Th2 cells but could not present antigen to Th1 cells. Increased Th2 cytokines such as IL-4, IL-5, IL-6, and IL-10 resulted, which reduced the presentation of antigens to T cells. Trans-urocanic acid is found in the outer layers of the skin and isomerizes to cis-urocanic acid following UVB exposure. Cis-urocanic acid can also decrease antigen presentation to T cells, in addition to inducing the formation of suppressor T cells.[21]

Free radicals can also contribute to immune suppression through peroxidation of lipid membranes. Generated free radicals cause release of platelet activating factor (PAF) from the epidermis. Free radicals and PAF attack mainly unsaturated fatty acids in the lipid membrane. Lipids are damaged through the direct oxidation of their double bonds or by free radical-induced chain reactions. The peroxidation of lipids impacts prostaglandin synthesis and cytokine release, which results in active regulatory T cells and immune suppression.[19,22]

## NONMELANOMA SKIN CANCER
### Epidemiology

Nonmelanoma skin cancer largely consists of BCC and SCC. Although NMSC is found mainly in elderly individuals,[23] the incidence has been increasing, especially among younger women.[24]

BCC is the most common NMSC, comprising about 80% of skin cancers. BCCs are slow-growing and locally invasive, reflected in the low mortality rate. Established risk factors for sporadic BCC include intermittent UV exposure in childhood and adolescence, skin types I and II, exposure to ionizing radiation, arsenic exposure, immunosuppression, family history, male sex, and older age.[25]

Increasing attention has focused on BCCs in younger individuals. Risk factors for BCC occurring in those under the age of 40 were examined by Bakos and colleagues.[26] They found that women were more likely than men to be affected, and that most tumors occurred on the neck and face. Tanning bed use and smoking were found to be associated with increased risk for sporadic BCC before the age of 40. Sunscreen use was found to be a protective factor. Although BCC incidence is increasing in this age group, the overall frequency of BCC in this age group remains low.

SCCs have a stronger link to cumulative UV exposure and tend to occur on sun-exposed surfaces, frequently the head and neck. Unlike BCC, they have a higher mortality rate and are more likely to metastasize if not treated.[27] Additional risk factors for developing SCC are similar to the risk factors for developing BCC, with immunosuppression

(including organ transplant) being a stronger risk factor for SCC than BCC.[28]

### Genetic Predisposition for NMSC

Some patients have an increased risk for NMSC because of genetic predisposition, which may be amplified by UV exposure. Nevoid basal cell carcinoma syndrome, or Gorlin syndrome, is inherited in an autosomal-dominant manner. In Gorlin syndrome, there is a mutation in patched (PTCH), a tumor suppressor gene; the product of this gene, Patched, inhibits the G protein-coupled receptor Smoothened (SMO) at baseline. Sonic Hedgehog can bind to Patched, which releases SMO from inhibition; downstream signaling results in activation of the transcription factor Gli, and subsequent cellular proliferation (Fig. 2).[29] Patients characteristically have palmoplantar pits, odontogenic keratocysts, calcification of the dura, rib anomalies, ovarian fibromas, and medulloblastomas.[30] There is no increase in photocarcinogenesis in Gorlin syndrome, although some disorders with increased skin cancers do have an increase in photocarcinogenesis.[31]

Another genetic disorder, xeroderma pigmentosum (XP), can predispose patients to BCC, SCC, and melanoma through increased photocarcinogenesis. The disorder is autosomal-recessive, and there are several types of XP (XPA-XPG) and XP variant. In XP, the mutations are related to excision repair, which is responsible for removing the 6,4 photoproducts and pyrimidine dimers induced by UVR. Inability or decreased efficacy in removing the DNA damage leads to mutations, which can then progress to carcinomas.[15] In a proof of concept study, application of liposomes containing DNA repair enzyme T4 endonuclease V to skin of patients with XP resulted in lower development of BCCs and AKs.[32]

### Sporadic Formation of NMSC

Acquired (noninherited) DNA mutations, such as those induced by UV, are responsible for sporadic NMSC. Sporadic BCCs arise when mutations accrue in the basal keratinocytes and give selective survival advantage to these cells. Sporadic SCCs occur when keratinocytes with the potential to proliferate acquire mutations that lead to malignant transformation. As discussed earlier, UVR can damage DNA directly or indirectly, interfere with cell-cycle arrest, alter apoptosis, and affect the immune system.[6] Prolonged and intermittent exposure to high levels of UVR are responsible for BCC development, with intermittent exposure being the most important. BCC most commonly develops on the head and neck.[33] The tumor

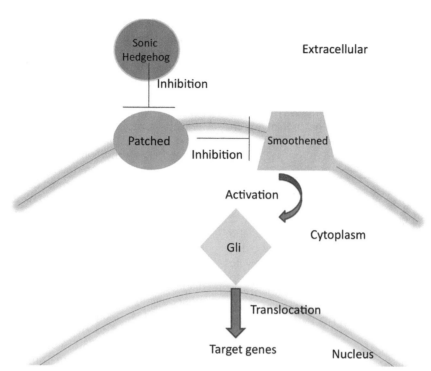

**Fig. 2.** Sonic hedgehog pathway. Under normal conditions, patched inhibits smoothened. When sonic hedgehog binds, it releases smoothened from inhibition of patched. Gli is then activated and translocated to the nucleus and acts on target genes resulting in proliferation. (*Data from* Bale AE, Yu K. The hedgehog pathway and basal cell carcinomas. Hum Mol Genet 2001;10(7):757–62.)

suppressor genes *PTCH* and *p53* are the most common mutations found in BCC, with *PTCH* mutations being the most prevalent.[6] The function of Patched protein is to relay growth regulatory signals to the nucleus of the cell.[26] Mutations found in BCC's *PTCH* gene are often C to T UVB signature mutations. It is thought that the mutation of *PTCH* is an earlier event in the initiation of BCC than the mutation of *p53*.[34]

Unlike BCC, SCC can be preceded by precursor lesions, such as AKs and Bowen's disease. Cumulative UV exposure seems to be important in SCC.[27] The rate of progression from AK to SCC in a given year ranges from 0.025% to 16%, whereas roughly 25% of AKs resolve in a given year.[35] Similar to BCC, SCC may develop *p53* mutations, as supported by studies that demonstrate increased mutated *p53* in normal sun-exposed skin compared with non-sun-exposed skin. This increase may predispose cells in sun-exposed skin to carcinogenesis. As many as 58% of SCC have UVB signature mutations in *p53*.[36]

## Occupational Exposure and NMSC

Although BCC is the most common cancer and UVR has been proven to contribute to its pathogenesis, little has been published in the literature regarding occupational exposure and preventative measures in the workplace. Stronger associations between workplace exposure and SCC have been established.[26]

A meta-analysis by Bauer and colleagues[37] included 23 epidemiologic studies and found a pooled odds ratio (OR) of 1.43 for the association between outdoor work and risk of BCC (95% confidence interval 1.23–1.66; $P = .0001$). An inverse relationship between geographic latitude and risk of BCC was also found. However, there were limitations including incomplete distinction in some studies between occupational and nonoccupational UV exposures, and classification of indoor and outdoor occupations. Some studies also failed to consider Fitzpatrick skin type, recall bias, and self-selection bias (ie, phenotypic characteristics of workers selecting outdoor occupations). The authors speculated the risk may be higher than what was found in the meta-analysis.

A meta-analysis of 18 studies was also performed on SCC and workplace UV exposure and found a pooled OR of 1.77 for the association between outdoor work and risk of SCC (95% confidence interval 1.40–2.22; $P<.001$).[27] The limitations of this meta-analysis were similar to the meta-analysis regarding BCC and workplace exposures in that many studies did not quantify the amounts of exposure, did not accurately classify indoor or outdoor work, and did not account for confounders such as age/sex/sensitivity to UV. Although some occupations with hazardous exposures have safety rules and preventative measures in place, there are currently no legal regulations on workplace exposure to UV light.

### Indoor Tanning and NMSC

Recreational UVR also contributes to the formation of BCC and SCC. Indoor tanning is popular among adolescents and young adults. Around 2 to 3 million indoor tanners are adolescents, and 24% of these are between 13 and 19 years old.[38] Tanning bed users are 1.5 times more likely to develop BCC[39] and 2.5 times more likely to develop SCC. In 2007, the IARC concluded that indoor tanning led to increased incidence of melanoma and SCC, but data on BCC were inconclusive at that time.[40]

Supporting evidence for the role of indoor tanning in BCC pathogenesis continues to accumulate. Ferrucci and colleagues[41] performed a case control study with 376 BCC patients and 390 control subjects under the age of 40 and found an increased risk for BCC with indoor tanning. The risk was stronger for female patients and those with multiple BCC and was associated with higher incidence of BCC on the trunk and extremities compared with BCC from incidental UV exposure. A dose-response effect between the number of burns received from indoor tanning and early-onset BCC was also illustrated. They were unable to examine the effect of indoor tanning in men because of insufficient numbers.

A recent cohort study by Zhang and colleagues[42] published in 2012 examined 73,494 patients in the Nurses' Health Study II cohort. Data were collected on how often the subjects tanned in a year, and what age subjects were when they tanned. It was found that the risk of BCC was increased in those who tanned in high school, college, or between the ages of 25 and 35. However, the risk for BCC was significantly higher for those who tanned during high school and college. Users who tanned indoors 4 times a year had a 15% increase in risk, and a dose-response relationship was detected. Confounders such as outdoor tanning and the UV index in the place of residence were controlled for in the study.

## MELANOMA

The incidence of melanoma is generally higher in men than in women in the United States.[43]

However, the epidemiology may be different for younger people.[44] In a 2008 study, there were 28.3 and 18.5 melanoma cases per 100,000 for men and women, respectively. For those under the age of 45, this trend was reversed with 8.2 cases for women compared with 5.3 cases for men.[44] This gender distribution reflects indoor tanning demographics. The increased tumors found in younger women are generally thin melanomas.[45] Disproportionate increase of BCC incidence has also been found in young women under the age of 40.[24] The most common locations for melanoma in men are the trunk and upper extremities. For women, most melanomas occur on the lower extremities.[40]

There is racial variation in the incidence of the types of melanoma. In African Americans, acral lentiginous melanoma is the most common type diagnosed, whereas superficial spreading is the most common type diagnosed in all other races.[46] From 2004 to 2006, the incidence of tumor types was found to be 57.2% melanoma not-otherwise-specified, 28.8% superficial spreading, 6.9% nodular, 6% lentigomaligna, and 1% acral lentiginous in Caucasians.[40]

There are known risk factors that predispose individuals to melanoma. The risks are attributed to genetic or phenotypic traits, as well as environmental factors. Those with fair skin, light eyes and hair, freckling, greater than 20 nevi, at least 3 atypical nevi, XP, or a family history of melanoma or dysplastic nevi are at increased risk for melanoma.[40] Individuals who are immunosuppressed, have experienced at least 3 sunburns, have periodic excessive UV exposure, or UV exposure in tanning salons are also at increased risk for melanoma.[40]

It has also been demonstrated that melanoma rates decrease in Caucasians with increasing distance from the equator. A notable exception is in Western Europe, where incidence is higher in the North compared with the South. This exception is thought to be due to Northern Europeans vacationing in the South, where they receive intermittent and intense sun exposure.[47] In the United States, melanoma incidence was associated with lower latitude and increased UV index only in Caucasians.[48] This correlation of UV index with city latitude persists in 2012 with updated analysis (**Fig. 3**).

An individual's current geographic location is not the only factor when considering UV exposure. It is important to consider migration and prior lifetime UV exposure in individuals. The importance of early sun exposure is illustrated in the study from Western Australia by Holman and Armstrong.[49] Migrants arriving from Great Britain and native

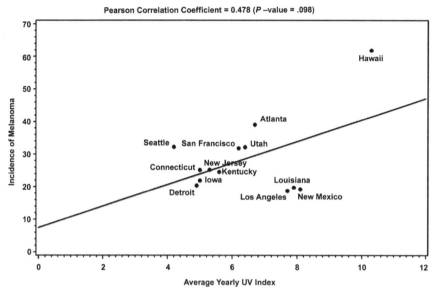

**Fig. 3.** Scatterplot of UV index versus age: adjusted melanoma incidence by registry in the white non-Hispanic population. (*From* Howlader N, Noone AM, Krapcho M, et al. SEER cancer statistics review, 1975-2008. Bethesda (MD): National Cancer Institute; 2011. Available at: http://seercancergov/csr/1975_2008/. Based on November 2010 SEER data submission, posted to the SEER web site. Accessed November 6, 2013.)

Australians were studied. Those who migrated before the age of 10 had a similar risk of melanoma compared with natives, whereas the incidence was lower in those arriving after the age of 15. The authors found that age of migration to Australia predicted melanoma risk better than duration of residence. Therefore, childhood exposure and not total exposure determined melanoma risk. Similarly, Mack and Floderus[50] studied 4611 cases of melanoma diagnosed in 1972 to 1982 among Caucasian residents of Los Angeles from known place of origin. Those who migrated to Los Angeles from higher US latitudes had less incidence of melanoma compared with natives. The time after migration did not seem to affect melanoma incidence. Similar migrant findings have been noted in other countries, including Israel.[51]

## Genetic Predisposition to Melanoma

Some individuals have an inherited genetic predisposition to melanoma, with about 5% to 11% of melanoma cases estimated to be hereditary.[52] Genetic syndromes that have defects in DNA repair, such as XP, predispose to melanoma through increased DNA mutations and malignant transformation of melanocytes.[15] Familial atypical multiple mole melanoma (FAMMM) syndrome results from a mutation in the tumor suppressor gene CDKN2A and is estimated to account for 25% to 40% of the inherited melanoma cases.[53]

The disorder has an autosomal-dominant inheritance with variable expressivity, which leads to a varied phenotype. Patients often have large, irregular nevi and a family history of melanoma. The most common visceral malignancy associated with FAMMM syndrome is pancreatic cancer, but other malignancies have also been reported. The gene encodes proteins p16, p15, and p18, which have a role in the G1/S checkpoint. When these protein products are impaired, the cell improperly moves from G1 to S phase and proliferation is uncontrolled.[53]

Recently, germline mutations in BAP1 have been discovered in families with hereditary melanoma. The hereditary BAP1 cancer predisposition syndrome includes uveal melanoma, cutaneous melanoma, mesothelioma, renal cell carcinoma, and melanocytic BAP1-mutated atypical intradermal tumors.[54] There have also been reports of ovarian carcinoma, hepatic cholangiocarcinoma, and possibly breast carcinoma in relatives of those with BAP1 mutations. Those who carry the mutation should get annual ophthalmologic examinations starting at age 11, get annual dermatologic examinations starting at age 22, and follow cancer screening guidelines as set forth by the American Cancer Society.[55] There are other families with melanoma that have unidentified mutations as of yet. It is especially important for those with a family history of melanoma to practice photoprotection.

## Sporadic Melanoma

Sporadic melanoma arises mostly with intense and intermittent exposure to high levels of UVR, especially in childhood.[13] Whiteman and colleagues[56] proposed a "divergent pathway" theory for sporadic melanomas, which may explain differences in anatomic location of melanoma. This theory proposes that melanomas may arise in individuals with inherently increased melanocyte proliferation. These individuals develop melanoma on sites such as the trunk, and history of exposure to sunlight is present early in life. The second possibility is that melanoma arises in individuals with less melanocyte proliferation, but on sites with chronic exposure to sunlight.

Melanin produced by melanocytes can protect the skin from some of the harmful effects of UVR. On exposure to UVR, melanocytes upregulate the melanocortin-1 receptor (MC1-R) and α-melanocytic stimulating hormone that leads to pigment production.[13] However, individuals with loss of function mutations in MC1-R produce pheomelanin instead of eumelanin and are thought to be at increased risk for melanoma. Pheomelanin is associated with increased oxidative stress in the skin following UVR by generating reactive oxygen species or consuming cellular antioxidant reserves.[57]

In addition to pigment production, stimulation of MC1-R leads to increased levels of cyclic AMP (cAMP), microphthalmia-associated transcription factor, protein kinase A, tyrosinase, and tyrosinase-related protein 1. Increased levels of cAMP can lead to increased levels of GTP-bound RAS, and activation of BRAF; this is significant because BRAF is a serine/threonine protein kinase that activates the mitogen-activated protein kinase (MAPK)/extracellular regulated kinase–signaling pathway. The pathway is responsible for functions such as differentiation, proliferation, and apoptosis.[58]

About 50% of melanomas express activating BRAF mutations. BRAFV600E occurs in about 90% of the BRAF mutations. BRAF mutations are mainly detected in skin exposed to intermittent UVR, such as the extremities and trunk.[52] Around 15% to 20% of melanomas have mutations in RAS, specifically, NRAS with mutations observed less in HRAS and KRAS.[59] Another pathway involved in the initiation and progression of melanoma is the phosphatidyl inositol 3-kinase (PI3K/Akt) pathway. PI3K is activated by growth factors and generates phosphatidyl inositol triphosphate (PIP3). PIP3 activates Akt, leading to decreased apoptosis and increased proliferation of cells. The levels of PIP3 are decreased by phosphatase

and tensin homolog (PTEN). Suppression of PTEN or activation of Akt decreases apoptosis of melanoma cells (Fig. 4).[60] The KIT oncogene is also found to be mutated in melanomas, most often in chronically sun-exposed skin and acral or mucosal melanomas. KIT is a tyrosine kinase that is involved in regulation of the MAPK pathway and PI3K/Akt pathway. Mutations lead to its constituent activation, resulting in proliferation and decreased apoptosis of cells.[61] Last, p53 can also be found to be mutated in melanoma but is thought to be a later occurring event when compared with p53 mutations in NMSC. p53 mutations have been found in up to 25% of melanomas.[62]

## Occupational Exposure and Melanoma

Workplace exposure to solar or artificial UV light is a source of concern with rising incidence of melanoma. Because of the rarity of melanoma compared with NMSC, less is known about the role of occupational UV exposure in melanoma development. Elwood and Jopson[63] reviewed 35 case control studies and found a small but significant positive association between melanoma incidence and intermittent UV workplace exposure. Individual studies within the review also showed a decrease in melanoma incidence with greater occupational exposure, but detailed analysis revealed a possible nonlinear relationship. It may be that short-term work with high amounts of UV exposure may increase melanoma risk, whereas chronic occupational UV exposure does not. However, several occupational epidemiology studies from Australia, France, and Spain found strong associations between melanoma incidence and both intermittent exposure and total exposure. The authors postulated that with very high total exposure to UVR, the distinction between chronic exposure and intermittent exposure may be lost. Although definitive data are evolving, it is important to consider occupational exposure to UVR and advocate for acceptable protective measures to be made available for workers.

## Indoor Tanning and Melanoma

A clear association between indoor tanning and melanoma has emerged. Although early studies found both a negative and a positive correlation between tanning and melanoma, a 2005 meta-analysis by Gallagher and colleagues[64] found a significant increased risk of melanoma with tanning bed exposure. The risk increased the younger a person was when initiating indoor tanning. The positive association of tanning bed use and melanoma has now been confirmed by several other

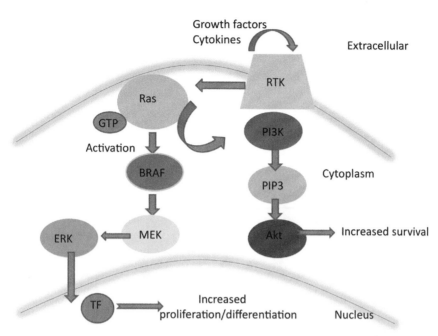

**Fig. 4.** Melanomagenesis. RTK is activated and activates RAS. Activation of BRAF leads to phosphorylation of transcription factors via extracellular-related kinases. PI3K is activated by growth factors and leads to accumulation of phosphatidyl inositol triphosphate, increased Akt activity, and decreased apoptosis. ERK, extracellular-related kinase; MEK, mitogen-activated protein kinase; PI3K, phosphatidyl inositol 3-kinase; PIP3, phosphatidyl inositol triphosphate; RTK, receptor tyrosine kinase; TF, transcription factors. (*Data from* Morgan AM, Lo J, Fisher DE. How does pheomelanin synthesis contribute to melanomagenesis? Bioessays 2013;35:672–6.)

studies.[65,66] Indoor tanning is now commonly recognized as a risk factor for melanoma.

Many claims were previously made that tanning was safer than natural exposure because of the relative lack of UVB. It should be noted that although tanning lamps emitted around 99% UVA and 1% UVB in the 1980s, the amount of UVB in tanning lamps has increased throughout the decades. Summer sunlight contains approximately 95% UVA and 5% UVB. However, UV emission can vary greatly between different tanning beds, and indoor tanners usually have a larger body surface exposed than with outdoor tanning.[67] In addition, the use of tanning booths and the training of tanning booth operators have not been well regulated, and the education of users before tanning sessions is currently lacking.

## UVR, VITAMIN D, AND SKIN CANCER

Although it is recognized that UVR can cause considerable increased risk for skin cancer, some individuals question whether the importance of UV exposure for vitamin D synthesis outweighs the risk of photocarcinogenesis. Vitamin D deficiency has been linked unquestionably to bone health. It also has drawn attention for a possible role in other diseases, including carcinomas of the colon, breast, and skin.[68]

Vitamin D plays an antiproliferative and tumor suppressive role in carcinogenesis. Vitamin D receptors (VDR) are found on melanocytes, keratinocytes, and immune cells of the skin, and VDR polymorphisms have been identified in melanoma and NMSC, as well as the vitamin D endocrine system.[68] Binding of 1,25-$(OH)_2$-D to VDR regulates the expression of vitamin D responsive genes in target tissues. The kidney is the main organ responsible for converting 25-OH-D to 1,25-$(OH)_2$-D.[69] However, it has recently been elucidated that many other tissues including the breast, prostate, colon, and skin can convert 25-OH-D to 1,25-$(OH)_2$D with 1,25 α-hydroxylase. The locally produced 1,25-$(OH)_2$-D has regulatory effects on the cells producing it. Therefore, individuals who are deficient in vitamin D not only experience deterioration of the musculoskeletal system but potentially can have higher rates of other diseases, such as colon cancer, breast cancer, skin cancer, autoimmune diseases, renal disease, and cardiovascular disease.[68]

Vitamin D can be synthesized in the skin by UV exposure. Vitamin D is formed when UVB converts 7-dehydrocholesterol (7DHC) to pre-vitamin D,

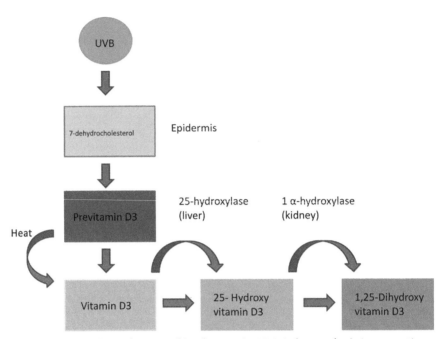

**Fig. 5.** Synthesis of vitamin D. (*Data from* Vanchinathan V, Lim HW. A dermatologist's perspective on Vitamin D. Mayo Clin Proc 2012;87(4):372–80.)

which then isomerizes to vitamin D (**Fig. 5**). However, less than 15% of 7DHC is converted in the skin.[63] Terushkin and colleagues[70] estimated the amount of sun exposure required to synthesize vitamin D production compared with oral supplementation in Boston and Miami. The time it took to synthesize vitamin D from UV exposure depended on location, time of year, body surface area (BSA) exposed, and time of day. Synthesis was found to be faster in summer, at noon, in lighter skin types, and in sunny geographic locations such as Miami. In Miami, synthesis of 400 international units (IU) was possible with short exposure times (3–6 minutes at noon with 25% BSA exposed). However, in Boston, it was estimated to take more than 2 hours during winter months to synthesize 400 IU, taking into account reduced BSA exposure. Because of variation in UV exposure for sufficient vitamin D synthesis and risk of photocarcinogenesis, oral supplementation with vitamin D is the recommended source for vitamin D at this time.[71] Currently, the Institute of Medicine recommends a daily intake of 600 IU per day for adults and children over 1 year of age.[72]

## SUMMARY

UV-induced photocarcinogenesis involves a complex interplay between UVR, cells of the skin, molecular pathways, DNA, and the immune system. With the incidence of skin cancers continuing to increase, photoprotective measures are important for the prevention of cutaneous photocarcinogenesis. Public health messages must emphasize the dangers of indoor tanning and safe ways to maintain adequate vitamin D levels.

## REFERENCES

1. American Cancer Society. Fact sheet on skin cancer. Available at: http://www.cancer.org/acs/groups/content/@nho/documents/document/skincancerpdf.pdf. Accessed October 20, 2013.
2. Lomas A, Leonardi-Bee J, Bath-Hextall F. A systematic review of worldwide incidence of non-melanoma skin cancer. Br J Dermatol 2012;166: 1069–80.
3. El Ghissassi F, Baan R, Straif K, et al. A review of human carcinogens—part D: radiation. Lancet Oncol 2009;10:751–2.
4. de Laat A, van Tilburg M, van der Leun JC, et al. Cell cycle kinetics following UVA irradiation in comparison to UVB and UVC irradiation. Photochem Photobiol 1996;63:492.
5. Lim HW, Hawk JL. Photodermatologic disorders. In: Bolognia J, Jorizzo JJ, Schaffer JV, editors. Dermatology. 3rd edition. St Louis (MO): Mosby/Elsevier; 2012. p. 1480–4.
6. Hussein MR. Ultraviolet radiation and skin cancer: molecular mechanisms. J Cutan Pathol 2005;32: 191–205.
7. Ikehata H, Kawai K, Komura J, et al. UVA1 genotoxicity is mediated not by oxidative damage but by

cyclobutane pyrimidine dimers in normal mouse skin. J Invest Dermatol 2008;128:2289–96.

8. Woo DK, Eide MJ. Tanning beds, skin cancer, and vitamin D: an examination of the scientific evidence and public health implications. Dermatol Ther 2010;23:61–71.

9. Ziegler A, Jonason AS, Leffell DJ, et al. Sunburn and p53 in the onset of skin cancer. Nature 1994; 372:773–6.

10. Jonason AS, Kunala S, Price GJ, et al. Frequent clones of p53-mutated keratinocytes in normal human skin. Proc Natl Acad Sci U S A 1996;93:14025.

11. Wilson GD. Radiation and the cell cycle, revisited. Cancer Metastasis Rev 2004;23:209–25.

12. Placzek M, Pryzbilla B, Kerkmann U, et al. Effect of ultraviolet (UV) A, UVB, or ionizing radiation on the cell cycle of human melanoma cells. Br J Dermatol 2007;156:843–7.

13. Jhappan C, Noonan FP, Merlino G. Ultraviolet radiation and cutaneous malignant melanoma. Oncogene 2003;22:3099–112.

14. Young AR, Chadwick CA, Harrison GI, et al. The in situ repair kinetics of epidermal thymine dimers and 6,4 photoproducts in human skin types I and II. J Invest Dermatol 1996;106:1307–13.

15. Black HS, deGruijl FR, Forbes PD, et al. Photocarcinogenesis: an overview. J Photochem Photobiol B 1997;40:29–47.

16. Morales-Ducret CR, van de Rijn M, Smoller BR. Bcl-2 expression in melanocytic nevi, Insights into the biology of dermal maturation. Arch Dermatol 1995;131:915.

17. Park K, Lee J. BCL-Xl protein is markedly decreased in UVB-irradiated basal cell carcinoma cell lines through proteasome mediated degradation. Oncol Rep 2009;21:689–92.

18. Kripke ML. Anitgenecity of murine skin tumors induced by ultraviolet light. J Natl Cancer Inst 1974;53(5):1333–6.

19. Ullrich SE. Mechanism underlying UV-induced immune suppression. Mutat Res 2005;571(1–2): 185–205.

20. Simon JC, Tigelaar RE, Bergstresser PR, et al. Ultraviolet B radiation converts Langerhans cells from immunogenic to tolerogenic antigen-presenting cells. Induction of specific clonal anergy in in CD4+ T helper 1 cells. J Immunol 1991;146(2): 485–91.

21. Kondo S, Sauder DN, McKenzie RC, et al. The role of cis-urocanic acid in UVB-induced suppression of contact hypersensitivity. Immunol Lett 1995;48: 181–6.

22. Garmyn M, Yarosh DB. The molecular and genetic effects of ultraviolet radiation exposure on skin cells. In: Lim HW, Honigsmann H, Hawk JL, editors. Photodermatology. New York: Informa Health Care; 2007. p. 41–54.

23. Rogers HW, Weinstock MA, Harris AR, et al. Incidence estimate of nonmelanoma skin cancer in the United States, 2006. Arch Dermatol 2010;146: 283–7.

24. Christenson LJ, Borrowman TA, Vachon CM, et al. Incidence of basal cell and squamous cell carcinomas in a population younger than 40 years. JAMA 2005;294(6):681–90.

25. Zak-Prelich M, Narbutt J, Sysa-Jedrzejowska A. Environamental risk factors predisposing to the development of basal cell carcinoma. Dermatol Surg 2004;30:248–52.

26. Bakos RM, Kriz M, Muhlstadt M, et al. Risk factors for early onset basal cell carcinoma in a German institution. Eur J Dermatol 2011;21(5):705–9.

27. Schmitt J, Seidler A, Diepgen TL, et al. Occupational ultraviolet light exposure increases the risk for the development of cutaneous squamous cell carcinoma: a systematic review and meta-analysis. Br J Dermatol 2011;164:291–307.

28. Ng JC, Cumming S, Leung V, et al. Accrual of non-melanoma skin cancer in renal transplant recipients: experience of a Victorian tertiary referral institution. Australas J Dermatol 2014;55(1):43–8. http://dx.doi.org/10.1111/ajd.12072.

29. Lesiak A. The role of sonic hedgehog pathway in skin carcinogenesis. Pol Merkur Lekarski 2010; 170:141–3.

30. Gorlin RJ. Nevoid basal cell carcinoma syndrome. Dermatol Clin 1995;13:113–25.

31. Brellier F, Valin A, Chevallier-Lagente O, et al. Ultraviolet responses of Gorlin syndrome primary skin cells. Br J Dermatol 2008;159(2):445–52.

32. Yarosh D, Klein J, O'Connor A, et al. Effect of topically applied T4 endonuclease V in liposomes on skin cancer in xeroderma pigmentosum: a randomised study. Xeroderma Pigmentosum Study Group. Lancet 2001;357(9260):926–9.

33. Rosso S, Zanetti R, Matinez C, et al. The multicenter south European study 'Helios'. II. Different sun exposure patterns in the aetiology of basal cell carcinoma and squamous cell carcinoma of the skin. Br J Cancer 1996;73:1447–54.

34. D'Errico M, Calcagnile A, Canzona F, et al. UV mutation signature in tumor suppressor genes involved in skin carcinogenesis in xeroderma pigmentosum patients. Oncogene 2000;19:463.

35. Marks R, Rennie G, Selwood TS. Malignant transformation of solar keratoses to squamous cell carcinoma. Lancet 1988;1(8589):795–7.

36. Ratushny V, Gober MD, Hick R, et al. From keratinocyte to cancer: the pathogenesis and modeling of cutaneous squamous cell carcinoma. J Clin Invest 2012;122(2):464–72.

37. Bauer A, Diepgen TL, Schmitt J. Is occupational solar ultraviolet irradiation a relevant risk factor for basal cell carcinoma? A systematic review and

meta-analysis of the epidemiological literature. Br J Dermatol 2011;165:612–25.

38. Lim HW, James WD, Rigel DS, et al. Adverse effects of ultraviolet radiation from the use of indoor tanning equipment: time to ban the tan. J Am Acad Dermatol 2011;64:51–60.

39. Karagas MR, Stannard VA, Mott LA, et al. Use of tanning devices and risk of basal cell and squamous cell skin cancers. J Natl Cancer Inst 2002; 94:224–6.

40. International Agency for Research on Cancer Working Group on artificial ultraviolet (UV) light and skin cancer. The association of use of sunbeds with cutaneous melanoma and other skin cancers: a systematic review. Int J Cancer 2007; 120:1116–22.

41. Ferrucci LM, Cartmel B, Molinaro AM, et al. Indoor tanning and risk of early-onset basal cell carcinoma. J Am Acad Dermatol 2011;67:552–62.

42. Zhang M, Qureshi AA, Geller AC, et al. Use of tanning beds and incidence of skin cancer. J Clin Oncol 2012;30:1588–93.

43. Little EG, Eide MJ. Update on the current state of melanoma incidence. Dermatol Clin 2012;30: 355–61.

44. Howlader N, Noone AM, Krapcho M, et al. SEER cancer statistics review, 1975-2008. Bethesda (MD): National Cancer Institute; 2011. Available at: http://seercancergov/csr/1975_2008/. Based on November 2010 SEER data submission, posted to the SEER Web site. Accessed November 6, 2013.

45. Jemal A, Saraiya M, Patel P, et al. Recent trends in cutaneous melanoma incidence and death rates in the United States, 1992-2006. J Am Acad Dermatol 2011;65:S17–25.

46. Wu XC, Eide MJ, King J, et al. Racial and ethnic variations in incidence and survival of cutaneous melanoma in the United States, 1999-2006. J Am Acad Dermatol 2011;65:S26–37.

47. De Vries E, Willem Coebergh J. Cutaneous malignant melanoma in Europe. Eur J Cancer 2004;40: 2355–66.

48. Eide MJ, Weinstock MA. Association of UV index, latitude, and melanoma incidence in nonwhite populations–US Surveillance, Epidemiology, and End Results (SEER) Program, 1992 to 2001. Arch Dermatol 2005;141:477–81.

49. Holman CD, Armstrong BK. Cutaneous malignant melanoma and indicators of total accumulated exposure to the sun: an analysis separating histogenetic types. J Natl Cancer Inst 1984;73:75–82.

50. Mack TM, Floderus B. Malignant melanoma risk by place of nativity, place of residence at diagnosis, and age at migration. Cancer Causes Control 1991;2:401–11.

51. Levine H, Afek A, Shamiss A, et al. Country of origin, age at migration and risk of cutaneous melanoma: a migrant cohort study of 1,100,000 Israeli men. Int J Cancer 2013;133(2):486–94.

52. Eckerle Mize D, Bishop M, Resse E, et al. Familial atypical multiple mole melanoma syndrome. In: Riegert-Johnson DL, Boardman LA, Hefferon T, et al, editors. Cancer syndromes [Internet]. Bethesda (MD): National Center for Biotechnology Information (US); 2009. Available at: http://www.ncbi.nlm.nih.gov/books/NBK7030/; 2009.

53. Goldstein AM, Chan M, Harland M, et al. High-risk melanoma susceptibility genes and pancreatic cancer, neural system tumors, and uveal melanoma across GenoMEL. Cancer Res 2006;66(20): 9818–28.

54. Abdel-Rahman MH, Pilarski R, Cebulla CM, et al. Germline BAP1 mutation predisposes to uveal melanoma, lung adenocarcinoma, meningioma, and other cancers. J Med Genet 2011;48:856–9.

55. Pilarski R, Cebulla CM, Massengill JB, et al. Expanding the clinical phenotype of hereditary BAP1 cancer predisposition syndrome, reporting three new cases. Genes Chromosomes Cancer 2014;53(2):177–82. http://dx.doi.org/10.1002/gcc.22129.

56. Whiteman DC, Watt P, Purdie DM, et al. Melanocytic nevi, solar keratoses, and divergent pathways to cutaneous melanoma. J Natl Cancer Inst 2003; 95(11):806–12.

57. Morgan AM, Lo J, Fisher DE. How does pheomelanin synthesis contribute to melanomagenesis? Bioessays 2013;35:672–6.

58. Sharma A, Shah SR, Illum H, et al. Vemurafenib: targeted inhibition of mutated BRAF for treatment of advanced melanoma and its potential in other malignancies. Drugs 2012;72(17): 2207–22.

59. Ball NJ, Yohn JJ, Morelli JG, et al. Ras mutations in human melanoma: a marker of malignant progression. J Invest Dermatol 1994;102(3):285–90.

60. Stahl JM, Sharma A, Cheung M, et al. Deregulated Akt3 activity promotes development of malignant melanoma. Cancer Res 2004;64(19):7002–10.

61. Curtin JA, Fridlyand J, Kageshita T, et al. Distinct sets of genetic alterations in melanoma. N Engl J Med 2005;353(20):2135–47.

62. Hussein MR, Hamel AK, Wood GS. Apoptosis and melanoma: molecular mechanisms. J Pathol 2003; 199:275.

63. Elwood JM, Jopson J. Melanoma and sun exposure: an overview of published studies. Int J Cancer 1997;73:198–203.

64. Gallagher RP, Spinelli JJ, Lee TK. Tanning beds, sunlamps, and risk of cutaneous malignant melanoma. Cancer Epidemiol Biomarkers Prev 2005; 14(3):562–6.

65. Lazovich D, Vogel RI, Berwick M, et al. Indoor tanning and risk of melanoma: a case control study in

a highly exposed population. Cancer Epidemiol Biomarkers Prev 2010;19(6):1557–68.

66. Boniol M, Autier P, Boyle P, et al. Cutaneous melanoma attributable to sunbed use: systematic review and meta-analysis. BMJ 2012;345:e4757.

67. Berwick M. Are tanning beds "safe"? Human studies of melanoma. Pigment Cell Melanoma Res 2008;21:517–9.

68. Mason RS, Reichrath J. Sunlight, vitamin D, and skin cancer. Anticancer Agents Med Chem 2013; 13:83–97.

69. Dusso AS, Tokumuto M. Defective renal maintenance of the vitamin D endocrine system impairs vitamin D renoprotection: a downward spiral in kidney disease. Kidney Int 2011;79:715–29.

70. Terushkin V, Bender A, Psaty EL, et al. Estimated equivalency of vitam D production from natural sun exposure versus oral vitamin D supplementation across seasons at two US latitudes. J Am Acad Dermatol 2010;62:929.e1–9.

71. World Health Organization: International Agency for Cancer Research. Vitamin D and Cancer. Available at: http://www.iarc.fr/en/Media-Centre/IARC-News/Vitamin-D-and-Cancer. Accessed November 14, 2013.

72. Report Brief. Dietary reference intakes for calcium and vitamin D. Available at: http://www.iom.edu/Reports/2010/Dietary-Reference-Intakes-for-Calcium-and-Vitamin-D/Report-Brief.aspx. Accessed December 1, 2013.

# Polymorphous Light Eruption
## Clinic Aspects and Pathogenesis

Alexandra Gruber-Wackernagel, MD[a], Scott N. Byrne, PhD[b],
Peter Wolf, MD[a],*

### KEYWORDS

- Polymorphous light eruption • Polymorphic • Photoantigen • Immune suppression • Cytokines
- Chemotaxis • Photoprotection • Skin cancer

### KEY POINTS

- PMLE is the most common form of photodermatosis, with a prevalence of up to approximately 20%, particularly among young women in temperate climates.
- PMLE is characterized by pruritic skin lesions of variable morphology, occurring in spring or early summer on sun-exposed body sites; although PMLE lesions are self-limited and nonscarring, patients can experience significant discomfort and loss of quality of life.
- A resistance to ultraviolet radiation–induced immunosuppression (ie, a physiologic phenomenon in healthy subjects) and a subsequent delayed-type hypersensitivity response to a photoantigen have been suggested as key factors in the disease.
- Standard management is based on prevention through medical photohardening with UVB radiation and protection by broad-band sunscreens and clothing, and treatment of symptoms with topical and/or systemic steroids.
- Novel prophylactic and/or therapeutic treatment includes substances with antioxidant and anti-inflammatory properties or those that interfere with melanization in the skin, DNA repair, or vitamin D pathway.

### INTRODUCTION

Polymorphous light eruption (PMLE) is the most common photodermatosis, with a prevalence of up to approximately 20%, particularly among young women in temperate climates.[1–5] Several hours to days after the first exposure to an intense dose of sunlight in spring or early summer, pruritic, nonscarring lesions of distinct morphology appear on sun-exposed skin. These usually subside in a few days if further exposure is avoided.[1,2] As summer progresses and after repetitive exposures to sunlight, many individuals experience a hardening effect. This means that skin lesions are less likely to occur, or may be less severe than they were in early spring, which permits patients with PMLE to tolerate prolonged sun exposure.[1] Whereas PMLE lesions are described to occur usually in spring or early summer after the first intense sun exposure,[1,4,6] Rhodes and colleagues[5] found

Funding Sources: P. Wolf was supported by the Oesterreichische Nationalbank Anniversary Fund project no. 13279 and FWF Austrian Science Fund no. KLI 132-B00.
Conflict of Interest: None.
[a] Research Unit for Photodermatology, Department of Dermatology, Medical University of Graz, Auenbruggerplatz 8, Graz A-8036, Austria; [b] Cellular Photoimmunology Group, Infectious Diseases and Immunology, Department of Dermatology, Sydney Medical School, Royal Prince Alfred Hospital, The University of Sydney, 676, Blackburn Building D06, Darlington, New South Wales 2006, Australia
* Corresponding author.
E-mail address: peter.wolf@medunigraz.at

that most patients suffered from flares during summer holidays. Sun-exposed areas, particularly those that are normally covered during the winter, such as the upper chest, the neck, and the extensor aspects of the arms, are most affected.[1,2] Presumably because of daily sun exposure and thus continuous natural hardening, the face and the hands of patients with PMLE are typically spared.[7]

## HISTORY

PMLE was described in 1942 by Epstein under the name of prurigo aestivalis.[8] He first hypothesized that PMLE represents a form of delayed-type hypersensitivity (DTH) response to photoantigens.[8]

## EPIDEMIOLOGY
### General Epidemiology

Similar to other autoimmune disorders, PMLE predominantly affects females and shows a mean disease onset in the second to third decade of life.[1,2] However, symptoms may also begin in early childhood or late adulthood.[1,2] Onset during childhood is less commonly seen in PMLE (20% of patients) than in actinic prurigo.[4] Women are affected 4 times more often than men.[1,2]

PMLE can affect all skin types and races, including Africans, Asians, and native Americans.[4,9,10] Rhodes and colleagues[5] reported the highest prevalence of PMLE (33.4% of women, 28.6% of men) in people with skin type I (Fitzpatrick classification), declining in skin types II (30.8%, 15.0%) and III (18.9%, 7.9%), with subjects of skin type IV or higher showing the lowest prevalence (11.2%, 4.0%). However, in a recent study from Detroit comparing pattern of photodermatoses between African American and white patients, Nakamura and colleagues[10] reported that PMLE was diagnosed in 86% of the African American and 54% of the white patients; this is consistent with the result of an earlier study from the same institution.[11]

PMLE has a wide geographic distribution, but is seen more frequently in temperate climates.[1] The incidence rate of PMLE in the United Kingdom, for instance, is approximately 15%, compared with less than 5% in sun-drenched Australia.[3] This difference is most likely attributed to the varied amounts of UV light in these geographic regions, rather than to cultural, dietary, or ethnic factors. The observation that PMLE increases in prevalence and severity toward higher northern latitudes, with greater relative differences in UVB between summer and winter, may indicate the importance of UV adaptation. Loss of adaptation

of the skin to UV radiation (UVR) during winter, making patients sun-sensitive in spring, may be of paramount importance in the disease.[12] In contrast, in a multicenter survey of countries on the Mediterranean Sea to Scandinavia, Rhodes and colleagues[5] found a prevalence of PMLE in 18% of Europeans with no correlation between PMLE incidence and increasing latitude. Although PMLE was found to be common across Europe, the highest prevalence was observed in the most southern city (Athens, 19.5%) and the lowest in the most northern (Turku/Finland, 13.6%).

## CLINICAL MANIFESTATIONS

As the name of the condition implies, the skin lesions are of variable morphology, including papular, papulo-vesicular, plaque, erythema multiforme (EM)-like, and insect bite–like (strophulus) forms (**Fig. 1**).[1,2] The most important differential diagnoses are solar urticaria, photosensitive erythema multiforme, and lupus erythematosus.[13]

However, in an individual patient, lesions are usually monomorphic.[1,2] Indeed, in a 7-year follow-up evaluation of 114 patients with PMLE, Jansen and Karvonen[14] found that 76% of patients reported consistent lesion morphology during the follow-up period. Most patients with PMLE experience a chronic course with little tendency to remit.[14,15] However, 64 patients (57%) described a diminution of sun-related skin complaints, including 12 patients who reported total remission from sun sensitivity during the previous 2 years.[14] Mallorca acne (see **Fig. 1**D),[16] characterized by acneiform lesions in sun-exposed areas of the upper chest, and juvenile spring eruption,[15,16] which presents with localized pruritic papulovesicular lesions of the ears in young boys, may be subtypes of PMLE that share a pathologic relationship.[17,18] Sometimes postherpetic erythema multiforme can mimic juvenile spring eruption (see **Fig. 1**F). Individuals with skin phototypes IV to VI most commonly present with the pinhead popular variant.[19] Solar purpura has been described as another rare variant of PMLE, with skin changes predominantly on the lower legs (see **Fig. 1**E).[20–25] In addition, a mild variant of PMLE, called benign summer light eruption, and another variant, called PMLE sine eruption with intense pruritus on sun-exposed skin but without visible skin changes, have been reported.[26–28] Recently, the existence of a localized variant of PMLE limited to the elbows has been suggested.[29] Systemic symptoms, such as headache, fever, chills, and nausea, are rare but may be associated with PMLE[4,30]; it is unclear whether systemic symptoms are directly related to PMLE itself or rather

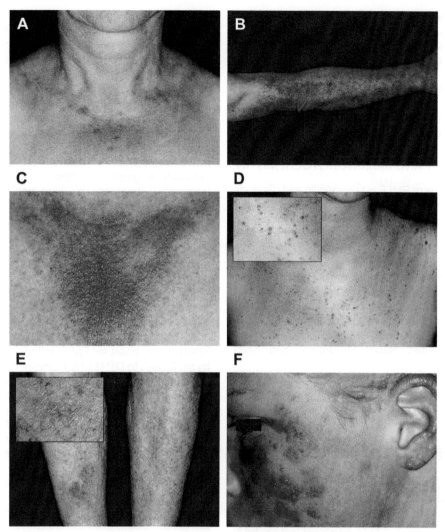

**Fig. 1.** Clinical forms of PMLE and variants. (*A*) Plaque type of PMLE. (*B*) Papular type of PMLE. (*C*) Vesicular type of PMLE. (*D*) Mallorca acne. Insert shows higher magnification. (*E*) Purpura solaris. Insert shows higher magnification. (*F*) Postherpetic erythema multiforme mimicking juvenile spring eruption.

result from an accompanying (severe) sunburn reaction. Indeed, systemic UV exposure can lead to the production and release of many cytokines, including interleukin (IL)-1 and IL-6, known for their endogenous pyrogenic activity.[31,32]

## Quality of Life

Patients with PMLE experience significant discomfort and loss of quality of life during spring and summer months.[33–38] High levels of anxiety and depression can occur in PMLE.[34] Young patients in particular, as well as patients with facial involvement, may need psychological management.[34,37] To quantify disease severity, PMLE severity scores have been established, based on questions concerning the occurrence of the rash

and quality of life during spring and summer months.[33] Other scores are more related to the severity of the disease over the season.[39–42]

## Relation to Lupus Erythematosus

In some cases, the photosensitive cutaneous manifestations of lupus erythematosus are virtually indistinguishable from PMLE.[43–46] The presence of antinuclear antibodies (ANA) in patients with lupus was an early criteria used to distinguish PMLE from lupus; however, several studies have demonstrated that patients with PMLE may also have elevated ANA titers in the absence of other apparent lupus symptoms.[14,15,47–49] The reported high prevalence of PMLE in patients with lupus, together with the clustering of PMLE among first-degree relatives of patients with subacute cutaneous lupus erythematosus and chronic cutaneous (discoid) lupus erythematosus, suggests a shared pathogenic basis for PMLE and cutaneous lupus.[45,46] PMLE lesions may precede the development of lupus,[45] and progression of PMLE to lupus has been proposed, although long-term follow-up studies of patients with PMLE have not shown an increased rate of transition to lupus.[14,15]

## HISTOLOGY AND IMMUNOHISTOCHEMISTRY

The histology of PMLE is nonspecific and depends on the clinical morphology (**Fig. 2**). In the papulovesicular type, spongiotic microvesicles are seen together with subepidermal edema and a mixed, predominantly lymphoid perivascular infiltrate in the superficial and deep dermis.[17,50] In contrast, in the erythema multiforme type of PMLE, vacuolar alterations of cells and liquefaction degeneration at the dermo-epidermal junction may be present.[17] Recently, a potential histologic variant of PMLE with unusual neutrophilic infiltration, resembling photodistributed Sweet syndrome, has been reported.[51]

An enhanced immune response has long been thought responsible for the pathogenesis of PMLE. The skin infiltrate of PMLE is composed mainly of activated Ia+ (HLA+) CD4+ T cells resembling the histopathologic characteristics of DTH reactions.[52] In 1984, Moncada and colleagues[53] found a predominance of T-helper (Th) cells and cells expressing high levels of Ia antigens in the dermal cell infiltrate, suggesting that an abnormal immune response is responsible for the tissue damage in PMLE. These features support the original hypothesis of Epstein in 1942 that PMLE represents a form of DTH to photo-induced antigens.[8] In 1989, Norris and colleagues[54] observed in immunohistochemical studies that UVB exposure of PMLE skin resulted in an initial influx of CD4+ T lymphocytes up to 72 hours in early lesions, followed by CD8+ T cells in established lesions, consistent with a cellular-mediated immune reactivity underlying the pathogenesis of PMLE. The predominantly lymphocytic perivascular cellular infiltrate was associated with increased numbers of dermal macrophages and dendritic cells (DCs), as well as epidermal Langerhans cells (LCs) 5 hours after UV exposure. An immunologic basis for PMLE is further supported by similarities to DTH in the expression of endothelial leukocyte adhesion molecule-1, intercellular adhesion molecule-1 (ICAM-1), and vascular cell adhesion molecule-1.[55,56] These results further support the concept that PMLE is not simply an aberrant reaction to UV exposure and provide additional insight into the underlying immunologic basis of PMLE.[55,56]

## PHOTOBIOLOGIC EVALUATION
### Waveband Aspects

The UV waveband action spectrum for PMLE induction is quite broad. Most patients with PMLE are sensitive to UVA, but lesions can be induced with UVB alone as well, whereas some patients are sensitive to both wavebands.[1] The observation that most patients with PMLE exhibit a sensitivity to sunlight through window glass and the lack of protection from pure UVB-absorbing sunscreens in most patients with PMLE substantiate the role of UVA in triggering the eruption.[13,57,58] Patients with PMLE also report that a sunburn is not mandatory for the development of a PMLE skin rash. This, together with the higher incidence of PMLE in subjects living in temperate areas where the levels of UVA are higher during the spring and autumn,[3] also supports the importance of UVA.

Patients with PMLE do not exhibit an abnormal sensitivity to develop (physiologic) erythema on UV exposure and show a normal value when tested for their UVB-induced or UVA-induced

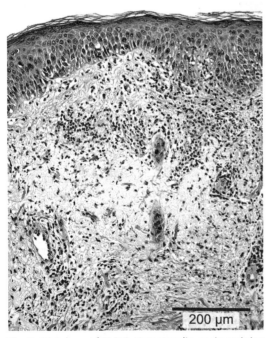

**Fig. 2.** Histology of PMLE. Hematoxylin-eosin staining shows subepidermal edema and a mixed, predominantly lymphoid perivascular infiltrate in the superficial and deep dermis. Note slight vacuolar alterations of cells and liquefaction degeneration at the dermo-epidermal junction.

200 µm

minimal erythema dose (MED). Epstein first reported that rather than a single exposure, repeated daily exposures of the same skin area to UVA or UVB are necessary to provoke PMLE lesions in situ.[59] This concept underlies the basis of photoprovocation in current clinical practice, a method that is widely accepted as a highly effective way of reproducing PMLE to confirm the diagnosis. The aim is to provoke the pathologic reaction by repeatedly exposing the skin at predilection sites in circumscribed areas to increasing suberythemal or near erythemal doses of UVR. UVA or UVB alone[4,48,60,61] or solar-simulated UVR (**Fig. 3**)[62,63] can all be used to photo-provoke PMLE. Various protocols are used but in general the principles of photoprovocation are as follows: 2 symmetrically located test areas, preferably on previously involved skin, are exposed daily for 4 to 5 days to UVA or UVB radiation. The time and site of photoprovocation are critical; exposure of previously uninvolved skin may yield false-negative results, whereas the same may occur when the test is done too late in a season (ie, late spring or summer) because of tolerance induction through natural photohardening.[4] Therefore, photoprovocation is best performed before the beginning of the sunny summer season, preferentially in early spring. Depending on the method, PMLE lesions can be reproduced in 60% to 90% of affected subjects, most of whom exhibit sensitivity to UVA and UVB.[4,48,60–64] To assess the severity of PMLE in the test areas of patients, a specific score has recently been introduced. Ranging from 0 to 12, the score is based on lesion area, degree of skin infiltration, and severity of pruritus in the test field(s).[62,63]

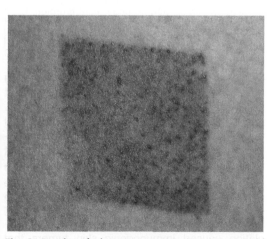

**Fig. 3.** Results of photoprovocation in a 44-year-old female patient. Typical papular PMLE is present in the test area after repeated suberythemal exposure to solar-simulated ultraviolet radiation.

## PATHOGENESIS
### Genetics

Genetic factors seem to play a role in PMLE.[1,46,65–68] Two studies have investigated the genetics of PMLE in greater detail and the results of these twin studies suggest that a polygenic model may explain PMLE inheritance.[65,66] For instance, a family history of PMLE in first-degree relatives was present in 12% of affected twins, compared with 4% in unaffected twins, providing evidence of familial clustering.[66] More recently, a reverse link to a glutathione-S-transferase GSTP1 allele was reported as the first genetic association in PMLE, supporting a potential role for reactive oxygen species in the pathogenesis.[69] However, this observation could not be confirmed in another study.[70]

### Potential Antigens in PMLE

A critical factor in the pathogenesis of PMLE is the effect of UVR on skin components. It has been hypothesized that in genetically predisposed subjects, UVR induces a modification of particular cutaneous molecules that renders them immunogenic (**Fig. 4**). The best evidence for this comes from experiments in which epidermal cells derived from the skin of patients with PMLE were exposed to high doses of UVA or UVB radiation. That these UV-irradiated cells can stimulate autologous peripheral blood mononuclear cells strongly suggests that an immune-sensitizing agent is induced by UVR in PMLE skin.[71] Although conclusive identification of the antigen remains elusive, that 10% to 20% of the adult population in Western countries report symptoms of PMLE[5] suggests that the putative (photo)antigen should be ubiquitous.

Given its importance in autoimmune processes, such as lupus, heat shock protein 65 (HSP65) has been suggested as a possible photoantigen in PMLE lesions.[72] Using skin biopsies from experimentally induced PMLE lesions, McFadden and colleagues[73] showed a significant increase in HSP expression by epidermal keratinocytes and dermal endothelial cells 1 hour postirradiation. Dermal dendritic cells also upregulated HSP from 5 hours to 6 days post UV. However, no increase in HSP65 labeling was observed in healthy subjects.

Herpes simplex virus (HSV) is commonly observed within EM lesions (see **Fig. 1**F), which like PMLE, is suspected to have an etiology involving cell-mediated (auto)immune reactivity. However, although the reactivity in EM manifests itself against pertinent antigens like HSV, the PMLE antigen remains unidentified.[17,74] Reports

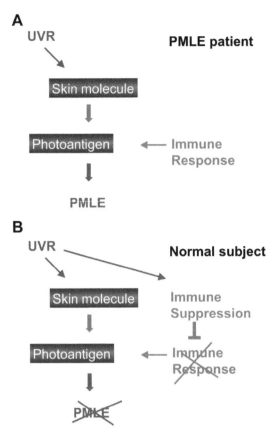

Fig. 4. Immune resistance to UVR in PMLE. (*A*) UVR hits a molecule in the skin that leads to the formation of a photoantigen. In patients with PMLE, an immune response is mounted against such a photoantigen that results in the formation of PMLE. (*B*) In healthy subjects, such an immune response is abrogated by simultaneous immune suppression induced by UVR.

of patients with PMLE who are free of PMLE symptoms while taking the antiviral acyclovir,[75] as well as cases in which PMLE episodes are followed by recurrent EM,[76] led to the suggestion that HSV may be the photoantigen in UV-exposed PMLE skin. However, polymerase chain reaction and Southern blot hybridization failed to show HSV DNA in PMLE skin samples, in contrast to presence in 32% of EM lesions.[77] Thus, a direct immune response to HSV antigens in the skin is unlikely to be involved in the pathogenesis of PMLE.[77]

## General Immunologic Aspects

The exact etiology and pathogenesis of PMLE are unknown, but a resistance to UV-induced immune suppression and subsequent immune reaction to UV-modified skin are suggested (see **Fig. 4**; **Box 1**). UVB radiation modifies cellular organic

---

**Box 1**
**Abnormalities in proposed models of potential significance for the pathogenesis of PMLE**

*Abnormality (model or method)*

Immune sensitization against autologous UVR-modified skin antigens (cell proliferation assay)[71]

Heat shock protein 65 as a possible photoantigen[73]

Resistance to UV-induced immune suppression (CHS model)[87,88]

Impaired UV-induced immune tolerance (CHS model)[89]

Resistance of LCs to UVR (immunohistochemical staining)[105]

Reduced cytokine expression related to LC migration and Th1 suppression (TNF-$\alpha$, IL-4, IL-10) in UVB-irradiated PMLE skin (immunohistochemical staining)[123]

Decreased skin infiltration of neutrophils after UVB irradiation (immunohistochemical staining)[117]

Abnormal but reversible (after photohardening) chemotactic response of neutrophils to chemoattractants (LTB4, fMLP) (flow cytometry, shape change assay)[119]

Abnormal T regulatory cell infiltration of the skin (immunohistochemical and immunofluorescence staining)[62,141]

Altered systemic cytokine levels in PMLE, modulated by photohardening (in particular IL-1$\beta$) (multiplex bead-array immunoassay)[183]

Decreased 25-hydroxyvitamin D3 serum levels (enzyme immunoassay)[172]

*Abbreviations:* CHS, contact hypersensitivity; LC, Langerhans cell; PMLE, polymorphous light eruption; UV, ultraviolet; UVR, ultraviolet radiation.
*Adapted from* Refs.[62,73,87–89,105,117,119,123,141,172,183]

---

molecules, such as proteins and DNA, creating new or potentially altered skin components that the immune system may recognize as foreign. Although these photoantigens have the potential to provoke (auto)-immune reactivity, the immunosuppressive properties of UVR may ensure that this adverse reaction is prevented in healthy subjects who do not have PMLE.[78–80]

Three decades ago, the immunosuppressive properties of UVR were demonstrated by Fisher and Kripke.[81] Exposure to UVR before tumor inoculation caused immunogenic skin tumors that would normally be rejected by naïve recipients to grow progressively.[81] In addition to the suppression of antitumor immune responses, UVR also inhibits cell-mediated immune reactions generated during allergic contact dermatitis.[78,80] In healthy human subjects, the ability of contact allergens to generate strong T-cell–mediated immune responses is significantly suppressed by UVR.[82–86] In addition to the failure to sensitize and mount a primary immune response, immunologic tolerance develops as individuals treated in this way cannot be resensitized against the same hapten even when topically applied at a later time point. This UV-induced tolerance is hapten specific, as the sensitization against another non-related hapten is not affected.

Thus, PMLE may be the result of reduced UV immunosuppression or tolerance induction to either aberrant antigen formation or increased immune reactivity to a universal cutaneous antigen. Two studies found that compared with healthy controls, patients with PMLE displayed no sign of an increased reaction to contact sensitization. However, patients with PMLE demonstrated a functional resistance to UV-induced immunosuppression, favoring a DTH response to potential UV-induced antigens under certain circumstances.[87,88] The work by van de Pas and colleagues[87] revealed that there was a narrow UV dose-response window for this resistance to immunosuppression, with a significant difference found between groups irradiated with 1 MED of solar-simulated UVR, but not those exposed to 0.6 or 2 MED. The highest UVR dose of 2 MED used in this study was highly immunosuppressive in both patients with PMLE and controls, leading to almost complete (90%) immunosuppression.[87] More recently, Koulu and colleagues[89] showed that UV-induced tolerance to a contact allergen is impaired in PMLE. In their study of 24 patients with PMLE and 24 healthy sex-matched and age-matched controls, they found that both groups had a diminished contact hypersensitivity response to diphenylcyclopropenone if they were earlier exposed to solar-simulated UVR.[89] However, only 1 (8%) of 13 patients with PMLE compared with 6 (55%) of 11 controls exhibited a state of UV-induced immunotolerance toward the same allergen 10 to 24 months later.[89] It was concluded that the impaired propensity to UVR-induced allergen-specific immunotolerance may promote recurrent PMLE.[89]

## Cell Migration Patterns and Cytokines

UVR-induced suppression of contact hypersensitivity (CHS) in healthy subjects[78] involves the release of cytokines, particularly tumor necrosis factor (TNF)-α, IL-4 and IL-10. The infiltration of a subset of HLA-DR+/CD11b+/CD1a− macrophages,

together with the emigration of LCs out of the epidermis, is another hallmark feature.[90] UVB radiation causes a temporal change in the cutaneous cytokine milieu, and the microenvironment becomes favorable to the development of type 2 helper (Th2) cell–like immune responses.[91]

Exposing skin of healthy individuals to UVR induces LC migration from the epidermis to the draining lymph nodes,[92,93] and it is thought that these DNA-damaged DCs are responsible for inducing immunologic tolerance.[94–97] IL-1β, TNF-α, and IL-18 release can modulate LC migration out of the skin.[98–104] Early work by Kölgen and colleagues[105] showed that in patients with PMLE, UVB radiation failed to deplete CD1a+ epidermal LCs,[105] indicating this defect as a key event in PMLE. This same group later demonstrated that in healthy human skin, UVB-induced LC depletion is mainly caused by migration and not by apoptosis.[106] Concurrently with the depletion of CD1a+ LCs after UV exposure, CD36+CD11b+CD1− cells appear in the dermis and infiltrate the epidermis in healthy subjects who do not have PMLE.[107] These CD11b+ macrophagelike cells play an important role in the induction of immune suppression and tolerance after UVB irradiation.[78,108,109]

Neutrophils expressing CD15 and CD11b also migrate into human skin after UV irradiation.[55,110–113] Teunissen and colleagues[110] showed that UVB radiation induces a transient appearance of IL-4+ neutrophils in normal human skin. This suggests that the presence of neutrophils and IL-4, a strong Th2-polarizing cytokine,[114] favors the development of Th2 over Th1 responses in UVB-exposed skin. This is relevant because IL-4 is shown to be involved in UV-induced suppression of both DTH[115] and CHS.[116]

Kölgen and colleagues[105] found that exposure to high doses of UVB recruited a different macrophage subset into the skin of patients with PMLE. Whereas macrophages that infiltrated the skin of healthy volunteers were mostly CD68 negative, the few CD11b+ cells that managed to infiltrate the skin of patients with PMLE were all CD68 positive.[105] This finding is consistent with that found by Schornagel and colleagues[117] who demonstrated in an immunohistochemical study that UVB exposure of PMLE skin fails to recruit CD11b+CD68− neutrophils. As neutrophils produce a variety of immunosuppressive cytokines (IL-4 and IL-10) and can regulate immune reactions,[110,113,118] these studies have led to the suggestion that the observed decreased infiltration of neutrophils after UVB irradiation of PMLE skin leads to activation of the skin immune response rather than suppression.[117] The abnormal cell migration patterns of PMLE and consequences are depicted in **Fig. 5**.

The reason why immune-suppressive neutrophils might fail to be recruited into PMLE skin is not entirely clear. In both patients with PMLE and healthy controls, the expression of adhesion molecules (ICAM-1 and E-selectin) on endothelial cells is critical to this migration; both are increased 6 hours after UVB irradiation.[117] Furthermore, neutrophil chemotactic responses to IL-8 and CD5a, as well as the expression of cell surface markers involved in adhesion and chemotaxis, is similar in patients with PMLE and healthy controls.[117] In contrast, Gruber-Wackernagel and colleagues[119] reported that patients with PMLE have an impaired neutrophil responsiveness to the chemoattractants leukotriene B4 and formylmethionyl-leucyl-phenylalanine that is restored after photohardening. Leukocytes also may be stimulated to enter skin tissue following the local release of lipid mediators, such as platelet-activating factor (PAF)[120,121] as well as leukotrienes.[122] Importantly, photochemotherapy as used for photohardening has been shown to be able to downregulate PAF.[121] Kolgen and colleagues[123] proposed that a lack of infiltrating neutrophils may explain the reduced expression of TNF-α, IL-4, and to a lesser extent, IL-10 in UV-exposed PMLE skin. There were no differences in the expression of Th1-related cytokines (IL-12, interferon [IFN]-γ and IL-6). The investigators

concluded that the reduced expression of neutrophil-derived TNF-α, IL-4 and IL-10 in UVB-irradiated PMLE skin is responsible for both reduced LC migration and a failure to suppress Th1 responses in these patients. In contrast, Wackernagel and colleagues[124] found that there was no significant difference in UV-induced cell migration (CD1a+ LCs, CD11b+ cells, CD68+ cells) or cutaneous cytokine expression (TNF-α, IL-1β, IL-10, or IL-12) between patients with PMLE and healthy controls. Explanations for the apparent differences in the results of these 2 studies may include spectra (narrowband UVB in the Kolgen and colleagues[123] study vs solar-simulated UV in the Wackernagel and colleagues[124] study), dose (6 MED vs 1, 2, and 3 MED) and kinetics (48–72 hours vs 6–24 hours).

A number of other cell types also may play a role in PMLE, including plasmacytoid DCs (pDCs). The pDCs are identical to the natural-type I IFN-producing cells,[125] a rare CD4+/major histocompatibility complex II+ population that is capable of synthesizing extremely high amounts of type I IFN on viral infection.[126] In addition to their classical antiviral and antiproliferative effects, type I IFNs like IFN-α also perform important immunomodulatory functions, including the promotion of Th1 cell survival and differentiation, the development of autoantibodies, and, thus, the promotion of autoimmunity.[127–129] Farkas and colleagues[130] first reported that pDCs accumulate in chronic

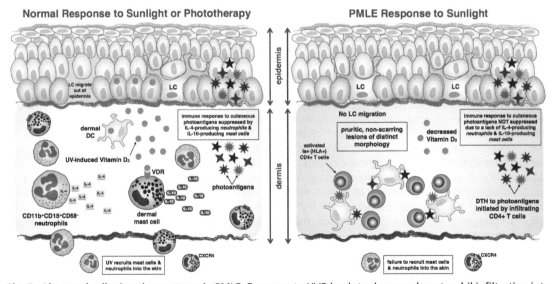

**Fig. 5.** Abnormal cell migration patterns in PMLE. Exposure to UVR leads to decreased neutrophil infiltration into the skin of patients with PMLE compared with healthy subjects. This lack of neutrophil infiltration (caused by decreased chemoattraction) is associated with reduced IL-4 and IL-10 production and release. In addition, mast cell infiltration is inhibited, whereas LCs are resistant to UV-induced migration triggers. Overall, this results in a nonimmune suppressive cutaneous microenvironment and subsequent DTH response to photoantigens in patients with PMLE but not healthy subjects. CXCR4, C-X-C motif receptor 4; VDR, vitamin D receptor.

cutaneous (discoid) lupus erythematosus and systemic LE skin lesions and that their density positively correlated with the high number of type I IFN-inducible protein MxA+ cells (a surrogate marker for IFN-α and IFN-β in such lesions). Increased levels of type I IFNs are often found in patients with lupus and correlate with disease activity and severity. In light of these findings, Wackernagel and colleagues[131] investigated whether pDCs populate the skin of UV-exposed patients with PMLE and participate in PMLE pathogenesis. Microscopic examination of the immunohistochemically stained sections confirmed the presence of CD68+/CD123+ pDCs in most specimens obtained from LE (10/11 [91%]) but in none obtained from patients with PMLE. The complete absence of pDCs in PMLE skin lesions suggests that these cells are not involved in cutaneous immune modulation of PMLE.

Mast cell is another immune cell that is required for UV-induced immune suppression, as mast cell–deficient mice are resistant to the effects of UVB.[132] Mast cells are responsible for transmitting the suppressive signal generated in UV-irradiated skin to the immune system.[133] UVB exposure induces a recruitment of mast cells into irradiated skin sites, followed by migration of these cells to the draining lymph nodes, required for the activation of regulatory cells.[133,134] When this migration is blocked, UV-induced immunosuppression[133] and subsequent development of skin cancer[135] are prevented. It has been confirmed in humans that UVB exposure induces a similar recruitment of mast cells into irradiated skin sites.[134] A recent study has suggested that low mast cell numbers in the skin of patients with PMLE may play a role in the pathogenesis of PMLE.[136] This is consistent with results in mast cell–deficient Kit$^{W-Sh/W-Sh}$ mice that were recently tested as a photodermatosis model.[137] Indeed, mast cell–derived cytokines, such as IL-10, may contribute to the recruitment of other immune cells, like Tregs, that could potentially protect against autoimmunity.[138–140] In PMLE, a low Treg infiltration of the skin has been observed, further supporting the potential role of mast cells in this disease.[62,141]

## Antimicrobial Peptides

Although UVR suppresses adaptive T-cell mediated immune responses,[142] its simultaneous induction of innate immune mechanisms, particularly antimicrobial peptides (AMP), may serve to counteract any potential increased risk of cutaneous infections.[143] These small peptides guard the body-environment interface and have potent antimicrobial activity.[144] They can also modulate inflammatory responses by stimulating the production of proinflammatory cytokines and chemokines,[145] or by suppressing cytokine release (TNF-α) from monocytes and macrophages.[146] AMPs may also act as chemoattractants for effector cells, including neutrophils, monocytes, macrophages, dendritic cells, and lymphocytes, and as activators of dendritic cells that modulate T-cell activation and function.[147–150] It was demonstrated that AMP (defensins) can contribute to immunosuppression via induction of regulatory T cells.[151] Felton and colleagues[152] suggested that dysregulated UVR induction of these proinflammatory proteins may play a role in the pathogenesis of certain immune-mediated diseases caused by sunlight. Whereas nonirradiated skin from both healthy individuals and patients with PMLE had no abnormalities in AMP expression, UVR induction of AMPs occurred in an atypical manner in those with PMLE, with greater upregulation and altered expression of AMPs, particularly in the early stages of the development of PMLE lesions.[152] Thus, it has been suggested that dysregulated AMP expression following UVR[152] could play some part in the relative failure of photoimmunosuppression that is described in PMLE.[88]

## Hormonal Factors

Compared with men, women are relatively resistant to the immunosuppressive effects of UV, requiring more than 3 times the amount to achieve the same level of immune suppression as men.[86] Although this may explain why men are more likely to get skin cancer,[153,154] it may also explain the disproportionately higher incidence of PMLE observed in women. The exact mechanism is unclear, although the female hormone 17β-estradiol, which can prevent UVR-induced suppression by limiting the release of immunosuppressive IL-10 from keratinocytes,[155,156] is likely to be involved. This hypothesis is supported by the groundbreaking study of Widyarini and colleagues,[157] who showed that signaling through the estrogen receptor (ER) "protects" women from UV-induced immune suppression. These investigators showed that blocking ERs significantly exacerbated the immunosuppression caused by solar-simulated UVR, suggesting a natural role for the ER in photoimmune protection.[157] Meanwhile, topical application of the 17-β-estradiol to mice provided dose-dependent photoimmune protection, which could be inhibited by an ER antagonist. This protection has been attributed to its antioxidant activities,[158] as well as inactivation of the downstream actions of cis-urocanic acid,[157] a key UV-induced photoproduct with potent immune suppressive capabilities.[157] Despite all this, the role of oral hormonal contraceptives is controversial,[159,160] and there is no clear link between their use and PMLE. In light of these gender differences, further studies are needed to address the question of whether resistance to UV-induced immune suppression lowers the skin cancer risk in patients with PMLE.

## Vitamin D

Beyond its effect on bone metabolism, calcium, and phosphorous homeostasis, vitamin D exerts profound modulating effects on the immune system. It can suppress T-cell activation, alter cytokine-secretion patterns, modulate cell proliferation, interfere with apoptosis, and even induce regulatory T cells.[161] Several studies have shown a link between the incidence of Th1-mediated autoimmune diseases, latitude, sun exposure, and vitamin D insufficiency.[162,163] It has been proposed that impaired vitamin D homeostasis can contribute to the autoimmune process, and that vitamin D is an environmental factor that can modulate the immune system affecting the development of autoimmunity.[162] Reduced serum 25-hydroxyvitamin-D (25[OH]D) levels, which are used to classify vitamin D status, have been observed in several autoimmune diseases and are a suspected risk factor for the development of autoimmunity.[164,165] However, whether this "cause and effect" is due to low vitamin D levels or insufficient amounts of sunlight exposure remains a contentious issue.[166] Similar to natural sunlight exposure, phototherapy of patients with psoriasis induces vitamin D production through the skin and increases serum 25(OH)D to normal levels.[167–170] As observed in other autoimmune diseases,[171] patients with PMLE have significantly lower 25(OH)D serum levels than healthy controls.[172] This is consistent with a recent report in which patients with increased photosensitivity were also found to be at high risk for low vitamin D status.[173] This is perhaps not all that surprising considering that basic photoprotective measures, such as avoiding sun exposure, are highly effective in preventing PMLE. Nevertheless, photohardening with 311-nm UVB phototherapy significantly increased vitamin D levels, leading to speculation that boosting levels of vitamin D may be important in ameliorating the adverse effects of PMLE.[172]

## Relation to Skin Carcinogenesis

Solar UVR is a major environmental cause of skin cancer, and patients with skin phototypes I and II are at greater risk for skin cancer than darker skin types.[174] In 1998, Kelly and colleagues[84]

demonstrated that a single exposure to solar-simulated UVR is highly immunosuppressive in all study subjects tested. Irradiating a small area of skin with a single exposure of 3 MEDs of solar-simulated UVR completely suppressed CHS both locally (12/12 volunteers) and systemically (10/12 volunteers).[84] In a subsequent study, the same group[175] reported that sensitivity to sunburn is associated with susceptibility to UVR-induced suppression of cutaneous cell-mediated immunity.[175] Whereas a single suberythemal exposure of either 0.25 or 0.5 MED suppressed CHS responses in skin types I and II by 50% and 80%, respectively, 2 to 4 times as much solar-simulated radiation (or 1 MED) was required to suppress CHS by 40% in skin types III/IV.[175] This enhanced sensitivity of skin types I/II for a given level of sunburn may play a role in their greater susceptibility to developing skin cancer.[175] It is difficult to reconcile this observation with the prevalence of PMLE among different skin types reported from the European study, where the highest prevalence of PMLE is in people with skin type I, declining in skin types II and III, with subjects of skin type IV or higher showing the lowest prevalence.[5]

Other studies in fair-skinned people have suggested that only 40% (12/32) of the studied subjects could be classified as "susceptible" to UVR immunosuppression.[80] In a 1990 study, Yoshikawa and colleagues[80] compared healthy human volunteers with patients who had a history of nonmelanoma skin cancer for their capacity to develop a CHS response to dinitrochlorobenzene (DNCB) following exposure to acute, low-dose UVB. Whereas approximately 60% of healthy volunteers developed a vigorous CHS response to a given dose of DNCB painted on the UV-irradiated test site (designated "UV resistant"), more than 90% of patients with skin cancer exposed to UVB and DNCB failed to develop CHS. Almost half of these "UVB-susceptible" patients remained unresponsive, implying that they had been rendered immunologically tolerant to the antigen. Hence, a patient's susceptibility to the immunosuppressive effects of UVB radiation is a risk factor for skin cancer development.[80] If patients with skin cancer have a general increased susceptibility to UV-induced immune suppression, this may make them less likely to develop PMLE. Such a hypothesis is supported by the work of Lembo and colleagues,[176] who reported a reduced prevalence of PMLE in people with skin cancer (including basal cell carcinoma, squamous cell carcinoma, and/or melanoma) of 7.5% compared with 21.4% for controls. They also found a trend for decreased skin cancer prevalence in patients with PMLE compared with gender-matched and age-matched controls (4% vs 7.1% respectively).[176] These combined studies provide strong support for the idea that resistance to UV-induced immune suppression is a likely risk factor for PMLE.

## MANAGEMENT
### Prevention

Prophylaxis is an important therapeutic approach to PMLE (**Table 1**), and mild cases respond well to basic photoprotective measures, such as avoiding sun exposure, the use of broad-spectrum sunscreens with high UVA protection capacity, and wearing protective clothing.[177] Bissonnette and colleagues[178] investigated the influence that the type of sunscreen and the amount of applied sunscreen had on protection against PMLE. The results showed that when applied at 2 mg/cm$^2$, none of the patients developed PMLE when high UVA protection sunscreen was used, whereas 73% exhibited PMLE when low UVA protection sunscreen was used.[178] At 1 mg/cm$^2$, 33% and 80% of patients presented a PMLE reaction with the high and low UVA protection sunscreen, respectively.[178] These results show that a high SPF sunscreen with a corresponding high UVA protection factor is able to protect most patients from the development of UV-induced PMLE reaction even at low concentration application.[178]

### Photohardening

In spring, just before the first intense sun exposure, prophylactic medical photohardening can be administered to patients with PMLE. The therapy works by significantly reducing subsequent PMLE eruptions that would occur during the summer months or on vacations in areas with high sun exposure. The phototherapeutic modalities used for hardening include broadband UVB (290–320 nm), narrow-band UVB (311 nm), or psoralen plus UVA photochemotherapy.[1] Photohardening is usually given 2 to 3 times per week for 4 to 6 weeks with suberythemal doses. The treatment stimulates the naturally occurring phenomenon of hardening and aims to induce photoadaption by using small, carefully regulated UV doses without inducing eruption.[1,2] However, not rarely, mild episodes of PMLE can occur during periods of medical photohardening (**Fig. 6**). If so, there may be a need to pause photohardening for a few days before it can be re-continued.

The mechanisms underlying the photohardening effect include melanization in the skin, thickening of the stratum corneum, and/or immunologic changes induced by UVR.[1,179–181] As described previously, the eruptions experienced by patients with PMLE may arise because of disturbed cell-migration patterns.[105,117] Another way in which photohardening may work is to restore the normal immune cell migration following exposure to UV.[105,182] For example, successful hardening therapy increased the migration of LCs from the epidermis 48 hours after exposure to 6 MED of UVB.[105] More recent work by Janssens and colleagues[182] showed that before hardening therapy, UV-induced LC depletion and neutrophil influx were impaired in patients with PMLE

| Table 1<br>Treatment concepts for PMLE | |
|---|---|
| **Agent** | **Mechanism** |
| Sunscreens | UVA+UVB photoprotection[178] |
| Photohardening | Melanization in the skin[1,179–181]<br>Restoring UV-induced LC depletion and neutrophil infiltration into skin[182]<br>Restoration of an abnormal chemotactic potential of neutrophils[119]<br>Increasing 25-hydroxyvitamin D3 serum levels[172] |
| Chloroquine | Immunomodulatory and anti-inflammatory properties[189] |
| Oral *Polypodium leucotomos* extract | Antioxidant and anti-inflammatory effects[61,190] |
| Nutritional supplement containing lycopene, β-carotene and *Lactobacillus johnsonii* | Antioxidant effects[191] |
| Topical DNA repair enzymes | Potential elimination of an antigenic trigger[63] |
| Topical vitamin D3 | Immunomodulating and -suppressive properties similar to UVR[62] |
| Afamelanotide | Melanization in the skin[200] |

*Abbreviations:* LC, Langerhans cell; PMLE, polymorphous light eruption; UV, ultraviolet; UVR, ultraviolet radiation.

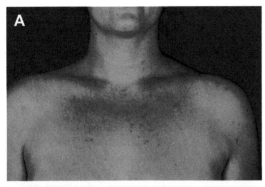

**Fig. 6.** Thirty-two-year-old female patient with PMLE. (A) Provocation of PMLE during a course of photohardening with 311-nm UVB irradiation after 14 exposures, resulting in PMLE in the V-neck area. (B) Higher magnification shows typical papulo-vesicular PMLE lesions.

compared with healthy controls. Following successful phototherapy, normal cell migratory responses were reestablished to levels that were not statistically different from healthy controls.[182] Photohardening-induced normalization of systemic cytokine levels (in particular IL-1β) and neutrophil chemotactic responsiveness may be the underlying key events of prophylactic efficacy (see **Table 1**).[119,183] Furthermore, because patients with PMLE are less likely to develop UV-induced immunosuppression, photohardening may result in sufficient immunosuppression that prevents the subsequent delayed hypersensitivity response to UV-induced antigen.[87–89]

### Established Treatments

After eruption of PMLE lesions, topical corticosteroids and occasionally oral antihistamines can be used to reduce the inflammation, alleviate itch, and shorten the duration of the eruption.[4,6,184] Further PMLE treatment depends on the severity of the disease and the impact of the treatment on lifestyle.[177,184] Short course of oral corticosteroids (prednisone, 0.6–1.0 mg/kg for 7–10 days)

can be used for PMLE flares, or given to patients prophylactically to prevent flares while they go to sunny locations for winter vacation.[185,186] In cases with severe symptoms, treatment can involve administration of azathioprine,[187] antimalarials,[13,188,189] or thalidomide.[13] These agents also can be administered to prevent the symptoms of the disease. Their exact mechanism of action in PMLE is not known.

### Experimental Approaches

The standard and experimental prevention approaches for PMLE are listed in **Table 1**. Tanew and colleagues[61] recently investigated the effect of oral administration of a hydrophilic extract of *Polypodium leucotomos* (PL). This natural extract from tropical fern leaves displays potent antioxidant and anti-inflammatory properties that were beneficial in the prevention of PMLE. In their study, 30 patients developed PMLE lesions after repeated irradiation with UVA. Of these, 18 also responded to UVB. After PL treatment, 9 (30%) and 5 (28%) patients, respectively, were unresponsive to repeated UVA und UVB exposure. In the remaining patients, the mean number of UVA and UVB irradiations required to elicit PMLE increased significantly from 1.95 to 2.62 and from 2.38 to 2.92, respectively.[61] In a separate study on 25 patients with PMLE, Caccialanza and colleagues[190] found that the administration of PL extract resulted in a relevant and statistically significant reduction of skin reactions and subjective symptoms. Together, these 2 studies indicate that oral PL treatment might be beneficial for the prevention of PMLE. Along this line, Marini and colleagues[191] recently found in a randomized, placebo-controlled, double-blinded study that the symptoms of PMLE could be diminished by a 12-week treatment course of oral administration of a nutritional supplement containing lycopene, β-carotene and *Lactobacillus johnsonii*.

Another novel approach is the administration of vitamin D3 analogs, such as calcipotriol. Topical treatment with calcipotriol leads to a dose-dependent decrease in the number and function of epidermal LCs. This effect of calcipotriol on LCs is comparable with that observed with the potent corticosteroid mometasone furoate.[192] It was also shown to be as powerful an immunosuppressant as UV exposure itself.[192,193] Considering that patients receiving phototherapy are theoretically at increased risk of developing skin cancer,[194] the use of vitamin D analogs (rather than UV) may be a promising, and potentially safer, prophylactic treatment for patients with PMLE. To that end, we recently described how topical treatment with calcipotriol significantly diminished the appearance and/or severity of PMLE.[62] In this randomized, placebo-controlled, intra-individual trial on topical treatment with calcipotriol in PMLE, 13 patients pretreated their skin test sites twice daily for 7 days before start of phototesting with solar-simulated irradiation. At 48, 72, and 144 hours after the first photoprovocation exposure, calcipotriol pretreatment resulted in a lower PMLE assessment score, including affected area, skin infiltration, and pruritus, in 58% to 83% of the 12 patients with PMLE. Considering all time points together, compared with placebo, calcipotriol diminished the PMLE assessment score in all 12 photoprovocable patients.[62] These results suggest a potential therapeutic benefit of topical 1,25 dihydroxyvitamin D analogs as a novel prophylactic treatment option in patients with PMLE.

Another promising approach is enhancing DNA repair by topical application of liposomal DNA repair enzymes, such as photolyase from *Anacystis nidulans* and endonucleases from *Micrococcus luteus* lysate.[195–199] These enzymes can be incorporated through liposomes in sunscreens or after-sun lotions. Enhancing DNA repair immediately after UV exposure significantly diminished PMLE symptoms in human volunteers on photoprovocation with artificial solar-simulated UVR.[63] This was unanticipated, as DNA damage is regarded as one of the triggers of UV-induced immune suppression.[196–199] Although the exact mechanism remains to be determined, it is possible that the enhanced removal of UV-induced DNA photoproducts may have eliminated the initial antigenic immune trigger in UV-exposed skin of patients with PMLE.[63]

Melanization in the skin induced by afamelanotide, an analog of $\alpha$-melanocyte–stimulating hormone, given as a subcutaneous implant, is currently undergoing phase II and III trials in Europe and the United States for skin diseases including PMLE.[200,201]

## SUMMARY AND PERSPECTIVES

Clinical and experimental evidence supports the hypothesis of an aberrant cellular immune response in UV-exposed PMLE skin. This suggests the formation of a photoantigen in PMLE skin and/or a failure of UV-induced immunosuppression. As yet, the presence of a possible photoantigen in PMLE skin has not been confirmed, but studies have shown a failure of UV-induced immunosuppression related to disturbed cell and cytokine shifts in PMLE skin. This is relevant for the pathogenesis of PMLE and the therapeutic efficacy of photohardening therapy. New local treatment opportunities with agents with antioxidative and anti-inflammatory properties, those that enhance DNA repair, or vitamin D have been recently demonstrated. A better understanding of the phenomenon of resistance to UV-induced immune suppression, together with any potential benefits (ie, reduced skin cancer risk) associated with PMLE, may help to develop novel strategies to treat and prevent the disease but also to establish mechanistic links to photocarcinogenesis.

## ACKNOWLEDGMENTS

The authors thank Werner Stieber, Department of Dermatology, Medical University of Graz, for his professional support in preparing the clinical photographs for this publication.

## REFERENCES

1. Gruber-Wackernagel A, Byrne SN, Wolf P. Pathogenic mechanisms of polymorphic light eruption. Front Biosci (Elite Ed) 2009;1:341–54.
2. Wolf P, Byrne SN, Gruber-Wackernagel A. New insights into the mechanisms of polymorphic light eruption: resistance to ultraviolet radiation-induced immune suppression as an aetiological factor. Exp Dermatol 2009;18(4):350–6.
3. Pao C, Norris PG, Corbett M, et al. Polymorphic light eruption: prevalence in Australia and England. Br J Dermatol 1994;130(1):62–4.
4. Stratigos AJ, Antoniou C, Katsambas AD. Polymorphous light eruption. J Eur Acad Dermatol Venereol 2002;16(3):193–206.
5. Rhodes LE, Bock M, Janssens AS, et al. Polymorphic light eruption occurs in 18% of Europeans and does not show higher prevalence with increasing latitude: multicenter survey of 6,895 individuals residing from the Mediterranean to Scandinavia. J Invest Dermatol 2010;130(2):626–8.
6. Naleway AL. Polymorphous light eruption. Int J Dermatol 2002;41(7):377–83.
7. Gonzalez E, Gonzalez S. Drug photosensitivity, idiopathic photodermatoses, and sunscreens. J Am Acad Dermatol 1996;35(6):871–85 [quiz: 886–7].
8. Epstein S. Studies in abnormal human sensitivity to light. IV. Photoallergic concept of prurigo aestivalis. J Invest Dermatol 1942;5:289–98.
9. Wadhwani AR, Sharma VK, Ramam M, et al. A clinical study of the spectrum of photodermatoses in dark-skinned populations. Clin Exp Dermatol 2013;38(8):823–9.
10. Nakamura M, Henderson M, Jacobsen G, et al. Comparison of photodermatoses in African-Americans and Caucasians: a follow-up study.

Photodermatol Photoimmunol Photomed 2013. [Epub ahead of print].

11. Kerr HA, Lim HW. Photodermatoses in African Americans: a retrospective analysis of 135 patients over a 7-year period. J Am Acad Dermatol 2007; 57(4):638–43.

12. van der Leun JC, van Weelden H. Light-induced tolerance to light in photodermatoses. J Invest Dermatol 1975;64:280.

13. Holzle E, Plewig G, von Kries R, et al. Polymorphous light eruption. J Invest Dermatol 1987; 88(Suppl 3):32s–8s.

14. Jansen CT, Karvonen J. Polymorphous light eruption. A seven-year follow-up evaluation of 114 patients. Arch Dermatol 1984;120(7):862–5.

15. Hasan T, Ranki A, Jansen CT, et al. Disease associations in polymorphous light eruption. A long-term follow-up study of 94 patients. Arch Dermatol 1998;134(9):1081–5.

16. Hjorth N, Sjolin KE, Sylvest B, et al. Acne aestivalis—Mallorca acne. Acta Derm Venereol 1972; 52(1):61–3.

17. Wolf P, Soyer HP, Fink-Puches R, et al. Recurrent post-herpetic erythema multiforme mimicking polymorphic light and juvenile spring eruption: report of two cases in young boys. Br J Dermatol 1994; 131(3):364–7.

18. Lava SA, Simonetti GD, Ragazzi M, et al. Juvenile spring eruption: an outbreak report and systematic review of the literature. Br J Dermatol 2013;168(5): 1066–72.

19. Isedeh P, Lim HW. Polymorphous light eruption presenting as pinhead papular eruption on the face. J Drugs Dermatol 2013;12(11):1285–6.

20. Wood BA, LeBoit PE. An 'inflammatory' variant of solar purpura: a simulant of leukocytoclastic vasculitis and neutrophilic dermatoses. Pathology 2013; 45(5):484–8.

21. Waters AJ, Sandhu DR, Green CM, et al. Solar capillaritis as a cause of solar purpura. Clin Exp Dermatol 2009;34(8):e821–4.

22. Kalivas J, Kalivas L. Solar purpura appearing in a patient with polymorphous light eruption. Photodermatol Photoimmunol Photomed 1995;11(1):31–2.

23. Guarrera M, Parodi A, Rebora A. Solar purpura is not related to polymorphous light eruption. Photodermatol 1989;6(6):293–4.

24. Ros AM. Solar purpura—an unusual manifestation of polymorphous light eruption. Photodermatol 1988;5(1):47–8.

25. Latenser BA, Hempstead RW. Exercise-associated solar purpura in an atypical location. Cutis 1985; 35(4):365–6.

26. Verheyen AM, Lambert JR, Van Marck EA, et al. Polymorphic light eruption—an immunopathological study of provoked lesions. Clin Exp Dermatol 1995;20(4):297–303.

27. Guarrera M, Cardo P, Rebora AE, et al. Polymorphous light eruption and benign summer light eruption in Italy. Photodermatol Photoimmunol Photomed 2011;27(1):35–9.

28. Dover JS, Hawk JL. Polymorphic light eruption sine eruption. Br J Dermatol 1988;118(1):73–6.

29. Molina-Ruiz AM, Sanmartin O, Santonja C, et al. Spring and summer eruption of the elbows: a peculiar localized variant of polymorphous light eruption. J Am Acad Dermatol 2013;68(2):306–12.

30. Jansen CT. Heredity of chronic polymorphous light eruptions. Arch Dermatol 1978;114(2):188–90.

31. Granstein RD, Sauder DN. Whole-body exposure to ultraviolet radiation results in increased serum interleukin-1 activity in humans. Lymphokine Res 1987;6(3):187–93.

32. Urbanski A, Schwarz T, Neuner P, et al. Ultraviolet light induces increased circulating interleukin-6 in humans. J Invest Dermatol 1990;94(6):808–11.

33. Ling TC, Richards HL, Janssens AS, et al. Seasonal and latitudinal impact of polymorphic light eruption on quality of life. J Invest Dermatol 2006; 126(7):1648–51.

34. Richards HL, Ling TC, Evangelou G, et al. Evidence of high levels of anxiety and depression in polymorphic light eruption and their association with clinical and demographic variables. Br J Dermatol 2008;159(2):439–44.

35. Richards HL, Ling TC, Evangelou G, et al. Psychologic distress in polymorphous light eruption and its relationship to patients' beliefs about their condition. J Am Acad Dermatol 2007;56(3):426–31.

36. Jong CT, Finlay AY, Pearse AD, et al. The quality of life of 790 patients with photodermatoses. Br J Dermatol 2008;159(1):192–7.

37. Rizwan M, Haylett AK, Richards HL, et al. Impact of photosensitivity disorders on the life quality of children. Photodermatol Photoimmunol Photomed 2012;28(6):290–2.

38. Rizwan M, Reddick CL, Bundy C, et al. Photodermatoses: environmentally induced conditions with high psychological impact. Photochem Photobiol Sci 2013;12(1):182–9.

39. Janssens AS, Pavel S, Ling T, et al. Susceptibility to UV-A and UV-B provocation does not correlate with disease severity of polymorphic light eruption. Arch Dermatol 2007;143(5):599–604.

40. Schornagel IJ, Knol EF, van Weelden H, et al. Diagnostic phototesting in polymorphous light eruption: the optimal number of irradiations. Br J Dermatol 2005;153(6):1234–6.

41. Palmer RA, van de Pas CB, Young AR, et al. Validation of the 'polymorphic light eruption severity index'. Br J Dermatol 2006;155(2):482–4.

42. Schornagel IJ, Guikers KL, Van Weelden H, et al. The polymorphous light eruption-severity assessment score does not reliably predict the results of

phototesting. J Eur Acad Dermatol Venereol 2008; 22(6):675–80.

43. Orteu CH, Sontheimer RD, Dutz JP. The pathophysiology of photosensitivity in lupus erythematosus. Photodermatol Photoimmunol Photomed 2001; 17(3):95–113.

44. Bickers DR. Sun-induced disorders. Emerg Med Clin North Am 1985;3(4):659–76.

45. Nyberg F, Hasan T, Puska P, et al. Occurrence of polymorphous light eruption in lupus erythematosus. Br J Dermatol 1997;136(2):217–21.

46. Millard TP, Lewis CM, Khamashta MA, et al. Familial clustering of polymorphic light eruption in relatives of patients with lupus erythematosus: evidence of a shared pathogenesis. Br J Dermatol 2001;144(2): 334–8.

47. Petzelbauer P, Binder M, Nikolakis P, et al. Severe sun sensitivity and the presence of antinuclear antibodies in patients with polymorphous light eruption-like lesions. A form fruste of photosensitive lupus erythematosus? J Am Acad Dermatol 1992;26(1):68–74.

48. Mastalier U, Kerl H, Wolf P. Clinical, laboratory, phototest and phototherapy findings in polymorphic light eruptions: a retrospective study of 133 patients. Eur J Dermatol 1998;8(8):554–9.

49. Murphy GM, Hawk JL. The prevalence of antinuclear antibodies in patients with apparent polymorphic light eruption. Br J Dermatol 1991;125(5): 448–51.

50. Epstein JH. Polymorphous light eruption. Dermatol Clin 1986;4(2):243–51.

51. Foroozan M, Balme B, Depaepe L, et al. Polymorphic light eruption with unusual neutrophilic infiltration. Eur J Dermatol 2012;22(2):262–3.

52. Lever WF, Schaumburg-Lever G. Noninfectious vesicular and bullous disease. 7th edition. Philadelphia: JB Lippincott; 1990.

53. Moncada B, Gonzalez-Amaro R, Baranda ML, et al. Immunopathology of polymorphous light eruption. T lymphocytes in blood and skin. J Am Acad Dermatol 1984;10(6):970–3.

54. Norris PG, Morris J, McGibbon DM, et al. Polymorphic light eruption: an immunopathological study of evolving lesions. Br J Dermatol 1989;120(2): 173–83.

55. Norris P, Poston RN, Thomas DS, et al. The expression of endothelial leukocyte adhesion molecule-1 (ELAM-1), intercellular adhesion molecule-1 (ICAM-1), and vascular cell adhesion molecule-1 (VCAM-1) in experimental cutaneous inflammation: a comparison of ultraviolet B erythema and delayed hypersensitivity. J Invest Dermatol 1991; 96(5):763–70.

56. Norris PG, Barker JN, Allen MH, et al. Adhesion molecule expression in polymorphic light eruption. J Invest Dermatol 1992;99(4):504–8.

57. Hönigsmann H. Polymorphous light eruption. In: Lim HW, Soter NA, editors. Clinical photomedicine. New York: Marcel Dekker Inc; 1993. p. 167–80.

58. Diffey BL, Farr PM. An evaluation of sunscreens in patients with broad action-spectrum photosensitivity. Br J Dermatol 1985;112(1):83–6.

59. Epstein JH. Polymorphous light eruptions: phototest technique studies. Arch Dermatol 1962;85: 502–4.

60. Ortel B, Tanew A, Wolff K, et al. Polymorphous light eruption: action spectrum and photoprotection. J Am Acad Dermatol 1986;14(5 Pt 1):748–53.

61. Tanew A, Radakovic S, Gonzalez S, et al. Oral administration of a hydrophilic extract of *Polypodium leucotomos* for the prevention of polymorphic light eruption. J Am Acad Dermatol 2012;66(1):58–62.

62. Gruber-Wackernagel A, Bambach I, Legat FJ, et al. Randomized double-blinded placebo-controlled intra-individual trial on topical treatment with a 1,25-dihydroxyvitamin D(3) analogue in polymorphic light eruption. Br J Dermatol 2011;165(1): 152–63.

63. Hofer A, Legat FJ, Gruber-Wackernagel A, et al. Topical liposomal DNA-repair enzymes in polymorphic light eruption. Photochem Photobiol Sci 2011; 10(7):1118–28.

64. van de Pas CB, Hawk JL, Young AR, et al. An optimal method for experimental provocation of polymorphic light eruption. Arch Dermatol 2004; 140(3):286–92.

65. McGregor JM, Grabczynska S, Vaughan R, et al. Genetic modeling of abnormal photosensitivity in families with polymorphic light eruption and actinic prurigo. J Invest Dermatol 2000;115(3):471–6.

66. Millard TP, Bataille V, Snieder H, et al. The heritability of polymorphic light eruption. J Invest Dermatol 2000;115(3):467–70.

67. Millard TP, Kondeatis E, Cox A, et al. A candidate gene analysis of three related photosensitivity disorders: cutaneous lupus erythematosus, polymorphic light eruption and actinic prurigo. Br J Dermatol 2001;145(2):229–36.

68. Millard TP, Kondeatis E, Vaughan RW, et al. Polymorphic light eruption and the HLA DRB1*0301 extended haplotype are independent risk factors for cutaneous lupus erythematosus. Lupus 2001; 10(7):473–9.

69. Millard TP, Fryer AA, McGregor JM. A protective effect of glutathione-S-transferase GSTP1*Val(105) against polymorphic light eruption. J Invest Dermatol 2008;128(8):1901–5.

70. Zirbs M, Purner C, Buters JT, et al. GSTM1, GSTT1 and GSTP1 gene polymorphism in polymorphous light eruption. J Eur Acad Dermatol Venereol 2013;27(2):157–62.

71. Gonzalez-Amaro R, Baranda L, Salazar-Gonzalez JF, et al. Immune sensitization against

epidermal antigens in polymorphous light eruption. J Am Acad Dermatol 1991;24(1):70–3.

72. Kaufmann SH. Heat shock proteins and the immune response. Immunol Today 1990;11(4): 129–36.

73. McFadden JP, Norris PG, Cerio R, et al. Heat shock protein 65 immunoreactivity in experimentally induced polymorphic light eruption. Acta Derm Venereol 1994;74(4):283–5.

74. Norris PG. The idiopathic photodermatoses: polymorphic light eruption, actinic prurigo and hydroa vacciniforme. In: Hawk JL, editor. Photodermatology. London: Arnold; 1999. p. 178–90.

75. Baby O. Polymorphous light eruption: is herpes virus the culprit? Photodermatol Photoimmunol Photomed 2002;18(3):162.

76. Fraser-Andrews EA, Morris-Jones R, Novakovic L, et al. Erythema multiforme following polymorphic light eruption: a report of two cases. Clin Exp Dermatol 2005;30(3):232–4.

77. Wackernagel A, Zochling N, Back B, et al. Presence of herpes simplex virus DNA in erythema multiforme but not polymorphic light eruption. Br J Dermatol 2006;155(5):1084–5.

78. Cooper KD, Oberhelman L, Hamilton TA, et al. UV exposure reduces immunization rates and promotes tolerance to epicutaneous antigens in humans: relationship to dose, CD1a-DR+ epidermal macrophage induction, and Langerhans cell depletion. Proc Natl Acad Sci U S A 1992;89(18): 8497–501.

79. Cooper KD. Cell-mediated immunosuppressive mechanisms induced by UV radiation. Photochem Photobiol 1996;63(4):400–6.

80. Yoshikawa T, Rae V, Bruins-Slot W, et al. Susceptibility to effects of UVB radiation on induction of contact hypersensitivity as a risk factor for skin cancer in humans. J Invest Dermatol 1990;95(5): 530–6.

81. Fisher MS, Kripke ML. Systemic alteration induced in mice by ultraviolet light irradiation and its relationship to ultraviolet carcinogenesis. Proc Natl Acad Sci U S A 1977;74(4):1688–92.

82. Damian DL, Barnetson RS, Halliday GM. Low-dose UVA and UVB have different time courses for suppression of contact hypersensitivity to a recall antigen in humans. J Invest Dermatol 1999;112(6): 939–44.

83. Wolf P, Hoffmann C, Quehenberger F, et al. Immune protection factors of chemical sunscreens measured in the local contact hypersensitivity model in humans. J Invest Dermatol 2003;121(5): 1080–7.

84. Kelly DA, Walker SL, McGregor JM, et al. A single exposure of solar simulated radiation suppresses contact hypersensitivity responses both locally and systemically in humans: quantitative studies with high-frequency ultrasound. J Photochem Photobiol B 1998;44(2):130–42.

85. Fourtanier A, Moyal D, Maccario J, et al. Measurement of sunscreen immune protection factors in humans: a consensus paper. J Invest Dermatol 2005; 125(3):403–9.

86. Damian DL, Patterson CR, Stapelberg M, et al. UV radiation-induced immunosuppression is greater in men and prevented by topical nicotinamide. J Invest Dermatol 2008;128(2):447–54.

87. van de Pas CB, Kelly DA, Seed PT, et al. Ultraviolet-radiation-induced erythema and suppression of contact hypersensitivity responses in patients with polymorphic light eruption. J Invest Dermatol 2004;122(2):295–9.

88. Palmer RA, Friedmann PS. Ultraviolet radiation causes less immunosuppression in patients with polymorphic light eruption than in controls. J Invest Dermatol 2004;122(2):291–4.

89. Koulu LM, Laihia JK, Peltoniemi HH, et al. UV-induced tolerance to a contact allergen is impaired in polymorphic light eruption. J Invest Dermatol 2010;130(11):2578–82.

90. Ullrich SE. Modulation of immunity by ultraviolet radiation: key effects on antigen presentation. J Invest Dermatol 1995;105(Suppl 1):30S–6S.

91. Duthie MS, Kimber I, Norval M. The effects of ultraviolet radiation on the human immune system. Br J Dermatol 1999;140(6):995–1009.

92. Noonan FP, Bucana C, Sauder DN, et al. Mechanism of systemic immune suppression by UV irradiation in vivo. II. The UV effects on number and morphology of epidermal Langerhans cells and the UV-induced suppression of contact hypersensitivity have different wavelength dependencies. J Immunol 1984;132(5):2408–16.

93. Toews GB, Bergstresser PR, Streilein JW. Epidermal Langerhans cell density determines whether contact hypersensitivity or unresponsiveness follows skin painting with DNFB. J Immunol 1980;124(1):445–53.

94. Vink AA, Strickland FM, Bucana C, et al. Localization of DNA damage and its role in altered antigen-presenting cell function in ultraviolet-irradiated mice. J Exp Med 1996;183(4):1491–500.

95. Vink AA, Moodycliffe AM, Shreedhar V, et al. The inhibition of antigen-presenting activity of dendritic cells resulting from UV irradiation of murine skin is restored by in vitro photorepair of cyclobutane pyrimidine dimers. Proc Natl Acad Sci U S A 1997; 94(10):5255–60.

96. Applegate LA, Ley RD, Alcalay J, et al. Identification of the molecular target for the suppression of contact hypersensitivity by ultraviolet radiation. J Exp Med 1989;170(4):1117–31.

97. Stingl G, Gazze-Stingl LA, Aberer W, et al. Antigen presentation by murine epidermal Langerhans

cells and its alteration by ultraviolet B light. J Immunol 1981;127(4):1707–13.

98. Cumberbatch M, Kimber I. Dermal tumour necrosis factor-alpha induces dendritic cell migration to draining lymph nodes, and possibly provides one stimulus for Langerhans' cell migration. Immunology 1992;75(2):257–63.

99. Cumberbatch M, Griffiths CE, Tucker SC, et al. Tumour necrosis factor-alpha induces Langerhans cell migration in humans. Br J Dermatol 1999; 141(2):192–200.

100. Cumberbatch M, Dearman RJ, Kimber I. Interleukin 1 beta and the stimulation of Langerhans cell migration: comparisons with tumour necrosis factor alpha. Arch Dermatol Res 1997;289(5):277–84.

101. Cumberbatch M, Dearman RJ, Kimber I. Langerhans cells require signals from both tumour necrosis factor-alpha and interleukin-1 beta for migration. Immunology 1997;92(3):388–95.

102. Boonstra A, Savelkoul HF. The role of cytokines in ultraviolet-B induced immunosuppression. Eur Cytokine Netw 1997;8(2):117–23.

103. Tominaga K, Yoshimoto T, Torigoe K, et al. IL-12 synergizes with IL-18 or IL-1beta for IFN-gamma production from human T cells. Int Immunol 2000; 12(2):151–60.

104. Byrne SN, Halliday GM, Johnston LJ, et al. Interleukin-1beta but not tumor necrosis factor is involved in West Nile virus-induced Langerhans cell migration from the skin in C57BL/6 mice. J Invest Dermatol 2001;117(3):702–9.

105. Kölgen W, Van Weelden H, Den Hengst S, et al. CD11b+ cells and ultraviolet-B-resistant CD1a+ cells in skin of patients with polymorphous light eruption. J Invest Dermatol 1999;113(1):4–10.

106. Kolgen W, Both H, van Weelden H, et al. Epidermal Langerhans cell depletion after artificial ultraviolet B irradiation of human skin in vivo: apoptosis versus migration. J Invest Dermatol 2002;118(5): 812–7.

107. Meunier L, Bata-Csorgo Z, Cooper KD. In human dermis, ultraviolet radiation induces expansion of a CD36+ CD11b+ CD1– macrophage subset by infiltration and proliferation; CD1+ Langerhans-like dendritic antigen-presenting cells are concomitantly depleted. J Invest Dermatol 1995;105(6): 782–8.

108. Hammerberg C, Duraiswamy N, Cooper KD. Reversal of immunosuppression inducible through ultraviolet-exposed skin by in vivo anti-CD11b treatment. J Immunol 1996;157(12):5254–61.

109. Kang K, Hammerberg C, Meunier L, et al. CD11b+ macrophages that infiltrate human epidermis after in vivo ultraviolet exposure potently produce IL-10 and represent the major secretory source of epidermal IL-10 protein. J Immunol 1994;153(11): 5256–64.

110. Teunissen MB, Piskin G, di Nuzzo S, et al. Ultraviolet B radiation induces a transient appearance of IL-4+ neutrophils, which support the development of Th2 responses. J Immunol 2002;168(8): 3732–9.

111. Hawk JL, Murphy GM, Holden CA. The presence of neutrophils in human cutaneous ultraviolet-B inflammation. Br J Dermatol 1988;118(1):27–30.

112. Gilchrest BA, Soter NA, Hawk JL, et al. Histologic changes associated with ultraviolet A–induced erythema in normal human skin. J Am Acad Dermatol 1983;9(2):213–9.

113. Piskin G, Bos JD, Teunissen MB. Neutrophils infiltrating ultraviolet B-irradiated normal human skin display high IL-10 expression. Arch Dermatol Res 2005;296(7):339–42.

114. Kopf M, Le Gros G, Bachmann M, et al. Disruption of the murine IL-4 gene blocks Th2 cytokine responses. Nature 1993;362(6417):245–8.

115. el-Ghorr AA, Norval M. The role of interleukin-4 in ultraviolet B light-induced immunosuppression. Immunology 1997;92(1):26–32.

116. Hart PH, Grimbaldeston MA, Jaksic A, et al. Ultraviolet B-induced suppression of immune responses in interleukin-4–/– mice: relationship to dermal mast cells. J Invest Dermatol 2000;114(3): 508–13.

117. Schornagel IJ, Sigurdsson V, Nijhuis EH, et al. Decreased neutrophil skin infiltration after UVB exposure in patients with polymorphous light eruption. J Invest Dermatol 2004;123(1):202–6.

118. Terui T, Tagami H. Mediators of inflammation involved in UVB erythema. J Dermatol Sci 2000; 23(Suppl 1):S1–5.

119. Gruber-Wackernagel A, Heinemann A, Konya V, et al. Photohardening restores the impaired neutrophil responsiveness to chemoattractants leukotriene B4 and formyl-methionyl-leucyl-phenylalanin in patients with polymorphic light eruption. Exp Dermatol 2011;20(6):473–6.

120. Wolf P, Nghiem DX, Walterscheid JP, et al. Platelet-activating factor is crucial in psoralen and ultraviolet A-induced immune suppression, inflammation, and apoptosis. Am J Pathol 2006;169(3):795–805.

121. Singh TP, Huettner B, Koefeler H, et al. Platelet-activating factor blockade inhibits the T-helper type 17 cell pathway and suppresses psoriasis-like skin disease in K5.hTGF-beta1 transgenic mice. Am J Pathol 2011;178(2):699–708.

122. Baggiolini M. Chemokines and leukocyte traffic. Nature 1998;392(6676):565–8.

123. Kolgen W, van Meurs M, Jongsma M, et al. Differential expression of cytokines in UV-B-exposed skin of patients with polymorphous light eruption: correlation with Langerhans cell migration and immunosuppression. Arch Dermatol 2004;140(3): 295–302.

124. Wackernagel A, Back B, Quehenberger F, et al. Langerhans cell resistance, CD11b+ cell influx, and cytokine mRNA expression in skin after UV exposure in patients with polymorphous light eruption as compared with healthy control subjects. J Invest Dermatol 2004;122(5):1342–4.

125. Siegal FP, Kadowaki N, Shodell M, et al. The nature of the principal type 1 interferon-producing cells in human blood. Science 1999;284(5421):1835–7.

126. Fitzgerald-Bocarsly P. Human natural interferon-alpha producing cells. Pharmacol Ther 1993; 60(1):39–62.

127. Bogdan C. The function of type I interferons in antimicrobial immunity. Curr Opin Immunol 2000;12(4): 419–24.

128. Akbar AN, Lord JM, Salmon M. IFN-alpha and IFN-beta: a link between immune memory and chronic inflammation. Immunol Today 2000;21(7):337–42.

129. Sinigaglia F, D'Ambrosio D, Rogge L. Type I interferons and the Th1/Th2 paradigm. Dev Comp Immunol 1999;23(7–8):657–63.

130. Farkas L, Beiske K, Lund-Johansen F, et al. Plasmacytoid dendritic cells (natural interferon- alpha/beta-producing cells) accumulate in cutaneous lupus erythematosus lesions. Am J Pathol 2001; 159(1):237–43.

131. Wackernagel A, Massone C, Hoefler G, et al. Plasmacytoid dendritic cells are absent in skin lesions of polymorphic light eruption. Photodermatol Photoimmunol Photomed 2007;23(1):24–8.

132. Hart PH, Grimbaldeston MA, Swift GJ, et al. Dermal mast cells determine susceptibility to ultraviolet B-induced systemic suppression of contact hypersensitivity responses in mice. J Exp Med 1998; 187(12):2045–53.

133. Byrne SN, Limon-Flores AY, Ullrich SE. Mast cell migration from the skin to the draining lymph nodes upon ultraviolet irradiation represents a key step in the induction of immune suppression. J Immunol 2008;180(7):4648–55.

134. Kim MS, Kim YK, Lee DH, et al. Acute exposure of human skin to ultraviolet or infrared radiation or heat stimuli increases mast cell numbers and tryptase expression in human skin in vivo. Br J Dermatol 2009;160(2):393–402.

135. Sarchio SN, Scolyer RA, Beaugie C, et al. Pharmacologically antagonizing the CXCR4-CXCL12 chemokine pathway with AMD3100 inhibits sunlight-induced skin cancer. J Invest Dermatol 2014;134(4):1091–100.

136. Wolf P, Gruber-Wackernagel A, Legat FJ, et al. Successful phototherapy of polymorphic light eruption patients is associated with a recruitment of mast cells into the skin [abstract]. J Invest Dermatol 2010;130(Suppl 2):50.

137. Schweintzger N, Gruber-Wackernagel A, Reginato E, et al. Mast cell-deficient KitW-sh/W-sh mice as a photodermatosis model [abstract]. J Invest Dermatol 2013;133:S33.

138. Lu LF, Lind EF, Gondek DC, et al. Mast cells are essential intermediaries in regulatory T-cell tolerance. Nature 2006;442(7106):997–1002.

139. Singh TP, Schon MP, Wallbrecht K, et al. 8-methoxypsoralen plus ultraviolet A therapy acts via inhibition of the IL-23/Th17 axis and induction of Foxp3+ regulatory T cells involving CTLA4 signaling in a psoriasis-like skin disorder. J Immunol 2010; 184(12):7257–67.

140. Singh TP, Schon MP, Wallbrecht K, et al. 8-Methoxypsoralen plus UVA treatment increases the proportion of CLA+ CD25+ CD4+ T cells in lymph nodes of K5.hTGFbeta1 transgenic mice. Exp Dermatol 2012;21(3):228–30.

141. Gambichler T, Terras S, Kampilafkos P, et al. T regulatory cells and related immunoregulatory factors in polymorphic light eruption following ultraviolet A1 challenge. Br J Dermatol 2013;169(6): 1288–94.

142. Schwarz T. 25 years of UV-induced immunosuppression mediated by T cells—from disregarded T suppressor cells to highly respected regulatory T cells. Photochem Photobiol 2008;84(1):10–8.

143. Glaser R, Navid F, Schuller W, et al. UV-B radiation induces the expression of antimicrobial peptides in human keratinocytes in vitro and in vivo. J Allergy Clin Immunol 2009;123(5):1117–23.

144. Zanetti M. Cathelicidins, multifunctional peptides of the innate immunity. J Leukoc Biol 2004;75(1): 39–48.

145. Niyonsaba F, Ushio H, Nakano N, et al. Antimicrobial peptides human beta-defensins stimulate epidermal keratinocyte migration, proliferation and production of proinflammatory cytokines and chemokines. J Invest Dermatol 2007;127(3): 594–604.

146. Mookherjee N, Brown KL, Bowdish DM, et al. Modulation of the TLR-mediated inflammatory response by the endogenous human host defense peptide LL-37. J Immunol 2006;176(4):2455–64.

147. Yang D, Chertov O, Bykovskaia SN, et al. Beta-defensins: linking innate and adaptive immunity through dendritic and T cell CCR6. Science 1999; 286(5439):525–8.

148. Biragyn A, Ruffini PA, Leifer CA, et al. Toll-like receptor 4-dependent activation of dendritic cells by beta-defensin 2. Science 2002;298(5595): 1025–9.

149. Wuerth K, Hancock RE. New insights into cathelicidin modulation of adaptive immunity. Eur J Immunol 2011;41(10):2817–9.

150. Morgera F, Pacor S, Creatti L, et al. Effects on antigen-presenting cells of short-term interaction with the human host defence peptide beta-defensin 2. Biochem J 2011;436(3):537–46.

151. Navid F, Boniotto M, Walker C, et al. Induction of regulatory T cells by a murine beta-defensin. J Immunol 2012;188(2):735–43.

152. Felton S, Navid F, Schwarz A, et al. Ultraviolet radiation-induced upregulation of antimicrobial proteins in health and disease. Photochem Photobiol Sci 2013;12(1):29–36.

153. Molife R, Lorigan P, MacNeil S. Gender and survival in malignant tumours. Cancer Treat Rev 2001;27(4):201–9.

154. Foote JA, Harris RB, Giuliano AR, et al. Predictors for cutaneous basal- and squamous-cell carcinoma among actinically damaged adults. Int J Cancer 2001;95(1):7–11.

155. Aubin F. Why is polymorphous light eruption so common in young women? Arch Dermatol Res 2004;296(5):240–1.

156. Hiramoto K, Tanaka H, Yanagihara N, et al. Effect of 17beta-estradiol on immunosuppression induced by ultraviolet B irradiation. Arch Dermatol Res 2004;295(8–9):307–11.

157. Widyarini S, Domanski D, Painter N, et al. Estrogen receptor signaling protects against immune suppression by UV radiation exposure. Proc Natl Acad Sci U S A 2006;103(34):12837–42.

158. Widyarini S, Domanski D, Painter N, et al. Photoimmune protective effect of the phytoestrogenic isoflavonoid equol is partially due to its antioxidant activities. Photochem Photobiol Sci 2012;11(7):1186–92.

159. Mentens G, Lambert J, Nijsten T. Polymorphic light eruption may be associated with cigarette smoking and alcohol consumption. Photodermatol Photoimmunol Photomed 2006;22(2):87–92.

160. Neumann R. Polymorphous light eruption and oral contraceptives. Photodermatol 1988;5(1):40–2.

161. May E, Asadullah K, Zugel U. Immunoregulation through 1,25-dihydroxyvitamin D3 and its analogs. Curr Drug Targets Inflamm Allergy 2004;3(4):377–93.

162. Cantorna MT. Vitamin D and autoimmunity: is vitamin D status an environmental factor affecting autoimmune disease prevalence? Proc Soc Exp Biol Med 2000;223(3):230–3.

163. Ponsonby AL, McMichael A, van der Mei I. Ultraviolet radiation and autoimmune disease: insights from epidemiological research. Toxicology 2002;181–182:71–8.

164. Shoenfeld N, Amital H, Shoenfeld Y. The effect of melanism and vitamin D synthesis on the incidence of autoimmune disease. Nat Clin Pract Rheumatol 2009;5(2):99–105.

165. Arnson Y, Amital H, Shoenfeld Y. Vitamin D and autoimmunity: new aetiological and therapeutic considerations. Ann Rheum Dis 2007;66(9):1137–42.

166. Hart PH, Gorman S, Finlay-Jones JJ. Modulation of the immune system by UV radiation: more than just the effects of vitamin D? Nat Rev Immunol 2011;11(9):584–96.

167. Czarnecki D. Narrowband ultraviolet B therapy is an effective means of raising serum vitamin D levels. Clin Exp Dermatol 2008;33(2):202.

168. Ryan C, Moran B, McKenna MJ, et al. The effect of narrowband UV-B treatment for psoriasis on vitamin D status during wintertime in Ireland. Arch Dermatol 2010;146(8):836–42.

169. Vahavihu K, Ala-Houhala M, Peric M, et al. Narrowband ultraviolet B treatment improves vitamin D balance and alters antimicrobial peptide expression in skin lesions of psoriasis and atopic dermatitis. Br J Dermatol 2010;163(2):321–8.

170. Vahavihu K, Ylianttila L, Kautiainen H, et al. Narrowband ultraviolet B course improves vitamin D balance in women in winter. Br J Dermatol 2010;162(4):848–53.

171. Kamen DL, Cooper GS, Bouali H, et al. Vitamin D deficiency in systemic lupus erythematosus. Autoimmun Rev 2006;5(2):114–7.

172. Gruber-Wackernagel A, Obermayer-Pietsch B, Byrne SN, et al. Patients with polymorphic light eruption have decreased serum levels of 25-hydroxyvitamin-D3 that increase upon 311 nm UVB photohardening. Photochem Photobiol Sci 2012;11(12):1831–6.

173. Reid SM, Robinson M, Kerr AC, et al. Prevalence and predictors of low vitamin D status in patients referred to a tertiary photodiagnostic service: a retrospective study. Photodermatol Photoimmunol Photomed 2012;28(2):91–6.

174. Armstrong BK, Kricker A. Skin cancer. Dermatol Clin 1995;13(3):583–94.

175. Kelly DA, Young AR, McGregor JM, et al. Sensitivity to sunburn is associated with susceptibility to ultraviolet radiation-induced suppression of cutaneous cell-mediated immunity. J Exp Med 2000;191(3):561–6.

176. Lembo S, Fallon J, O'Kelly P, et al. Polymorphic light eruption and skin cancer prevalence: is one protective against the other? Br J Dermatol 2008;159(6):1342–7.

177. Fesq H, Ring J, Abeck D. Management of polymorphous light eruption: clinical course, pathogenesis, diagnosis and intervention. Am J Clin Dermatol 2003;4(6):399–406.

178. Bissonnette R, Nigen S, Bolduc C. Influence of the quantity of sunscreen applied on the ability to protect against ultraviolet-induced polymorphous light eruption. Photodermatol Photoimmunol Photomed 2012;28(5):240–3.

179. Norris PG, Hawk JL. Polymorphic light eruption. Photodermatol Photoimmunol Photomed 1990;7(5):186–91.

180. Wolf R, Oumeish OY. Photodermatoses. Clin Dermatol 1998;16(1):41–57.

181. Ferguson J, Ibbotson S. The idiopathic photodermatoses. Semin Cutan Med Surg 1999;18(4): 257–73.

182. Janssens AS, Pavel S, Out-Luiting JJ, et al. Normalized ultraviolet (UV) induction of Langerhans cell depletion and neutrophil infiltrates after artificial UVB hardening of patients with polymorphic light eruption. Br J Dermatol 2005;152(6):1268–74.

183. Wolf P, Gruber-Wackernagel A, Rinner B, et al. Phototherapeutic hardening modulates systemic cytokine levels in patients with polymorphic light eruption. Photochem Photobiol Sci 2013;12(1): 166–73.

184. Millard TP. Treatment of polymorphic light eruption. J Dermatol Treat 2000;11:195–9.

185. Molin L, Volden G. Treatment of polymorphous light eruption with PUVA and prednisolone. Photodermatol 1987;4(2):107–8.

186. Patel DC, Bellaney GJ, Seed PT, et al. Efficacy of short-course oral prednisolone in polymorphic light eruption: a randomized controlled trial. Br J Dermatol 2000;143(4):828–31.

187. Norris PG, Hawk JL. Successful treatment of severe polymorphous light eruption with azathioprine. Arch Dermatol 1989;125(10):1377–9.

188. Corbett MF, Hawk JL, Herxheimer A, et al. Controlled therapeutic trials in polymorphic light eruption. Br J Dermatol 1982;107(5):571–81.

189. Murphy GM, Hawk JL, Magnus IA. Hydroxychloroquine in polymorphic light eruption: a controlled trial with drug and visual sensitivity monitoring. Br J Dermatol 1987;116(3):379–86.

190. Caccialanza M, Percivalle S, Piccinno R, et al. Photoprotective activity of oral polypodium leucotomos extract in 25 patients with idiopathic photodermatoses. Photodermatol Photoimmunol Photomed 2007;23(1):46–7.

191. Marini A, Jaenicke T, Grether-Beck S, et al. Prevention of polymorphic light eruption by oral administration of a nutritional supplement containing lycopene, ss-carotene and *Lactobacillus johnsonii*: results from a randomized, placebo-controlled, double-blinded study. Photodermatol Photoimmunol Photomed 2013. [Epub ahead of print].

192. Dam TN, Moller B, Hindkjaer J, et al. The vitamin D3 analog calcipotriol suppresses the number and antigen-presenting function of Langerhans cells in normal human skin. J Investig Dermatol Symp Proc 1996;1(1):72–7.

193. Hanneman KK, Scull HM, Cooper KD, et al. Effect of topical vitamin D analogue on in vivo contact sensitization. Arch Dermatol 2006;142(10):1332–4.

194. Dawe RS. There are no 'safe exposure limits' for phototherapy. Br J Dermatol 2010;163(1):209–10.

195. Yarosh DB, O'Connor A, Alas L, et al. Photoprotection by topical DNA repair enzymes: molecular correlates of clinical studies. Photochem Photobiol 1999;69(2):136–40.

196. Yarosh D, Klein J, O'Connor A, et al. Effect of topically applied T4 endonuclease V in liposomes on skin cancer in xeroderma pigmentosum: a randomised study. Xeroderma Pigmentosum Study Group. Lancet 2001;357(9260):926–9.

197. Wolf P, Maier H, Mullegger RR, et al. Topical treatment with liposomes containing T4 endonuclease V protects human skin in vivo from ultraviolet-induced upregulation of interleukin-10 and tumor necrosis factor-alpha. J Invest Dermatol 2000; 114(1):149–56.

198. Wolf P, Yarosh DB, Kripke ML. Effects of sunscreens and a DNA excision repair enzyme on ultraviolet radiation-induced inflammation, immune suppression, and cyclobutane pyrimidine dimer formation in mice. J Invest Dermatol 1993;101(4): 523–7.

199. Wolf P, Cox P, Yarosh DB, et al. Sunscreens and T4N5 liposomes differ in their ability to protect against ultraviolet-induced sunburn cell formation, alterations of dendritic epidermal cells, and local suppression of contact hypersensitivity. J Invest Dermatol 1995;104(2):287–92.

200. Fabrikant J, Touloei K, Brown SM. A review and update on melanocyte stimulating hormone therapy: afamelanotide. J Drugs Dermatol 2013; 12(7):775–9.

201. Langan EA, Nie Z, Rhodes LE. Melanotropic peptides: more than just 'Barbie drugs' and 'sun-tan jabs'? Br J Dermatol 2010;163(3):451–5.

# Actinic Prurigo

Martha C. Valbuena, MD[a],*, Sandra Muvdi, MD, MSc[b], Henry W. Lim, MD[c]

## KEYWORDS

- Actinic prurigo • Polymorphic light eruption • Thalidomide • Human leukocyte antigen

## KEY POINTS

- Actinic prurigo is a chronic photosensitivity disorder, which is more prevalent in Amerindians and Latin American mestizos and has a strong association with human leukocyte antigen DR4, especially the DRB1*0407 subtype.
- Clinical features are typical, but sometimes could be similar to a persistent form of polymorphic light eruption or photosensitive atopic dermatitis.
- Biopsies of lips and conjunctivae, in conjunction with clinical findings, help to confirm the diagnosis.
- Repetitive exposure to ultraviolet A and B could reproduce lesions.
- Thalidomide is the treatment of choice but should be used with caution, especially in women of childbearing age.

## INTRODUCTION

Actinic prurigo (AP) is an uncommon, immunologically mediated photosensitivity disorder,[1] usually beginning in childhood or before 20 years of age, although it can start later in life.[2] It is characterized by a chronic course, with development of intensely pruritic papules, plaques, and nodules, mainly over sun-exposed skin.[3,4] Involvement of lips and conjunctivae is frequent in North American and Latin American patients, and sometimes can be the only feature of the disease. Human leukocyte antigen (HLA) DR4, especially the HLA DRB1*0407 subtype, is associated with most cases of AP,[5–7] suggesting an autoimmune basis for this disorder.

Some investigators, based on cases seen in the United Kingdom, consider AP as a clinical variant of polymorphic light eruption with a different genetic background.[8] However, because of its unique clinical presentation, most Latin American dermatologists consider AP to be a distinct entity.[3]

Because of the intense pruritus that can lead to scarring, and owing to the need for sun avoidance, AP has a great impact on the quality of life of affected patients (Dermatology Life Quality Index scores >10 [moderate effect]).[9]

## HISTORY

Robert Willan (1798) was the first author to describe a skin disease caused by sun, which he called "eczema solaris."[10] This report was probably the earliest of patients suffering from AP. However, most investigators consider Jonathan Hutchinson's report about "summer prurigo" in 1878 as the primary reference to this disease,[11] although the cases he described did not correspond completely with all clinical features of AP.[12]

In 1956, Robert Brandt was the first to identify familial involvement in AP patients after staying in a Navajo reservation and finding individuals of this community with clinical features of AP, which he called "solar prurigo."[13]

Conflict of Interest: None declared.
[a] Photodermatology Unit, Centro Dermatológico Federico Lleras Acosta, Avda. 1 No. 13A-61, Bogotá, Colombia; [b] Research and Education Department, Research and Education Office, Centro Dermatológico Federico Lleras Acosta, Avda. 1 No. 13A-61, Bogotá, Colombia; [c] Department of Dermatology, Henry Ford Health System, Henry Ford Medical Center - New Center One, 3031 West Grand Boulevard, Detroit, MI 48202, USA
* Corresponding author.
E-mail address: marvalbuen@yahoo.com

Dermatol Clin 32 (2014) 335–344
http://dx.doi.org/10.1016/j.det.2014.03.010
0733-8635/14/$ – see front matter © 2014 Elsevier Inc. All rights reserved.

derm.theclinics.com

The first use of the term "actinic prurigo" was by Londoño from Colombia,[14] who used it in a 1960 publication in Spanish. He reported a series of 31 cases, establishing the frequent eczema-like component of AP, which should be differentiated from photoallergic contact dermatitis mediated by photosensitizers. In 1966, Londoño and colleagues[15] also pointed out the possible familial character of this disease in 6 families.

In 1977 Calnan and Meara[16] were the first English-speaking investigators to use the current term actinic prurigo to refer to a group of British patients who had the disease; they stated that AP should be clearly differentiated from polymorphic light eruption.

Even before Londoño, other Spanish-speaking investigators made important contributions to the characterization of AP: López González, an Argentinian dermatologist, presented 3 cases of this disease in 1950 under the name *prurigo de verano*[17]; Escalona, in the first edition of his Dermatology textbook (1954),[18] described the clinical features of *prurigo solar*. Other investigators from Central and South America studied the disease and used different names to identify AP: *syndrome cutáneo guatemalense* (Cordero, 1960), *dermatitis solar* (Saúl, 1972), *dermatitis polimorfa a la luz* (Corrales Padilla, 1973), *erupción polimorfa lumínica, tipo prúrigo* (Hojyo and Dominguez, 1975), and *prurigo solar de altiplanicie* (Flores, 1975).[19]

## EPIDEMIOLOGY

AP predominantly affects indigenous tribes from North,[20–22] Central,[23] and South America,[24] and Latin American mestizos (individuals with a mixed Caucasian and Amerindian ancestry), particularly those from Mexico, Colombia, Peru, Bolivia, Ecuador, Guatemala, Honduras, and northern Argentina.[3,25] It is far less frequently seen in Europe (United Kingdom,[16,26] France,[27] Albania,[28] Greece,[29] Germany[30]), Oceania (Australia[31]), and Asia (Thailand,[32] Singapore,[33] Japan[34,35]).

Prevalence of AP varies depending on the studied population; in Canadian Aboriginals it is 0.1%,[22] in Mexican mestizos 1.3% to 3.5%,[36] in Trujillo (Peru) 3.4%,[25] in Chimila Indians of Colombia 8%,[37] and in Scotland 0.003%.[38] This disease probably represents less than 5% of referrals to photodermatology clinics.[29]

A family history is commonly found in closed communities; it has been reported in 75% of American Indian cases,[20,39] 50% in the United Kingdom,[26] and 4.3% to 25% in Mexico.[40,41] Some investigators have found personal and family history of atopy in AP patients,[26] even though sometimes it is difficult to clearly differentiate between photoaggravated atopic dermatitis and AP.[42] The disease predominates in skin phototypes III to V, and is more common in women than in men with a ratio of between 2:1 and 4:1[26,31,43]; notable exceptions are the Chimila indigenous tribe of Colombia[37] and in Asians,[44] in whom more men are affected. The effects of 17β-estradiol in preventing ultraviolet radiation (UVR)-induced immunosuppression[45,46] may explain why the disease is more frequent in females, as has been suggested in polymorphic light eruption, another immunologically mediated photodermatosis that is more common in women.[47]

AP is usually described in Latin American patients living at high altitudes (>1000 m), but has also been reported in patients residing at sea level in Colombia,[37] Canada,[21,22] and Peru.[25] Most of the patients from high-altitude locations improve when they move to lower-altitude locales.[48,49]

## PATHOGENESIS

The pathogenesis of AP is unknown, but is clearly related to sun exposure as reflected by the distribution of the skin lesions, the differences in the behavior of the disease between the summer and winter, and the reproduction of lesions with artificial UVR sources.[2,3,26] At present, the most accepted theory on the pathogenesis of AP is a delayed hypersensitivity reaction to an unidentified autoantigen induced by UVR, occurring in genetically susceptible individuals.[5,43,50,51] This hypothesis is supported by observations that there are activated CD4-positive T cells and memory T lymphocytes in the infiltrate of the biopsies of AP patients,[52,53] there is abnormal reactivity of AP lymphocytes against ultraviolet (UV)-irradiated keratinocytes,[54] there is higher autoantibody reactivity on the skin, and there are more intense proliferative responses to isolated autologous skin antigens in AP patients in comparison with controls.[50]

Torres-Alvarez and colleagues[55] showed persistence of Langerhans cells in the epidermis of AP patients on UV exposure, whereas in healthy individuals these cells decrease in number in the irradiated skin. This result suggests that there is persistence of antigen-presenting cells, which could result in enhanced inflammatory response and resistance to UVR-induced immunosuppression. A study comparing the density of Langerhans cells in lesional and nonlesional skin showed that there was a lower density of Langerhans cells in lesional skin.[56] Arrese and colleagues[57] found high tumor necrosis factor α (TNFα) immunoreactivity in keratinocytes in the suprabasal layer of AP patients. Therefore, they proposed that UVR in subjects genetically predisposed to AP could trigger excessive TNFα production by these cells, leading to the development of lesions.

## ASSOCIATION WITH HLA

There is a significant association of AP with HLA subtypes. The first studies were made with HLA class I antigens (Table 1), then with class II antigens. A strong association was found with HLA DR4 (Table 2), particularly with the subtype DRB1*0407 (Tables 3 and 4). Menagé and colleagues[58] postulate that HLA antigens may modify the patient's response to sunlight-induced antigens, and may contribute to the expression of the disease. It should be noted that HLA association is not essential for the development of AP lesions.[59]

Whereas HLA DRB1*0407 is commonly observed in the Americas, it is uncommon in European Caucasians (4.4%–6.7% of DR4-positive individuals)[58] and in other regions of the world, as described by Solberg and colleagues.[60] The geographic distribution of this allele may explain why AP is more common in some regions of North, Central, and South America.

The haplotype DRB1*0407/DQB1*0302/ DPB1*0402 was found in 68.8% of Colombian patients (odds ratio 15.4; 95% confidence interval 6.7–35.9) and only in 12.5% of the controls.[49] Zuloaga-Salcedo and colleagues[61] proposed the existence of an HLA B39/DRB1*0407 haplotype, which includes class I and class II HLA alleles located in the sixth chromosome, as a susceptibility region for this disease in Mexican patients. Some possible protective alleles have also been described, including HLA DRB1*0802 in Mexicans[61] and HLA DRB1*01 and DRB1*13 in Colombians.[5]

Although AP is strongly associated with HLA DR4, the disease may occur in the absence of this HLA subtype, leading Grabczynska and colleagues[62] to propose that there are other genes in the HLA DR region or its vicinity that may contribute to AP susceptibility. Some investigators proposed that AP is a persistent variant of polymorphic light eruption, in the presence of predisposing haplotypes and precipitation by environmental factors.[8,63] This view is supported by reported cases of coexistence of polymorphic light eruption and AP, or progression of polymorphic light eruption to AP and vice versa.[8] However, it should be noted that the combination of polymorphic light eruption, HLA DR4, and a family history of AP is not always associated with the development of AP.[64] Therefore, Latin American dermatologists consider AP as a distinct entity.[3,25]

## CLINICAL MANIFESTATIONS

AP is characterized by intensely pruritic lesions located almost exclusively on sun-exposed facial areas (eyebrows, malar region, distal half of the nose, lips, ears) (Fig. 1), neck, V area of the chest (Fig. 2), extensor areas of the arms and forearms, the dorsum of the hands (Fig. 3), and lower legs.[4,15,26,65] Involvement of covered sites has been described in 35% to 40% of AP patients in the United Kingdom,[26,59] in Canadian Aboriginals,[2] and in patients seen in Thailand and Singapore[38,65]; however, this presentation is distinctly uncommon in Latin American patients.

Characteristic lesions of AP are flat, shiny, and polygonal papules (especially on the face, neck, and hands); alternatively, cone-shaped papules with small hemorrhagic crusts can be seen, mainly in extensor areas of forearms. Papules coalesce to form lichenified plaques with crusts; excoriated nodules and hyperpigmented or hypopigmented pitted scars may be present. Vesicles can be found in cases of eczematization or secondary infection (Fig. 4).[3,43,59] In severe and chronic cases, prominent areas of the face are thickened and eyebrow alopecia may appear, giving the appearance of a leonine facies.[3,4]

**Table 1**
**HLA class I in cases of actinic prurigo**

| Country | Allele | Patients (%) | Controls (%) | OR | 95% CI |
|---|---|---|---|---|---|
| Colombia[24,97] | Cw4 | 53.5 | 21 | 4.3 | 1.8–10.2 |
| | B40 | 41.9 | 13 | 5.2 | 2.1–13.5 |
| Mexico[6,61] | A28 | 86.2 | 23 | 20.9 | 8.31–48.5 |
| | B39 | 72.4 | 28 | 6.7 | 3.11–13.2 |
| Canada[21] | Cw4 | 62.5 | 25 | 5.0 | 1.4–14.6 |
| | A24 | 65.6 | 21.9 | 6.8 | 2.2–20.7 |

Abbreviations: CI, confidence interval; HLA, human leukocyte antigen; OR, odds ratio.
Data from Refs.[6,21,24,61,97]

**Table 2**
**HLA class II DR4 in cases of actinic prurigo**

| Country | n | Patients (%) | n | Controls (%) | OR | 95% CI |
|---|---|---|---|---|---|---|
| Mexico[6,61] | 29 | 92.8 | 100 | 57 | 10.1 | 2.3–91.8 |
| Colombia[5] | 40 | 97.5 | 40 | 35 | 8.2 | 5–13.5 |
| Great Britain[58] | 26 | 100 | 177 | 39.5 | — | — |
| Great Britain[8] | 66 | 80 | 126 | 39 | — | — |
| Scotland[7] | 24 | 96 | — | — | — | — |
| Australia[31] | 21 | 85.7 | — | — | — | — |

*Abbreviations:* CI, confidence interval; HLA, human leukocyte antigen; OR, odds ratio.
*Data from* Refs.[5–8,31,58,61]

Cheilitis is reported in 33% to 85% of the patients, affecting mainly the lower lip or the central area of the upper lip; swelling, scaling, fissures, crust formation, hyperpigmentation, and ulceration may also occur (**Fig. 5**).[2,40,66,67] Involvement of the eyes occurs in up to 62% of the Latin American cases, beginning with hyperemia, photophobia, and increased lacrimation, and progressing to brown pigmentation, papillae hypertrophy, and pseudopterygium (**Fig. 6**).[3,22,66,68] In some patients, lip lesions may be the only clinical manifestation of the disease.

AP usually begins in childhood (6–8 years of age) or before 20 years of age. In sunny parts of the world, the disease runs a persistent and chronic course[3]; in other latitudes, it shows exacerbations in the spring and summer,[2,20,69,70] and the relationship to sun exposure may not be as clearly apparent. An adult-onset form of AP has been described, and these cases tend to be more persistent.[2,12] Spontaneous remission may occur, particularly in early-onset cases; however, in general AP is usually perennial with acute flares.[2,59]

## HISTOLOGY

Skin biopsies of AP patients are not specific. Hematoxylin and eosin–stained specimens show hyperkeratosis with orthokeratosis or parakeratosis, regular acanthosis, focal or multifocal spongiosis, thickening of the basal membrane, dense perivascular lymphocytic infiltrate in superficial and mid dermis, and papillary dermal edema. Eosinophils, melanophages, and extravasation of red blood cells can be observed within the infiltrate (**Fig. 7**).[3,30,36,71–73]

Histopathologic changes in lip biopsy include epidermal ulceration with crusts, hyperkeratosis with parakeratosis, acanthosis, spongiosis, vacuolar degeneration of the basal layer, and dense dermal lymphocytic or lymphoplasmacytic infiltrate, forming well-defined lymphoid follicles, with variable numbers of eosinophils and melanophages (**Fig. 8**).[3,40,66] These findings, known as follicular cheilitis, have sensitivity of 74.3% and specificity of 36.4% as predictors of AP.[66]

The affected conjunctivae show epithelial hyperplasia alternating with atrophy, vacuolization of the basal layer, and dilated capillaries in the dermis. Similar to mucosal lip biopsy, dense lymphocytic infiltrate forming lymphoid follicles are frequently observed (in up to 88% of cases).[3,68]

Lymphoid follicles seen in mucosal biopsy consist of T cells in the periphery and B cells in the center.[57,74] Direct immunofluorescence of skin samples to immunoglobulin (Ig)G, IgA, IgM, and C3 is negative.[30]

## LABORATORY FINDINGS

Complete blood count, metabolic profile, porphyrin levels, antinuclear antibodies, and

**Table 3**
**HLA class II DR4 subtypes in cases of actinic prurigo in the Americas**

| | Allele | Patients Allele (%) | Controls Allele (%) | OR | 95% CI |
|---|---|---|---|---|---|
| Mexico[61] | DRB1*0407 | 60.5 | 10.6 | 12.9 | 6.4–26 |
| Colombia[5] | DRB1*0407 | 63.8 | 14.5 | 9.9 | 4.3–23.3 |
| Canada: Inuit[22] | DRB1*14 | 51.2 | 26.2 | 3.0 | 1.19–7.86 |

*Abbreviations:* CI, confidence interval; HLA, human leukocyte antigen; OR, odds ratio.
*Data from* Refs.[5,22,61]

| Table 4 HLA class II DRB1*0407 in cases of actinic prurigo in other countries | | | | |
|---|---|---|---|---|
| Country | No. of Patients | % | No. of Controls | % |
| Great | 20 | 60 | 20 | 0 |
| Britain[8,58] | 66 | 56 | 126 | 2 |
| Scotland[7] | 18 | 72 | — | — |
| Australia[31] | 21 | 71.4 | — | — |

*Abbreviation:* HLA, human leukocyte antigen.
  *Data from* Refs.[7,8,31,58]

anti-Ro and anti-La levels are normal or negative.[48,59] Patch and photopatch tests are regularly negative,[48,75] unless the patient has developed a contact dermatitis or a photoallergic contact dermatitis. HLA typing is useful for the diagnosis, especially in populations where HLA DR4 is not prevalent, as in European Caucasians,[58] particularly if the subtype DRB1*0407 is present. However, not all AP patients exhibit these HLA alleles.[64]

## PHOTOBIOLOGICAL EVALUATION

Minimal erythema doses for ultraviolet A (UVA) and ultraviolet B (UVB) (MED-A and MED-B) may be normal or lowered (**Fig. 9**, **Table 5**). Photoprovocation with repeated exposure to UVA and/or UVB is able to reproduce AP lesions in most cases (75%–100%).[43,76]

## TREATMENT

Management of AP consists of avoidance of sun exposure, wearing protective clothing, widebrimmed hats, and sunglasses, and application

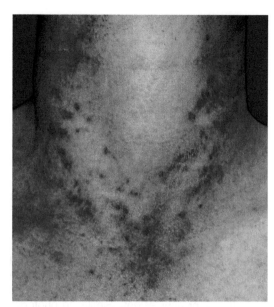

**Fig. 2.** Excoriated erythematous papules over sunexposed area of the neck.

of photoprotective lip balms and high–sun-protection factor, broad-spectrum sunscreens. Because UVA can be transmitted through window glass, and UVA could be an action spectrum of AP, patients should avoid working or standing by windows so as to minimize UVA exposure.[43,49,59,77] Application of a UV-protective film, if available, on home and car windows is helpful.[78]

Topical potent corticosteroids are effective in some AP patients for the control of pruritus and treatment of eczematous lesions; however, they should not be used chronically because of potential side effects with long-term use.[79] Topical calcineurin inhibitors, with a better safety profile, may be preferred for longer use in mild cases.[80] Short courses of oral corticosteroids (0.5–1 mg/kg) provide relief in acute episodes but usually do not completely clear the lesions.[31,43,59]

Phototherapy, particularly narrow-band UVB, has been used successfully in some patients, but

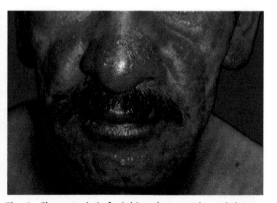

**Fig. 1.** Characteristic facial involvement in actinic prurigo (AP), with erythema on the cheeks, erythema and superficial erosions on the nose, and relative sparing of nasolabial folds.

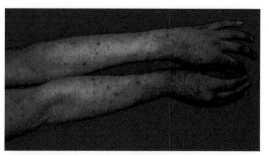

**Fig. 3.** Erythematous excoriated papules on sunexposed sites of upper extremities.

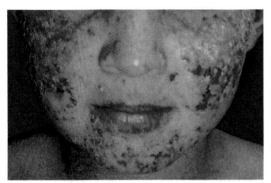

Fig. 4. Erosions covered with crusts in a patient with secondary infection. Note the relative sparing of naso-labial folds.

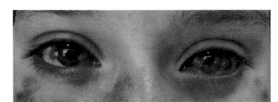

Fig. 6. Pseudopterygium formation in a patient with AP.

the effect is, unfortunately, limited.[81–83] The initial radiation dose is typically 50% of MED, with 20% increment increase at each visit if there is no erythema or new lesions. Similar to photode-sensitization in polymorphic light eruption, sessions 3 times weekly for 5 weeks is the standard treatment; afterward patients must be exposed to sunlight on a regular basis to maintain light tolerance. In addition, topical corticosteroids, or a 5- to 7-day course of oral corticosteroids, may be needed to manage flares.[84]

At present, the best available treatment for AP is thalidomide, a synthetic derivative of glutamic acid, with immunomodulatory and anti-inflammatory effects.[85] Thalidomide inhibits TNFα production in peripheral monocytes,[86] modulates the production of interferon-γ by CD3 cells,[87] and suppresses the ability of Langerhans cells to present antigens to T-helper 1 lymphocytes,[88] among other actions. In 1973, Londoño was the first author to report the use of thalidomide for the treatment of AP. Thirty-two of 34 treated patients achieved significant improvement in a mean time of 50 days, with doses of 100 to 300 mg per day.[89] These results have been confirmed by studies in different countries.[90–93]

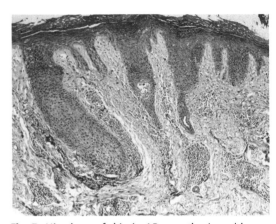

Fig. 7. Histology of skin in AP: acanthosis and hyper-keratosis with orthokeratosis, dense perivascular lymphocytic infiltrate in superficial and mid dermis, and some papillary dermal edema (Hematoxylin-eosin, original magnification ×10).

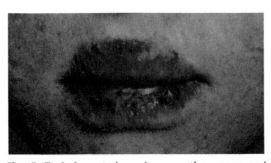

Fig. 5. Typical crusted erosions on the upper and lower lips of a patient with AP.

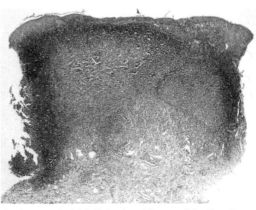

Fig. 8. Lymphoid follicles in a biopsy of the lip of a patient with AP (Hematoxylin-eosin, original magnification ×4).

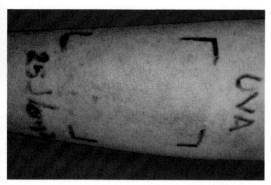

**Fig. 9.** Erythematous and excoriated papules 24 hours after a single dose of 25 J/cm² of ultraviolet A.

For this reason, the response of AP lesions to thalidomide may be used as a diagnostic marker of the disease. However, as lesions may recur on the withdrawal of the drug, it is recommended to taper the dose slowly. Many patients are controlled with a dose of 25 to 50 mg a week with few adverse effects.[43] Because of its well-known teratogenicity and peripheral neuropathy, thalidomide is not easily available in many countries.

Pentoxifylline, which demonstrates anti-TNF properties, has been reported to be effective in only one uncontrolled study, using 1200 mg/d for 6 months, with improvement in pruritus and cutaneous lesions; however, the disease relapsed after discontinuation of therapy.[94] Although the newer forms of injectable TNFα inhibitors (ie, etanercept, adalimumab, and infliximab) theoretically should be helpful for these patients, as of this writing there have been no reported cases.

Oral cyclosporine (2.5 mg/kg/d for 6–8 months)[53] and azathioprine (50–100 mg/d for 8 months)[44] have been used with some success in a few refractory cases. Efficacy of topical 2% cyclosporine ophthalmic solution has been reported for the treatment of ocular AP lesions, with a dosage of 2 or 3 drops daily for 3 months.[95,96]

## SUMMARY

AP is a chronic, immunologically mediated photodermatosis associated with HLA DRB1*0407, a common allele in Central America and some regions of North and South America. The characteristic pruritic, crusted papules and pitted scars of sun-exposed areas, involvement of eyes and lips (especially in Latin American mestizos and Amerindians), and the frequent onset in childhood help to diagnose this disease. Patient counseling and adequate treatment (photoprotection and thalidomide) will help patients to improve their quality of life.

## REFERENCES

1. Gambichler T, Al-Muhammadi R, Boms S. Immunologically mediated photodermatoses: diagnosis and treatment. Am J Clin Dermatol 2009;10(3): 169–80.
2. Lane PR, Hogan DJ, Martel MJ, et al. Actinic prurigo: clinical features and prognosis. J Am Acad Dermatol 1992;26(5 Pt 1):683–92.
3. Hojyo-Tomoka T, Vega-Memije E, Granados J, et al. Actinic prurigo: an update. Int J Dermatol 1995; 34(6):380–4.
4. López González G. Prurigo solar. Arch Argent Dermatol 1961;XI(3):301–18.
5. Suárez A, Valbuena MC, Rey M, et al. Association of HLA subtype DRB10407 in Colombian patients with actinic prurigo. Photodermatol Photoimmunol Photomed 2006;22(2):55–8.
6. Hojyo-Tomoka T, Granados J, Vargas-Alarcón G, et al. Further evidence of the role of HLA-DR4 in the genetic susceptibility to actinic prurigo. J Am Acad Dermatol 1997;36(6 Pt 1):935–7.
7. Dawe RS, Collins P, Ferguson J, et al. Actinic prurigo and HLA-DR4. J Invest Dermatol 1997; 108(2):233–4.
8. Grabczynska SA, McGregor JM, Kondeatis E, et al. Actinic prurigo and polymorphic light eruption: common pathogenesis and the importance of HLA-DR4/DRB1*0407. Br J Dermatol 1999;140(2): 232–6.
9. Jong CT, Finlay AY, Pearse AD, et al. The quality of life of 790 patients with photodermatoses. Br J Dermatol 2008;159(1):192–7.
10. Rasch C. Some historical and clinical remarks on the effect of light on the skin and skin diseases. Proc R Soc Med 1926;20(1):11–30.
11. Young P, Finn BC, Pellegrini D, et al. Hutchinson (1828-1913), su historia, su tríada y otras tríadas de la medicina. Rev Med Chil 2010;138(3):383–7.

**Table 5**
**Summary of phototesting in cases of actinic prurigo**

| Country | N | Lowered MEDs (%) | | |
| --- | --- | --- | --- | --- |
| | | UVA | UVB | UVA/UVB |
| Australia[31] | 20 | 40 | 0 | 20 |
| United Kingdom[70] | 53 | 9 | 32 | 34 |
| Singapore[98] | 11 | 55 | 9 | 36 |
| Canada[2] | 19 | 32 | 0 | 37 |

*Abbreviations:* MED, minimal erythema dose; N, number; UVA, ultraviolet A; UVB, ultraviolet B.
*Data from* Refs.[2,31,70,98]

12. Magaña M. Prurigo solar. Bol Med Hosp Infant Mex 2001;58(6):409–19.

13. Brandt R. Dermatologic observations on the Navajo Reservation. Arch Dermatol 1958;77(5):581–5.

14. Londoño F. Prúrigo-eczema actínico. Instant Med Colombia Mundo 1961(Enero-Febrero).

15. Londoño F, Muvdi F, Giraldo F, et al. Familial actinic prurigo. Arch Argent Dermatol 1966;16(4):290–307 [in Spanish].

16. Calnan CD, Meara RH. Actinic prurigo (Hutchinson's summer prurigo). Clin Exp Dermatol 1977; 2(4):365–72.

17. Driban NE. La dermatología en Mendoza. Revista Médica Universitaria Facultad de Ciencias Médicas UNCuyo 2008;4(1). Available at: http://revista.medicina.edu.ar/vol04_01/01/vol04_01_Art01.pdf. Accessed November 16, 2013.

18. Escalona E. Dermatología, lo esencial para el estudiante. 1st edition. Mexico: Impresiones Modernas; 1954.

19. Dominguez-Soto L. Prúrigo Actínico. Historia y situación actual. Dermatologia Rev Mex 1993; 37(Suppl 1):292.

20. Birt AR, Davis RA. Photodermatitis in North American Indians: familial actinic prurigo. Int J Dermatol 1971;10(2):107–14.

21. Sheridan DP, Lane PR, Irvine J, et al. HLA typing in actinic prurigo. J Am Acad Dermatol 1990; 22(6 Pt 1):1019–23.

22. Wiseman MC, Orr PH, Macdonald SM, et al. Actinic prurigo: clinical features and HLA associations in a Canadian Inuit population. J Am Acad Dermatol 2001;44(6):952–6.

23. Johnsons J, Fusaro R. Fotosensibilidad en indios americanos. Rev Mex Dermatol 1993;37(Suppl 1): 326–7.

24. Bernal JE, Duran de Rueda MM, Ordonez CP, et al. Actinic prurigo among the Chimila Indians in Colombia: HLA studies. J Am Acad Dermatol 1990;22(6 Pt 1):1049–51.

25. Tincopa Wong O, Tincopa Montoya L, Valverde Lopez J, et al. Solar prurigo in Trujillo. Clinical, histologic and epidemiologic study. 1973-1995. Dermatol Peru 2002;12(2):114–21.

26. Addo HA, Frain-Bell W. Actinic prurigo—a specific photodermatosis? Photodermatol 1984;1(3): 119–28.

27. Batard ML, Bonnevalle A, Ségard M, et al. Caucasian actinic prurigo: 8 cases observed in France. Br J Dermatol 2001;144(1):194–6.

28. Stefanaki C, Valari M, Antoniou C, et al. Actinic prurigo in an Albanian girl. Pediatr Dermatol 2006; 23(1):97–8.

29. Stratigos AJ, Antoniou C, Papathanakou E, et al. Spectrum of idiopathic photodermatoses in a Mediterranean country. Int J Dermatol 2003;42(6): 449–54.

30. Worret WI, Vocks E, Frias G, et al. Actinic prurigo. An assessment of current status. Hautarzt 2000; 51(7):474–8 [in German].

31. Crouch R, Foley P, Baker C. Actinic prurigo: a retrospective analysis of 21 cases referred to an Australian photobiology clinic. Australas J Dermatol 2002; 43(2):128–32.

32. Akaraphanth R, Gritiyarangsan P. A case of actinic prurigo in Thailand. J Dermatol 2000;27(1):20–3.

33. Khoo SW, Tay YK, Tham SN. Photodermatoses in a Singapore skin referral centre. Clin Exp Dermatol 1996;21(4):263–8.

34. Aoki T, Fujita M. Actinic prurigo: a case report with successful induction of skin lesions. Clin Exp Dermatol 1980;5(1):47–52.

35. Kuno Y, Sato K, Hasegawa K, et al. A case of actinic prurigo showing hypersensitivity of skin fibroblasts to ultraviolet A (UVA). Photodermatol Photoimmunol Photomed 2000;16(1):38–41.

36. Hojyo-Tomoka MT, Dominguez-Soto L, Vargas-Ocampo F. Actinic prurigo: clinical-pathological correlation. Int J Dermatol 1978;17(9):706–10.

37. Duran de Rueda MM, Bernal JE, Ordonez CP. Actinic prurigo at sea level in Colombia. Int J Dermatol 1989;28(4):228–9.

38. Dawe R. Abstract No. 2. Prevalences of the chronic idiopathic and metabolic photodermatoses in Scotland. Br J Dermatol 2006;155(4):866.

39. Orr PH, Birt AR. Hereditary polymorphic light eruption in Canadian Inuit. Int J Dermatol 1984;23(7): 472–5.

40. Vega-Memije ME, Mosqueda-Taylor A, Irigoyen-Camacho ME, et al. Actinic prurigo cheilitis: clinicopathologic analysis and therapeutic results in 116 cases. Oral Surg Oral Med Oral Pathol Oral Radiol Endod 2002;94(1):83–91.

41. Ibarra G, Mena-Cedillos C, Pérez-Garrigós M. Prurigo actinico: el aspecto familiar. Revisión de 10 aos en el HIM FG. Dermatologia Rev Mex 1993; 37(Suppl 1):300–2.

42. Rébora I. El prurigo actínico. Características clínicas, histopatológicas y consideraciones sobre su inmunología, fotobiología y genética Parte I. Arch Argent Dermatol 2009;59(3):89–95.

43. Hojyo-Tomoka MT, Vega-Memije ME, Cortes-Franco R, et al. Diagnosis and treatment of actinic prurigo. Dermatol Ther 2003;16(1):40–4.

44. Lestarini D, Khoo LS, Goh CL. The clinical features and management of actinic prurigo: a retrospective study. Photodermatol Photoimmunol Photomed 1999;15(5):183–7.

45. Hiramoto K, Tanaka H, Yanagihara N, et al. Effect of 17 beta-estradiol on immunosuppression induced by ultraviolet B irradiation. Arch Dermatol Res 2004;295(8–9):307–11.

46. Widyarini S, Domanski D, Painter N, et al. Estrogen receptor signaling protects against immune

suppression by UV radiation exposure. Proc Natl Acad Sci U S A 2006;103(34):12837–42.

47. Wolf P, Byrne SN, Gruber-Wackernagel A. New insights into the mechanisms of polymorphic light eruption: resistance to ultraviolet radiation-induced immune suppression as an aetiological factor. Exp Dermatol 2009;18(4):350–6.

48. Tincopa-Wong OW, Valverde-López J, Aguilar-Vargas M. Prúrigo Actínico. In: Rondón-Lugo A, Roberto-Antonio J, Piquero-Martín J, et al, editors. Dermatología Iberoamericana Online. Caracas: Fundación Piel Latinoamericana; 2013. Available from: http://piel-l.org/libreria/item/493. Accessed November 20, 2013.

49. Valbuena MC, Lim HW. Actinic prurigo. In: Heymann WR, Anderson BE, Hivnor CM, et al, editors. Clinical decision support: dermatology. Wilmington (DE): Decision Support in Medicine, LLC; 2012.

50. Gómez A, Umana A, Trespalacios AA. Immune responses to isolated human skin antigens in actinic prurigo. Med Sci Monit 2006;12(3):BR106–13.

51. Santos-Martínez L, Llorente L, Baranda L, et al. Profile of cytokine mRNA expression in spontaneous and UV-induced skin lesions from actinic prurigo patients. Exp Dermatol 1997;6(2):91–7.

52. Moncada B, González-Amaro R, Baranda ML, et al. Immunopathology of polymorphous light eruption. T lymphocytes in blood and skin. J Am Acad Dermatol 1984;10(6):970–3.

53. Umaña A, Gómez A, Durán MM, et al. Lymphocyte subtypes and adhesion molecules in actinic prurigo: observations with cyclosporin A. Int J Dermatol 2002;41(3):139–45.

54. González-Amaro R, Baranda L, Salazar-Gonzalez JF, et al. Immune sensitization against epidermal antigens in polymorphous light eruption. J Am Acad Dermatol 1991;24(1):70–3.

55. Torres-Alvarez B, Baranda L, Fuentes C, et al. An immunohistochemical study of UV-induced skin lesions in actinic prurigo. Resistance of Langerhans cells to UV light. Eur J Dermatol 1998;8(1):24–8.

56. Calderón-Amador J, Flores-Langarica A, Silva-Sánchez A, et al. Epidermal Langerhans cells in Actinic Prurigo: a comparison between lesional and non-lesional skin. J Eur Acad Dermatol Venereol 2009;23(4):438–40.

57. Arrese JE, Dominguez-Soto L, Hojyo-Tomoka MT, et al. Effectors of inflammation in actinic prurigo. J Am Acad Dermatol 2001;44(6):957–61.

58. Menagé H duP, Vaughan RW, Baker CS, et al. HLA-DR4 may determine expression of actinic prurigo in British patients. J Invest Dermatol 1996;106(2):362–7.

59. Ferguson J, Ibbotson S. The idiopathic photodermatoses. Semin Cutan Med Surg 1999;18(4):257–73.

60. Solberg OD, Mack SJ, Lancaster AK, et al. Balancing selection and heterogeneity across the classical human leukocyte antigen loci: a meta-analytic review of 497 population studies. Hum Immunol 2008;69(7):443–64.

61. Zuloaga-Salcedo S, Castillo-Vazquez M, Vega-Memije E, et al. Class I and class II major histocompatibility complex genes in Mexican patients with actinic prurigo. Br J Dermatol 2007;156(5):1074–5.

62. Grabczynska SA, Carey BS, McGregor JM, et al. Tumour necrosis factor alpha promoter polymorphism at position -308 is not associated with actinic prurigo. Clin Exp Dermatol 2001;26(8):700–4.

63. Hawk J. Benign summer light eruption and polymorphic light eruption: genetic and functional studies suggest that a revised nomenclature is required. J Cosmet Dermatol 2004;3(3):173–5.

64. Dawe RS, Ferguson J. A family with actinic prurigo and polymorphic light eruption. Br J Dermatol 1997;137(5):827–9.

65. Hojyo MT, Vega E, Romero A, et al. Actinic prurigo. Int J Dermatol 1992;31(5):372–3.

66. Herrera-Geopfert R, Magaña M. Follicular cheilitis. A distinctive histopathologic finding in actinic prurigo. Am J Dermatopathol 1995;17(4):357–61.

67. Birt AR, Hogg GR. The actinic cheilitis of hereditary polymorphic light eruption. Arch Dermatol 1979;115(6):699–702.

68. Magaña M, Mendez Y, Rodriguez A, et al. The conjunctivitis of solar (actinic) prurigo. Pediatr Dermatol 2000;17(6):432–5.

69. Fusaro RM, Johnson JA. Hereditary polymorphic light eruption of American Indians: occurrence in non-Indians with polymorphic light eruption. J Am Acad Dermatol 1996;34(4):612–7.

70. Grabczynska SA, Hawk JL. What is actinic prurigo in Britain? Photodermatol Photoimmunol Photomed 1997;13(3):85–6.

71. Lane PR, Murphy F, Hogan DJ, et al. Histopathology of actinic prurigo. Am J Dermatopathol 1993;15(4):326–31.

72. Vega-Memije M. Características histopatológicas del prúrigo actínico. Dermatologia Rev Mex 1993;37(Suppl 1):295–7.

73. Magaña M, Cervantes M. Histopathology of sun prurigo. Rev Invest Clin 2000;52(4):391–6 [in Spanish].

74. Guevara E, Hojyo-Tomoka M, Vega-Memije M, et al. Estudio inmunohistoquímico para demostrar la presencia de linfocitos T y B en el infiltrado inflamatorio de las biopsias de piel, labio y conjuntiva de pacientes con prúrigo actínico. Dermatol Rev Mex 1997;41(6):223–6.

75. Lane PR, Harms VL, Hogan DJ. Patch testing in actinic prurigo. Contact Dermatitis 1989;21(4):249–54.

76. Akaraphanth R, Sindhavananda J, Gritiyarangsan P. Adult-onset actinic prurigo in Thailand. Photodermatol Photoimmunol Photomed 2007;23(6):234–7.

77. Ross G, Foley P, Baker C. Actinic prurigo. Photodermatol Photoimmunol Photomed 2008;24(5): 272–5.

78. Kerr AC, Ferguson J. Actinic prurigo deterioration due to degradation of DermaGard window film. Br J Dermatol 2007;157(3):619–20.

79. Lane PR, Moreland AA, Hogan DJ. Treatment of actinic prurigo with intermittent short-course topical 0.05% clobetasol 17-propionate. A preliminary report. Arch Dermatol 1990;126(9):1211–3.

80. González-Carrascosa Ballesteros M, De la Cueva DP, Hernanz Hermosa JM, et al. Tratamiento del prúrigo actínico con tacrolimus al 0,1%. Med Cutan Ibero Lat Am 2006;34(5):233–6.

81. Collins P, Ferguson J. Narrow-band UVB (TL-01) phototherapy: an effective preventative treatment for the photodermatoses. Br J Dermatol 1995; 132(6):956–63.

82. Farr PM, Diffey BL. Treatment of actinic prurigo with PUVA: mechanism of action. Br J Dermatol 1989; 120(3):411–8.

83. Las DY, Youn JI, Park MH, et al. Actinic prurigo: limited effect of PUVA. Br J Dermatol 1997;136(6): 972–3.

84. Ferguson J. Diagnosis and treatment of the common idiopathic photodermatoses. Australas J Dermatol 2003;44(2):90–6.

85. Jacobson J. Thalidomide: a remarkable comeback. Expert Opin Pharmacother 2000;1(4):849–63.

86. Sampaio E, Sarno E, Galilly R, et al. Thalidomide selectively inhibits tumor necrosis alpha production by stimulated human monocytes. J Exp Med 1991; 173(3):699–703.

87. Estrada-G I, Garibay-Escobar A, Núñez-Vázquez A, et al. Evidence that thalidomide modifies the immune response of patients suffering from actinic prurigo. Int J Dermatol 2004;43(12): 893–7.

88. Deng L, Ding W, Granstein R. Thalidomide inhibits tumor necrosis factor alpha production and antigen presentation by Langerhans cells. J Invest Dermatol 2003;121(5):1060–5.

89. Londoño F. Thalidomide in the treatment of actinic prurigo. Int J Dermatol 1973;12(5):326–8.

90. Crouch RB, Foley PA, Ng JC, et al. Thalidomide experience of a major Australian teaching hospital. Australas J Dermatol 2002;43(4):278–84.

91. Lovell CR, Hawk JL, Calnan CD, et al. Thalidomide in actinic prurigo. Br J Dermatol 1983;108(4):467–71.

92. Yong-Gee SA, Muir JB. Long-term thalidomide for actinic prurigo. Australas J Dermatol 2001;42(4): 281–3.

93. Vega M, Hojyo-Tomoka M, Domínguez-Soto L. Tratamiento del prurigo actínico con talidomida. Estudio de 30 pacientes. Dermatol Rev Mex 1993; 37(Suppl 1):342–3.

94. Torres-Alvarez B, Castanedo-Cazares JP, Moncada B. Pentoxifylline in the treatment of actinic prurigo. A preliminary report of 10 patients. Dermatology 2004; 208(3):198–201.

95. McCoombes JA, Hirst LW, Green WR. Use of topical cyclosporin for conjunctival manifestations of actinic prurigo. Am J Ophthalmol 2000;130(6): 830–1.

96. Ortiz-Castillo JV, Boto-de-los-Bueis A, De-Lucas-Laguna R, et al. Topical cyclosporine in the treatment of ocular actinic prurigo. Arch Soc Esp Oftalmol 2006;81(11):661–4 [in Spanish].

97. Bernal JE, Duran de Rueda MM, de Brigard D. Human lymphocyte antigen in actinic prurigo. J Am Acad Dermatol 1988;18(2 Pt 1):310–2.

98. Ker KJ, Chong WS, Theng CT. Clinical characteristics of adult-onset actinic prurigo in Asians: a case series. Indian J Dermatol Venereol Leprol 2013; 79(6):783–8.

# Hydroa Vacciniforme and Solar Urticaria

Rattanavalai Nitiyarom, MD[a], Chanisada Wongpraparut, MD[b],*

## KEYWORDS

- Hydroa vacciniforme • Epstein-Barr virus • Photosensitivity • Photodermatoses
- Lymphoproliferative disorder • Solar urticaria • Phototherapy • Plasmapheresis

## KEY POINTS

- Hydroa vacciniforme (HV) is characterized by a vesiculopapular eruption and necrotic lesions that heal with varioliform scars.
- HV has been reported to be associated with latent Epstein-Barr virus infection, raising the possibility of increased risk of lymphoproliferative malignancy.
- The mainstay of therapy in HV is adequate photoprotection.
- Solar urticaria (SU) is characterized by skin erythema, swelling, and whealing immediately after sun exposure.
- Treatments for SU include photoprotection, medical therapy, phototherapy, photochemotherapy, and plasmapheresis.

## HYDROA VACCINIFORME

Hydroa vacciniforme (HV) is a rare photosensitivity disorder predominantly affecting children. It is characterized by recurrent vesiculopapular eruptions that evolve into necrotic crusts and varioliform scars on sun-exposed areas. Latent Epstein-Barr virus (EBV) infection has been suggested to have a role in the underlying pathogenesis. HV has clinically been classified into classic HV and severe HV-like eruption. The latter, described in adults, may be associated with systemic symptoms and an increased risk of lymphoproliferative disorders. Classic HV tends to remit by adolescence or early adulthood. This disease significantly affects quality of life, causing both psychosocial and emotional morbidity.

### History

HV was first reported by Bazin in 1862.[1] The term "hydroa" possibly derives from the Greek for "water eggs," a reference to the vesicular eruption. "Vacciniforme" means "poxlike" scar, which is characteristic of this condition when the lesions heal.

### Epidemiology

The rarity of HV and lack of universally diagnostic criteria make the precise prevalence difficult to establish. The estimated prevalence of HV is 0.34 cases per 100,000 population.[1] Although well recognized globally, it predominantly affects Caucasians.[2,3] A bimodal distribution has been described with peaks presenting at ages 1 to 7 and 12 to 16 years. Several cases of adult-onset classic HV have also been reported.[3–5] The proportion of female to male patients varies depending on the studies, ranging from 1:1 to 1:2.[1–3] Male patients tend to have a later onset, longer duration, and more severe symptoms than female patients.[1] Although HV is usually sporadic, familial cases have also been noted.[6]

Disclosure Statement: No conflict of interest.
[a] Department of Pediatrics, Faculty of Medicine, Siriraj Hospital, Mahidol University, 2 Wanglang Road, Bangkoknoi, Bangkok 10700, Thailand; [b] Department of Dermatology, Faculty of Medicine, Siriraj Hospital, Mahidol University, 2 Wanglang Road, Bangkoknoi, Bangkok 10700, Thailand
* Corresponding author.
E-mail address: ctuchinda@yahoo.com

Dermatol Clin 32 (2014) 345–353
http://dx.doi.org/10.1016/j.det.2014.03.013
0733-8635/14/$ – see front matter © 2014 Elsevier Inc. All rights reserved.

## Pathogenesis

The precise pathophysiology of HV remains unknown. Sunlight, especially ultraviolet A (UVA), is known to play an important role, because the characteristic lesions of HV can be reproduced after artificial UVA exposure.[7–10] EBV infections may also play a role in the pathogenesis of the disease, as EBV has been detected in the lymphocytic infiltrate of HV lesions from both pediatric and adult patients. Elevated levels of EBV DNA copies in the peripheral blood and EBV-encoded small nuclear ribonucleic acid (EBER) in cutaneous lesions have been found in both classic HV and severe HV-like eruptions.[11–13] Thus, both conditions have been suggested to be variants within the same disease spectrum. Higher copies of EBV are associated with symptom severity and worse prognosis for patients.[14,15] In addition to HV, chronic EBV infection is also known to be related to other heterogeneous disorders including lymphoproliferative disorders, hemophagocytic syndrome, and hypersensitivity to mosquito bites.[16–18] Therefore, patients with the severe variant of HV may be at risk of progression to various EBV-associated malignant lymphomas.[2,19–24]

## Clinical Manifestations

HV patients experience various clinical signs and symptoms related to their disease. HV is classified into two types: classic or typical HV, and severe HV-like eruption.[12]

### Mucocutaneous manifestations
Classic HV usually presents with recurrent erythematous papules and vesicles (**Fig. 1**) associated with itching or stinging sensation within hours or days after sun exposure. Subsequently, the lesions progress to ulceration with necrotic crusts, and eventually heal over a period of 1 to 6 weeks with varioliform atrophic scars (**Fig. 2**). The distribution tends to be symmetric. The eruptions typically develop on sun-exposed areas, such as the face and dorsal hands, in the summer. Unlike classic HV, the lesions of severe HV-like eruption are larger and deeper; this variant occurs more commonly in adults. The lesions are distributed extensively, including on sun-protected areas, and may not always be associated with photosensitivity.[19,22] Facial swelling is also common. Seasonal variation is not observed in the severe form. Disfigurement of the ears and nose, in addition to contracture of the fingers, has been reported.[22] Heat may provoke the symptoms in some of these patients.[3]

Ocular and oral mucosal involvement has been reported in HV. Ophthalmic complications include mild photophobia, chemosis, keratoconjunctivitis, corneal ulcer and erosion, iritis, uveitis, and scleritis[25]; these were observed in 6.3% of patients in a study from Japan.[25,26] The same study also reported oral lesions, including aphthous stomatitis and ulcerative gingivitis, in 17.5% of the patients. Oral lesions were seen predominantly in severe HV-like eruptions rather than in classic HV. Classic HV spontaneously resolves during adolescence or young adulthood, whereas severe HV-like eruptions tend to have a relatively longer clinical course and usually become more severe with age.[22]

### Systemic manifestations
Classic HV is considered a benign disease with rare complications. However, severe HV-like

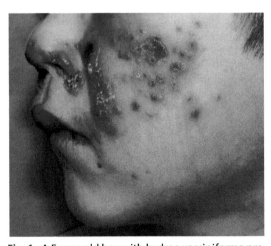

**Fig. 1.** A 5-year-old boy with hydroa vacciniforme presenting with papules, vesicles, and necrotic lesions of the left cheek. (*Courtesy of* Tor Shwayder, MD, Henry Ford Hospital, Detroit, MI.)

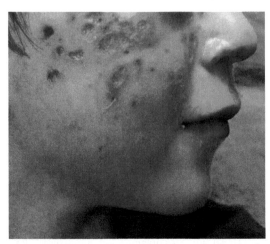

**Fig. 2.** Atrophic poxlike scars on the right cheek of a 5-year-old boy with hydroa vacciniforme after 10 days of treatment. (*Courtesy of* Tor Shwayder, MD, Henry Ford Hospital, Detroit, MI.)

eruptions may have systemic manifestations, such as fever, malaise, weight loss, hypersensitivity to mosquito bites, lymphadenopathy, hepatomegaly, splenomegaly, abdominal pain, headache, abnormal liver function testing, leukopenia, and thrombocytopenia.[19] Erosions in the esophagus and colon have also been noted.[26] Furthermore, patients with severe disease may progress to EBV-associated malignancy, including T-cell and/or natural killer cell lymphoma.[12]

## Histology

Histology of early lesions reveals epidermal spongiosis, focal keratinocyte degeneration, and a perivascular lymphohistiocytic infiltrate. Intraepidermal vesicles, confluent epidermal necrosis, and ulceration are demonstrated in older lesions. Both classic HV and the severe variant share similar histology.[12] However, the severe form usually reveals a denser lymphocytic infiltrate with few atypical cells, which extend into the subcutaneous fat.[27] Immunohistochemical study of the infiltrates usually demonstrates T-cell–expressing cytotoxic molecules, such as T-cell intracellular antigen 1 and granzyme B.[12] Direct immunofluorescence study is usually nonspecific.

## Differential Diagnosis

Several conditions need to be considered in the differential diagnosis. Erythropoietic protoporphyria and porphyria cutanea tarda can be differentiated by their characteristic porphyrin profiles. The vesicular form of polymorphous light eruption resolves without significant scarring. Actinic prurigo most commonly occurs in Amerindians or mestizos (individuals with a mixed Amerindian and European extraction). Antinuclear antibody (ANA) panel and skin biopsy should differentiate bullous systemic lupus erythematosus from HV. Herpes simplex virus infection can be diagnosed by viral culture, and contact dermatitis by the history of exposure to contactants.

## Laboratory Findings

The diagnosis is generally based on clinical findings and pathognomonic histologic features. In suspicious cases blood, urine, and stool porphyrins may be obtained to exclude cutaneous porphyria. Autoantibody evaluation may be assessed to exclude the low possibility of cutaneous lupus erythematosus. Circulating EBV DNA load may be checked in select cases. Previous reports have proposed that the most useful test to differentiate the two variants of HV is monoclonality of the T-cell receptor genes.[19,28]

## Photobiological Evaluation

Although most patients show increased sensitivity to UVA radiation, they may demonstrate normal minimal erythema dose (MED) to UVA. Repetitive UVA doses have been found to provoke characteristic lesions of HV.[9] The action spectrum for induction of skin lesions ranges from 320 to 390 nm.[8]

## Management

An important part of therapeutic management is strict photoprotection, including sun avoidance, use of photoprotective clothing and a wide-brimmed hat, and application of broad-spectrum sunscreen with sun-protection factor higher than 30. Unfortunately, no treatment has been universally successful.[3] Chloroquine, β-carotene, dietary fish oils, prophylactic ultraviolet B (UVB), and psoralen plus UVA (PUVA) have been effective in some cases while thalidomide, azathioprine, and cyclosporine are of uncertain efficacy. In severe cases, systemic corticosteroids can also be used. In cases of chronic EBV infection, antiviral therapy was reported to reduce the severity and frequency of eruptions in a small case series.[29] Because of the potential risk of systemic lymphoma in patients with HV and chronic EBV infection, close monitoring and systemic evaluation should be considered.

The negative impact on the quality of life in HV patients is significant. Psychosocial and emotional impairment in HV patients results from the disfiguring effect of scarring, and the necessity for sun avoidance and consequent restriction of daily activities.[3]

## SOLAR URTICARIA

Solar urticaria (SU) is a rare skin condition characterized by skin erythema, swelling, and whealing immediately after exposure to diverse wavelengths of sunlight. It is estimated that SU accounts for less than 1% of all causes of urticaria.[30,31] SU most commonly develops in women in the third decade of life. Though uncommon, it has a profound effect on individual quality of life.

## History

The term "solar urticaria" was first proposed by Duke in 1923 when he described a 43-year-old woman who developed itching, skin erythema, and edema while she was exposed to the sun during outdoor swimming.[32] In 1923, Wucherpfennig demonstrated that different wavelengths of light could produce urticarial lesions.[32] In 1942, Rajka successfully reproduced urticarial lesions on intradermal injection of an affected patient's serum into a normal subject.[32] Subsequent information obtained from the serum transfer test helped to clarify the pathogenesis of this condition.

## Epidemiology

SU accounts for less than 1% of all causes of urticaria.[30,31] The prevalence of idiopathic SU in Tayside, Scotland was reported to be 3.1 per 100,000.[33] The frequency of SU in photodermatology referral centers worldwide ranges from 1% to 18%.[34,35]

## Clinical Manifestations

Patients with SU characteristically develop urticarial lesions within 5 to 10 minutes of exposure to the sun; the lesions resolve within 24 hours, usually within 1 to 3 hours. In addition to pruritus, erythema, and edema of the skin, patients may also experience systemic symptoms, such as nausea, dizziness, headache, wheezing, syncope, or, rarely, anaphylactic shock.[32,36] Whereas most patients develop lesions during direct sun exposure, a minority of patients only develop urticarial lesions immediately or a few minutes after returning to the shade. This latter group was found to have a specific portion of sunlight that acts as an inhibition spectrum. SU commonly affects the upper chest, arms, and forearms, whereas areas that are regularly exposed to the sun, such as the face and hands, are infrequently involved. In highly sensitive patients, SU may occur in covered areas of skin via light penetration through thin clothing.[36]

In addition, there is a rare and less severe form of SU called fixed solar urticaria (FSU). In these patients, the wheals develop exclusively in a fixed area of skin and can be reproduced only at the same site. To date, only 7 patients with this condition have been reported.[37–41] Recently Wessendorf and colleagues[41] reported a case of delayed-onset FSU, with urticarial wheal development 6 hours after ultraviolet exposure. The pathogenesis of FSU has not been elucidated, but may involve a difference in mast-cell population and distribution in the skin.[40]

## Associated Conditions

SU usually occurs in healthy individuals, but has been reported to coexist with other photodermatoses such as polymorphous light eruption, chronic actinic dermatitis, actinic prurigo, and porphyria cutanea tarda.[42–44] Medications, including benoxaprofen, repirinast, oral contraceptive pills, and tetracycline, have also been reported to induce SU-like reactions.[36,45–47]

## Differential Diagnosis

The clinical manifestations of SU may resemble other photodermatoses. Detailed history, physical examination, phototesting, and other investigations are essential in arriving at the diagnosis. The onset of eruption within a few minutes of sun exposure and the resolution within a few hours are key in differentiating SU from polymorphous light eruption. Erythropoietic protoporphyria, which may present with urticarial lesions following exposure to sunlight, can be differentiated by its characteristic elevation of protoporphyrin in biological specimens. Systemic lupus erythematosus can be differentiated by ANA panel, and lesions of chronic idiopathic urticaria develop without any correlation with sun exposure. Chronic actinic dermatitis characteristically presents with lichenification on sun-exposed areas. HV heals with scars. Actinic prurigo mainly occurs in Amerindians and mestizos, presenting with persistent papules, cheilitis, and conjunctivitis.

## Pathogenesis and Classification

SU results from a type I hypersensitivity reaction. Once skin is exposed to sunlight, a previously inactive cutaneous chromophore is likely converted to a photoallergen. The photoallergen then interacts with immunoglobulin E (IgE)-specific mast cells, causing mast-cell degranulation and clinically apparent wheal and flare.

Studies in the past with passive transfer test, currently considered unethical, have provided significant information on the pathogenesis of SU. This procedure involves intradermal injection of an affected patient's serum into the skin of a normal subject, followed by irradiation with the causative wavelengths. The reverse passive transfer test involves irradiation of the skin of a healthy individual, followed by injection of serum from the affected patient.

According to Leenutaphong and colleagues,[48] SU is classified into 2 types. In type I, the patient demonstrates an IgE-mediated hypersensitivity to specific photoallergens, which are present only in patients with SU. A patient who has type I SU will have a variably positive passive transfer test and a negative reverse passive transfer test. In type II SU, the patient has abnormal IgE antibodies against a normal chromophore. Patients with type II SU will always have a positive passive transfer test and a variable or negative reverse passive transfer test.

## Action Spectrum

The action spectrum in SU refers to the specific wavelength that can produce an urticarial response. The action spectrum of SU varies by geographic and ethnic background, and can range from UVB to infrared wavelength.[36,49] In a study of 61 patients in France, UVA was the most common action spectrum.[50] In a study of 84 patients in Scotland, 41% of patients reacted to UVA and visible light while 30.9% reacted to visible light alone.[33] A study from Belgium demonstrated that the most common action spectra were UVA alone or UVA and visible light, followed by visible light alone and then UVB alone. In Asians, the most common action spectrum appears to be visible light, followed by a combination of visible light and UVA and UVB. Studies from Japan and Singapore demonstrated that most patients developed urticarial reactions from visible light alone.[31,36] The infrared spectrum can, in rare instances, precipitate SU; however, in such instances differentiation from heat urticaria could present a challenge because infrared is known to generate heat. The wide range of action spectra may be due to the diversity of photoallergens. Identifying the action spectrum for SU in each patient will allow an individualized treatment plan for photoprotection.

## Inhibition Spectrum

Some patients with SU display a delayed urticarial reaction after sun exposure but not while in direct sunlight. This phenomenon can be explained by the theory of inhibition spectrum, which has mainly been reported in the Japanese literature and was first described in 1982 by Hasei and Ichihashi.[51] This landmark study reported a 42-year-old woman who developed urticaria from visible light in the range of 400 to 500 nm, but this reaction was inhibited by immediate re-irradiation with a spectrum longer than 530 nm. In a clinical and photobiological study of 40 patients with SU in Japan, the inhibition spectrum was detected in 68% of patients.[52] In most cases, the wavelength of the inhibition spectrum was longer than that of the action spectrum. The mechanism of the inhibition spectrum is unclear; however, several hypotheses have been proposed, including mast-cell stabilization, photoallergen inactivation, competitive IgE blockade, and blockage between photoallergen and IgE mast cells.[32,53,54]

## Augmentation Spectrum

After the discovery of the inhibition spectrum, Horio and Fujigaki[55] observed that irradiation with specific wavelengths before irradiation with the action spectrum enhanced the urticarial reaction in a patient with SU. Soon thereafter, Danno and Mori[56] also reported enhanced urticarial response with irradiation of the augmentation spectrum following exposure to the action spectrum, and proposed that the augmentation spectrum may amplify production of photoallergen after irradiation.

## Photobiological Evaluation

The purpose of phototesting in patients with SU is to identify the action spectrum of minimal urticarial dose (MUD). Assessment of the phototest sites should be done immediately after irradiation, and ideally up to 1 hour after. The light sources for phototesting should include UVA, broadband UVB, and visible light (usually a slide projector). To eliminate the heat generated by a visible light source, a water filter should be placed between the light source and the irradiated sites. Fig. 3 illustrates an urticarial reaction after visible light exposure. If phototesting results are negative but SU is still suspected, natural sunlight exposure should be considered. In addition, FSU should be considered in patients with recurrent urticarial lesions in a specified area. For FSU, phototesting will only be positive if performed on the previously affected site.

As appropriate, serum ANA and porphyrin analyses should be carried out to exclude lupus erythematosus and porphyrias.

## Management

There are several treatment options for SU, including photoprotection, medical therapy, phototherapy, photochemotherapy, and plasmapheresis. As many patients with SU are sensitive to visible light, sunscreens alone are not particularly efficacious. In severe cases, a combination of several treatment modalities should be considered.

### Medical therapy
**Antihistamines** H1-receptor antagonists are the first-line treatment of SU. Similar to chronic idiopathic urticaria, high doses (as tolerated) of antihistamines may be needed to suppress the

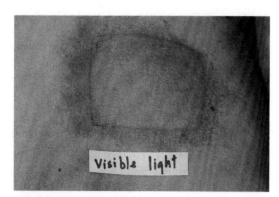

**Fig. 3.** Urticarial reaction at 20 minutes after phototesting with visible light.

development of SU. H1 antagonists that have been reported to effectively control this condition are hydroxyzine, astemizole, terfenadine, cetirizine, and fexofenadine.[32] However, astemizole and terfenadine have been withdrawn from the market because of the risk of cardiogenic toxicity. Cimetidine, an H2-receptor antagonist, and doxepin, an H1/H2-receptor antagonist, have also been reported to control this condition.[57,58]

**Cyclosporine** Cyclosporine was effectively used in one recalcitrant case of SU. At a dose of 4.5 mg/kg/d of cyclosporine, the patient tolerated 1 hour of sunlight compared with only a few minutes previously. However, the wheals recurred after the drug was discontinued.[59] Cyclosporine may be an option for patients who live in countries with short summer months.

**Methotrexate** Although the use of methotrexate for SU has not been reported, it is an established treatment for recalcitrant chronic urticaria.[60] Therefore, in resistant cases of SU it is reasonable to use methotrexate as another treatment option.

**Intravenous immunoglobulin** Intravenous immunoglobulin (IVIG) is a blood product containing polyvalent immunoglobulin G. Through its immunomodulatory effects, IVIG has demonstrated efficacy in the treatment of various types of recalcitrant urticaria, such as chronic, autoimmune, and delayed pressure, as well as SU.[61–65] A survey conducted of French photodermatology units reported that 5 of 7 patients with SU who were treated with IVIG obtained complete remission. The IVIG doses are in the range of 1.4 to 2.5 g/kg with infusion over 2 to 5 days. The number of courses varies from 1 to 3, with time between infusions typically 2 to 9 months. Remission was maintained for a duration from 4 months to more than a year.[66] IVIG is generally safe; however, it has been associated with an increased risk of viral infections and anaphylaxis.

**Omalizumab** Omalizumab is a recombinant humanized monoclonal anti-IgE antibody primarily indicated for the treatment of asthma. Recently there have been several reports of successful use of omalizumab for recalcitrant chronic urticaria, cold urticaria, cholinergic urticaria, and SU.[67–70] The dosage of omalizumab ranges from 150 mg every 2 weeks to 150 to 300 mg per month. Omalizumab may be an option for SU patients with elevated levels of IgE who fail other treatment modalities.

**α–Melanocyte stimulating hormone analogue** α–Melanocyte stimulating hormone (α-MSH) analogue, also known as afamelanotide, [NIe⁴-D-Phe⁷]-α-MSH, is a super-potent agonist of the melanocortin-1 receptor. Exogenous administration of this agent increases melanization via the melanogenesis pathway. A recent study published in the United Kingdom demonstrated potential benefits of α-MSH analogue for SU patients.[71] Five patients with SU received a single dose of 16 mg afamelanotide implant subcutaneously during the winter months. The investigators found that following day 7 after implantation the melanin index progressively increased, peaking at 15 days and persisting until 60 days. At 60 days postimplantation, the MUD was increased in comparison with baseline, along with significantly decreased whealing.[71] Afamelanotide is also currently under investigation for the treatment of erythropoietic protoporphyria. Although it may be a promising therapeutic option for SU in the future, the potential risk of dysplastic nevi and melanoma from this new agent, which has not been observed thus far, should also be taken into consideration.

### Procedural therapy

**Phototherapy and photochemotherapy** The concept of induction of a tolerant state or "hardening" by the causative wavelength may be used to treat various photosensitive diseases, including SU. Phototherapy for SU may involve either the traditional non–rush-hardening or newer rush-hardening protocols. The non–rush-hardening technique uses the action spectrum identified by phototesting to induce whealing of the skin, starting lower than the minimal whealing dose (MWD) and gradually increasing the dose. The frequency is 2 to 4 times per week. A drawback of this method is the very short period of remission.[72] Compared with phototherapy, photochemotherapy (PUVA) provides longer-lasting effects.[73]

The rush-hardening protocol is used for rapid tolerance to light. UVA rush hardening is performed by exposing the patient to half of the MWD of UVA to a quadrant and then to half of the body at increasing doses of UVA at 1-hour intervals over 2 to 3 days.[74,75] With this technique, the patient will gain a higher MWD within several days. Maintenance UVA irradiations are scheduled every 1 to 2 weeks. Remissions for at least 5 months to 1 year have been reported after treatment with the UVA rush-hardening protocol.[74,75] Finally, wavelengths outside the action spectra may induce tolerance. Recently, narrow-band UVB as an inhibition spectrum was successfully used in a patient with SU who had the action spectrum in the UVA and visible-light range.[76]

At the Phototherapy Unit at Henry Ford Hospital in Detroit, Michigan, a variation of rush hardening with UVA is commonly performed, with success.

The protocol involves exposing the patient to 50% of MWD of UVA, and increasing it by 10% to 20% as tolerated 3 times per week for a total of 30 treatments. Tapering then follows to 2 times weekly for 3 to 4 weeks, and then to once weekly as maintenance for the remaining duration of the summer months.

**Plasmapheresis** As the pathogenesis of SU likely implicates a photoallergen, removal via plasma exchange may be a therapeutic option. Ten recalcitrant SU patients have received this procedure to date.[77–83] Six of the patients responded well to the therapy; 4 had remission, 1 had relapse at 2 weeks, and the other had relapse at 2 months. Most patients who responded well to the treatment had a positive serum factor.

## Prognosis

SU is a chronic condition. Most patients require long-term antihistamines and/or combination treatments. Nevertheless, there have been reports of spontaneous remission over time. For solitary SU, the probability of clinical resolution is 15%, 24%, and 46% at 5, 10, and 15 years from onset, respectively.[33] Patients who are older than 40 years and with long duration of disease activity have a worse prognosis.[33]

## REFERENCES

1. Gupta G, Man I, Kemmett D. Hydroa vacciniforme: a clinical and follow-up study of 17 cases. J Am Acad Dermatol 2000;42(2 Pt 1):208–13.
2. Bennion SD, Johnson C, Weston WL. Hydroa vacciniforme with inflammatory keratitis and secondary anterior uveitis. Pediatr Dermatol 1987;4(4): 320–4.
3. Huggins RH, Leithauser LA, Eide MJ, et al. Quality of life assessment and disease experience of patient members of a web-based hydroa vacciniforme support group. Photodermatol Photoimmunol Photomed 2009;25(4):209–15.
4. De Pietro U, Simoni R, Barbieri C, et al. Hydroa vacciniforme persistent in a 60-year-old man. Eur J Dermatol 1999;9(4):311–2.
5. Wong SN, Tan SH, Khoo SW. Late-onset hydroa vacciniforme: two case reports. Br J Dermatol 2001;144(4):874–7.
6. Gupta G, Mohamed M, Kemmett D. Familial hydroa vacciniforme. Br J Dermatol 1999;140(1):124–6.
7. Halasz CL, Leach EE, Walther RR, et al. Hydroa vacciniforme: induction of lesions with ultraviolet A. J Am Acad Dermatol 1983;8(2):171–6.
8. Sonnex TS, Hawk JL. Hydroa vacciniforme: a review of ten cases. Br J Dermatol 1988;118(1): 101–8.
9. Sunohara A, Mizuno N, Sakai M, et al. Action spectrum for UV erythema and reproduction of the skin lesions in hydroa vacciniforme. Photodermatol 1988;5(3):139–45.
10. Wisuthsarewong W, Leenutaphong V, Viravan S. Hydroa vacciniform with ocular involvement. J Med Assoc Thai 1998;81(10):807–11.
11. Iwatsuki K, Ohtsuka M, Akiba H, et al. Atypical hydroa vacciniforme in childhood: from a smoldering stage to Epstein-Barr virus-associated lymphoid malignancy. J Am Acad Dermatol 1999;40(2 Pt 1): 283–4.
12. Iwatsuki K, Satoh M, Yamamoto T, et al. Pathogenic link between hydroa vacciniforme and Epstein-Barr virus-associated hematologic disorders. Arch Dermatol 2006;142(5):587–95.
13. Verneuil L, Gouarin S, Comoz F, et al. Epstein-Barr virus involvement in the pathogenesis of hydroa vacciniforme: an assessment of seven adult patients with long-term follow-up. Br J Dermatol 2010;163(1):174–82.
14. Au WY, Pang A, Choy C, et al. Quantification of circulating Epstein-Barr virus (EBV) DNA in the diagnosis and monitoring of natural killer cell and EBV-positive lymphomas in immunocompetent patients. Blood 2004;104(1):243–9.
15. Gotoh K, Ito Y, Shibata-Watanabe Y, et al. Clinical and virological characteristics of 15 patients with chronic active Epstein-Barr virus infection treated with hematopoietic stem cell transplantation. Clin Infect Dis 2008;46(10):1525–34.
16. Kimura H. Pathogenesis of chronic active Epstein-Barr virus infection: is this an infectious disease, lymphoproliferative disorder, or immunodeficiency? Rev Med Virol 2006;16(4):251–61.
17. Mendoza N, Diamantis M, Arora A, et al. Mucocutaneous manifestations of Epstein-Barr virus infection. Am J Clin Dermatol 2008;9(5):295–305.
18. Ohshima K, Kimura H, Yoshino T, et al. Proposed categorization of pathological states of EBV-associated T/natural killer-cell lymphoproliferative disorder (LPD) in children and young adults: overlap with chronic active EBV infection and infantile fulminant EBV T-LPD. Pathol Int 2008; 58(4):209–17.
19. Cho KH, Lee SH, Kim CW, et al. Epstein-Barr virus-associated lymphoproliferative lesions presenting as a hydroa vacciniforme-like eruption: an analysis of six cases. Br J Dermatol 2004;151(2):372–80.
20. Magana M, Sangueza P, Gil-Beristain J, et al. Angiocentric cutaneous T-cell lymphoma of childhood (hydroa-like lymphoma): a distinctive type of cutaneous T-cell lymphoma. J Am Acad Dermatol 1998;38(4):574–9.
21. Oono T, Arata J, Masuda T, et al. Coexistence of hydroa vacciniforme and malignant lymphoma. Arch Dermatol 1986;122(11):1306–9.

22. Quintanilla-Martinez L, Ridaura C, Nagl F, et al. Hydroa vacciniforme-like lymphoma: a chronic EBV+ lymphoproliferative disorder with risk to develop a systemic lymphoma. Blood 2013;122(18):3101–10.

23. Ruiz-Maldonado R, Parrilla FM, Orozco-Covarrubias ML, et al. Edematous, scarring vasculitic panniculitis: a new multisystemic disease with malignant potential. J Am Acad Dermatol 1995; 32(1):37–44.

24. Sangueza M, Plaza JA. Hydroa vacciniforme-like cutaneous T-cell lymphoma: clinicopathologic and immunohistochemical study of 12 cases. J Am Acad Dermatol 2013;69(1):112–9.

25. Trikha S, Turnbull A, Srikantha N, et al. Anterior keratouveitis secondary to hydroa vacciniforme: a role for ophthalmic slit-lamp examination in this condition? BMJ Case Rep 2011;2011.

26. Yamamoto T, Hirai Y, Miyake T, et al. Oculomucosal and gastrointestinal involvement in Epstein-Barr virus-associated hydroa vacciniforme. Eur J Dermatol 2012;22(3):380–3.

27. Lee HY, Baek JO, Lee JR, et al. Atypical hydroa vacciniforme-like Epstein-Barr virus associated T/NK-cell lymphoproliferative disorder. Am J Dermatopathol 2012;34(8):e119–24.

28. Barrionuevo C, Anderson VM, Zevallos-Giampietri E, et al. Hydroa-like cutaneous T-cell lymphoma: a clinicopathologic and molecular genetic study of 16 pediatric cases from Peru. Appl Immunohistochem Mol Morphol 2002;10(1):7–14.

29. Lysell J, Wiegleb Edstrom D, Linde A, et al. Antiviral therapy in children with hydroa vacciniforme. Acta Derm Venereol 2009;89(4):393–7.

30. Champion RH. Urticaria: then and now. Br J Dermatol 1988;119(4):427–36.

31. Chong WS, Khoo SW. Solar urticaria in Singapore: an uncommon photodermatosis seen in a tertiary dermatology center over a 10-year period. Photodermatol Photoimmunol Photomed 2004;20(2): 101–4.

32. Botto NC, Warshaw EM. Solar urticaria. J Am Acad Dermatol 2008;59(6):909–20 [quiz: 21–2].

33. Beattie PE, Dawe RS, Ibbotson SH, et al. Characteristics and prognosis of idiopathic solar urticaria: a cohort of 87 cases. Arch Dermatol 2003;139(9): 1149–54.

34. Kerr HA, Lim HW. Photodermatoses in African Americans: a retrospective analysis of 135 patients over a 7-year period. J Am Acad Dermatol 2007; 57(4):638–43.

35. Nakamura M, Henderson M, Jacobsen G, et al. Comparison of photodermatoses in African-Americans and Caucasians: a follow-up study. Photodermatol Photoimmunol Photomed 2013. [Epub ahead of print].

36. Horio T. Solar urticaria—idiopathic? Photodermatol Photoimmunol Photomed 2003;19(3):147–54.

37. Reinauer S, Leenutaphong V, Holzle E. Fixed solar urticaria. J Am Acad Dermatol 1993;29(2 Pt 1): 161–5.

38. Patel GK, Gould DJ, Hawk JL, et al. A complex photodermatosis: solar urticaria progressing to polymorphic light eruption. Clin Exp Dermatol 1998;23(2):77–8.

39. Schwarze HP, Marguery MC, Journe F, et al. Fixed solar urticaria to visible light successfully treated with fexofenadine. Photodermatol Photoimmunol Photomed 2001;17(1):39–41.

40. Tuchinda C, Leenutaphong V, Sudtim S, et al. Fixed solar urticaria induced by UVA and visible light: a report of a case. Photodermatol Photoimmunol Photomed 2005;21(2):97–9.

41. Wessendorf U, Hanneken S, Haust M, et al. Fixed solar urticaria with delayed onset. J Am Acad Dermatol 2009;60(4):695–7.

42. Beattie PE, Dawe RS, Ibbotson SH, et al. Co-existence of chronic actinic dermatitis and solar urticaria in three patients. Br J Dermatol 2004;151(2): 513–5.

43. Yu RC, King CM, Vickers CF. A case of actinic prurigo and solar urticaria. Clin Exp Dermatol 1990; 15(4):289–92.

44. Dawe RS, Clark C, Ferguson J. Porphyria cutanea tarda presenting as solar urticaria. Br J Dermatol 1999;141(3):590–1.

45. Kurumaji Y, Shono M. Drug-induced solar urticaria due to repirinast. Dermatology 1994;188(2): 117–21.

46. Yap LM, Foley PA, Crouch RB, et al. Drug-induced solar urticaria due to tetracycline. Australas J Dermatol 2000;41(3):181–4.

47. Morison WL. Solar urticaria due to progesterone compounds in oral contraceptives. Photodermatol Photoimmunol Photomed 2003;19(3):155–6.

48. Leenutaphong V, Holzle E, Plewig G. Pathogenesis and classification of solar urticaria: a new concept. J Am Acad Dermatol 1989;21(2 Pt 1):237–40.

49. Mekkes JR, de Vries HJ, Kammeyer A. Solar urticaria induced by infrared radiation. Clin Exp Dermatol 2003;28(2):222–3.

50. Du-Thanh A, Debu A, Lalheve P, et al. Solar urticaria: a time-extended retrospective series of 61 patients and review of literature. Eur J Dermatol 2013;23(2):202–7.

51. Hasei K, Ichihashi M. Solar urticaria. Determinations of action and inhibition spectra. Arch Dermatol 1982;118(5):346–50.

52. Uetsu N, Miyauchi-Hashimoto H, Okamoto H, et al. The clinical and photobiological characteristics of solar urticaria in 40 patients. Br J Dermatol 2000; 142(1):32–8.

53. Watanabe M, Matsunaga Y, Katayama I. Solar urticaria: a consideration of the mechanism of inhibition spectra. Dermatology 1999;198(3):252–5.

54. Fukunaga A, Horikawa T, Yamamoto A, et al. The inhibition spectrum of solar urticaria suppresses the wheal-flare response following intradermal injection with photo-activated autologous serum but not with compound 48/80. Photodermatol Photoimmunol Photomed 2006;22(3):129–32.

55. Horio T, Fujigaki K. Augmentation spectrum in solar urticaria. J Am Acad Dermatol 1988;18(5 Pt 2):1189–93.

56. Danno K, Mori N. Solar urticaria: report of two cases with augmentation spectrum. Photodermatol Photoimmunol Photomed 2000;16(1):30–3.

57. Neittaanmaki H, Jaaskelainen T, Harvima RJ, et al. Solar urticaria: demonstration of histamine release and effective treatment with doxepin. Photodermatol 1989;6(1):52–5.

58. Tokura Y, Takigawa M, Yamauchi T, et al. Solar urticaria: a case with good therapeutic response to cimetidine. Dermatologica 1986;173(5):224–8.

59. Edstrom DW, Ros AM. Cyclosporin A therapy for severe solar urticaria. Photodermatol Photoimmunol Photomed 1997;13(1–2):61–3.

60. Perez A, Woods A, Grattan CE. Methotrexate: a useful steroid-sparing agent in recalcitrant chronic urticaria. Br J Dermatol 2010;162(1):191–4.

61. Mitzel-Kaoukhov H, Staubach P, Muller-Brenne T. Effect of high-dose intravenous immunoglobulin treatment in therapy-resistant chronic spontaneous urticaria. Ann Allergy Asthma Immunol 2010;104(3):253–8.

62. Hughes R, Cusack C, Murphy GM, et al. Solar urticaria successfully treated with intravenous immunoglobulin. Clin Exp Dermatol 2009;34(8):e660–2.

63. Correia I, Silva J, Filipe P, et al. Solar urticaria treated successfully with intravenous high-dose immunoglobulin: a case report. Photodermatol Photoimmunol Photomed 2008;24(6):330–1.

64. Klote MM, Nelson MR, Engler RJ. Autoimmune urticaria response to high-dose intravenous immunoglobulin. Ann Allergy Asthma Immunol 2005;94(2):307–8.

65. Dawn G, Urcelay M, Ah-Weng A, et al. Effect of high-dose intravenous immunoglobulin in delayed pressure urticaria. Br J Dermatol 2003;149(4):836–40.

66. Adamski H, Bedane C, Bonnevalle A, et al. Solar urticaria treated with intravenous immunoglobulins. J Am Acad Dermatol 2011;65(2):336–40.

67. Waibel KH, Reese DA, Hamilton RG, et al. Partial improvement of solar urticaria after omalizumab. J Allergy Clin Immunol 2010;125(2):490–1.

68. Guzelbey O, Ardelean E, Magerl M, et al. Successful treatment of solar urticaria with anti-immunoglobulin E therapy. Allergy 2008;63(11):1563–5.

69. Fromer L. Treatment options for the relief of chronic idiopathic urticaria symptoms. South Med J 2008;101(2):186–92.

70. Metz M, Altrichter S, Ardelean E, et al. Anti-immunoglobulin E treatment of patients with recalcitrant physical urticaria. Int Arch Allergy Immunol 2011;154(2):177–80.

71. Haylett AK, Nie Z, Brownrigg M, et al. Systemic photoprotection in solar urticaria with alpha-melanocyte-stimulating hormone analogue [Nle4-D-Phe7]-alpha-MSH. Br J Dermatol 2011;164(2):407–14.

72. Roelandts R. Diagnosis and treatment of solar urticaria. Dermatol Ther 2003;16(1):52–6.

73. Roelandts R. Pre-PUVA UVA desensitization for solar urticaria. Photodermatol 1985;2(3):174–6.

74. Masuoka E, Fukunaga A, Kishigami K, et al. Successful and long-lasting treatment of solar urticaria with ultraviolet A rush hardening therapy. Br J Dermatol 2012;167(1):198–201.

75. Beissert S, Stander H, Schwarz T. UVA rush hardening for the treatment of solar urticaria. J Am Acad Dermatol 2000;42(6):1030–2.

76. Wolf R, Herzinger T, Grahovac M, et al. Solar urticaria: long-term rush hardening by inhibition spectrum narrow-band UVB 311 nm. Clin Exp Dermatol 2013;38(4):446–7.

77. Duschet P, Leyen P, Schwarz T, et al. Solar urticaria—effective treatment by plasmapheresis. Clin Exp Dermatol 1987;12(3):185–8.

78. Duschet P, Schwarz T, Gschnait F. Plasmapheresis in light urticaria. A rational therapy concept in cases with a proven serum factor. Hautarzt 1989;40(9):553–5 [in German].

79. Leenutaphong V, Holzle E, Plewig G, et al. Plasmapheresis in solar urticaria. Dermatologica 1991;182(1):35–8.

80. Hudson-Peacock MJ, Farr PM, Diffey BL, et al. Combined treatment of solar urticaria with plasmapheresis and PUVA. Br J Dermatol 1993;128(4):440–2.

81. Collins P, Ahamat R, Green C, et al. Plasma exchange therapy for solar urticaria. Br J Dermatol 1996;134(6):1093–7.

82. Bissonnette R, Buskard N, McLean DI, et al. Treatment of refractory solar urticaria with plasma exchange. J Cutan Med Surg 1999;3(5):236–8.

83. Insawang M, Wongpraparut C. Recalcitrant solar urticaria induced by UVA and visible light: a case report. J Med Assoc Thai 2010;93(10):1238–41.

# Chronic Actinic Dermatitis

So Yeon Paek, MD*, Henry W. Lim, MD

## KEYWORDS

- Chronic actinic dermatitis • Actinic reticuloid • Photosensitive eczema • Photosensitivity dermatitis
- Persistent light reaction • Photodermatosis

## KEY POINTS

- Chronic actinic dermatitis (CAD) is an immunologically mediated photodermatosis characterized by pruritic eczematous lesions of sun-exposed areas.
- Evaluation should include histologic examination, phototesting, and laboratory workup, including human immunodeficiency virus (HIV) test and Sezary count.
- The most common action spectrum is ultraviolet B (UVB) plus ultraviolet A (UVA), although CAD may also be seen with UVB or UVA alone, or with a combination of UVB, UVA, and visible light.
- Management begins with strict photoprotection, topical corticosteroids, and topical calcineurin inhibitors. Other treatments with noted efficacy include oral prednisone, cyclosporine, azathioprine, and mycophenolate mofetil.
- Proper diagnosis and management are essential, as CAD can have a moderate to large impact on quality of life.

## HISTORY

Chronic actinic dermatitis (CAD), previously known as actinic reticuloid, photosensitivity dermatitis, photosensitive eczema, and persistent light reaction, is an immunologically mediated photodermatosis characterized by pruritic eczematous lesions of areas exposed to the sun.[1–5] Haxthausen[6] first described this condition in 1933 in a patient with hypersensitivity to light after intravenous trypaflavine, a photosensitizing dye. Actinic reticuloid and two milder forms of CAD, referred to as photosensitive eczema and photosensitivity dermatitis, were reported in 1969.[7,8] By 1979, Hawk and Magnus[9] had introduced the term "chronic actinic dermatitis," but it was not until 1990, when Lim and colleagues[10] suggested unifying the variants under the same name, that the term became widely accepted.[11]

## EPIDEMIOLOGY

CAD has been reported in the United States, Europe, Asia, and Africa, with increased incidence in the summertime when sun exposure is greatest.[12–16] It commonly affects men older than 50 years who work or enjoy the outdoors. This condition can affect individuals of all skin types, although in the United States it is more commonly reported in persons with Fitzpatrick skin types V and VI.[17–20] In patients seen in the United Kingdom, but not those examined in the United States or Japan, CAD can be associated with contact allergy or photocontact allergy to *Compositae* oleoresins, a group of airborne plant allergens, presumably caused by exposure through gardening.[21–24] There is no familial inheritance. Association with human immunodeficiency virus (HIV) infection has been reported; as a group,

Disclosure Statement: No conflicts of interest.
Department of Dermatology, Henry Ford Hospital, 3031 West Grand Boulevard, Suite 800, Detroit, MI 48202, USA
* Corresponding author.
E-mail address: soyeon.paek@aya.yale.edu

Dermatol Clin 32 (2014) 355–361
http://dx.doi.org/10.1016/j.det.2014.03.007

these patients tend to be younger than CAD patients without HIV infection.[25]

## PATHOGENESIS

The pathogenesis of CAD has not been completely elucidated. The clinical and histologic features, the presence of mostly CD8[+] T cells in the dermis, and the pattern of adhesion molecule activation in CAD resemble allergic contact dermatitis.[26] Thus, a mechanism of delayed-type hypersensitivity can be inferred. However, rather than an exogenous agent, the cutaneous antigen is likely endogenous and photoinduced. Though not proven, it is possible that a pathophysiology similar to that described in polymorphous light eruption (PMLE) also occurs in CAD.[27] In normal healthy individuals, exposure to sunlight results in localized immunosuppression; therefore, there are no obvious clinical lesions even in the presence of photoinduced neoantigens in the skin. However, similarly to PMLE, it is possible that patients with CAD are less likely to be photoimmunosuppressed, resulting in a brisk response to the presence of ultraviolet (UV)-induced neoantigens in the skin, which manifest as cutaneous lesions. The antigenic molecule in CAD has been theorized to be DNA, which absorbs UV radiation and is the molecule thought to be involved in sunburn.[27,28] The action spectrum for CAD is similar to that for sunburn, but at lower doses.[29]

## DIAGNOSIS
### Clinical Manifestations

Skin findings of CAD include eczematous and often lichenified pruritic patches and confluent plaques limited to sun-exposed areas of the scalp, face, neck, chest, arms, hands, and back, with notable sparing of sun-protected areas, such as nasolabial folds, submental chin, upper eyelids, retroauricular areas, skin creases, and finger web spaces (**Fig. 1**). Acute flares are associated with erythematous patches and papules with fine scale on sun-exposed areas (**Fig. 2**). In severe cases, papules and plaques may occur on sun-protected sites, albeit to a lesser extent than on sun-exposed areas; rarely, erythroderma and hyperkeratosis of palms and soles may be observed (**Fig. 3**).[30]

### Differential Diagnoses

Conditions that may mimic CAD include drug eruption, allergic or photoallergic contact dermatitis, cutaneous T-cell lymphoma (CTCL),[31] and connective tissue diseases (such as acute or subacute cutaneous lupus erythematosus). Careful history taking, examination of morphology and distribution of lesions, and appropriate photobiological and laboratory investigations are essential in arriving at the correct diagnosis (**Table 1**).[32]

### Histology

Pathologic examination of CAD demonstrates spongiotic dermatitis with lymphohistiocytic infiltrate and variable acanthosis. Atypical lymphocytes and exocytosis seen in some specimens may mimic histologic changes of CTCL. Papillary dermal fibrosis and a brisk infiltrate, both histologic signs of chronicity, may also be found. In severe cases the biopsy may show focal epidermal necrosis, papillary dermal collagen, fibrin deposition in the dermal-epidermal junction, and erosions.

### Photobiological Evaluation

Phototesting is recommended for further evaluation of suspected CAD. If a monochromator or

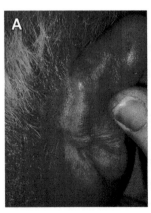
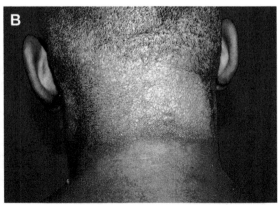

**Fig. 1.** Clinical features of chronic actinic dermatitis (CAD). (*A*) Erythema, lichenification, and scale on sun-exposed skin. Note sparing of postauricular area. (*B*) Lichenification of sun-exposed sites, with sharp cutoff of sun-protected areas of the skin.

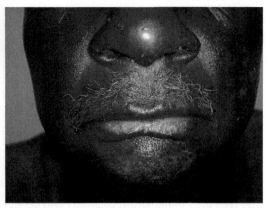

**Fig. 2.** Acute flare 24 hours after inadvertent sun exposure in a patient with CAD. Note diffuse erythema on the face and superficial erosions on the nose.

solar simulator is unavailable, testing with ultraviolet A (UVA; 320–400 nm) or ultraviolet B (UVB; 290–320 nm) therapy units and a slide projector (to test visible light) may be considered.[33] The most common action spectrum for CAD is UVB plus UVA, resulting in a decreased minimal erythema dose (MED) for both UVB and UVA in most patients.[29,34] However, CAD may be seen with decreased MED-B or MED-A alone (12%–25%), or with a combination of sensitivity to UVB, UVA, and visible light. A study conducted by Eadie and colleagues[35] also found that compact fluorescent lamps (CFLs),

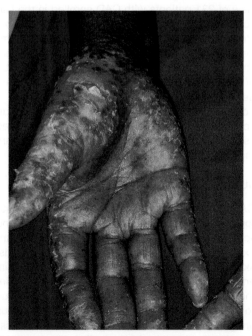

**Fig. 3.** Hyperkeratosis and scale on palms of a patient with CAD.

which are set to replace common incandescent lamps in Europe, may be a potential harmful source of UV radiation with prolonged exposure in patients with photosensitive conditions. These lamps contain mercury, which activates the phosphor-coated walls, emitting UV radiation in the UVB and UVA range. Patch testing and photo-patch testing may also be considered if warranted by the history of the patient. Patients with CAD in the United Kingdom often demonstrate positive patch testing to relevant *Compositae*, presumably resulting from exposure from gardening.

## Laboratory Evaluation

Lupus serologies, such as antinuclear antibody (ANA) and anti-Ro/anti-La antibodies, may be obtained and should be negative. Sezary-like cells may be seen in erythrodermic CAD, but the CD4:CD8 ratio will be low and T-cell clonality will be absent.[36] In addition, testing for HIV is recommended, especially in younger patients, in whom CAD may be a presenting sign of HIV.[25]

## MANAGEMENT

Strict photoprotection is key in the management of CAD.[37] Patients should be advised to wear broad-spectrum (UVA and UVB) sunscreen with a minimum sun-protection factor of 30, long-sleeved clothing, and wide-brimmed hats, and to seek shade during peak hours (between 10 AM and 4 PM). Clear museum films or UVA filters may be applied to windows to block most UV transmission.[38] It should be noted that there is no evidence that television and computer screens might exacerbate this condition.

In addition to photoprotection, patients may use topical corticosteroids or topical calcineurin inhibitors as first-line therapy. Mid-potency to high-potency topical corticosteroids are effective for the control of disease flare. However, the potential risks of skin atrophy, striae, and dyspigmentation preclude their long-term use. Many case reports and case series support the therapeutic benefit of topical tacrolimus 0.1% ointment, daily to twice daily, for CAD.[39–46] Tacrolimus (Protopic) binds to FK506-binding protein, blocking dephosphorylation of nuclear factor of activated T cells, and preventing transcription of interleukin-2 and other inflammatory cytokines. In CAD, this seems to work by inhibiting T-lymphocyte activation by suppressing Langerhans cells.[47] Similar results have been achieved with topical pimecrolimus (Elidel) cream for CAD.[48] Patients must be informed of the black-box warning for increased risk of cutaneous malignancy and lymphoma with topical

**Table 1**
**Evaluation of chronic actinic dermatitis**

| | Test | Results in CAD | Comments |
|---|---|---|---|
| Histology | Punch biopsy | Epidermal spongiosis with moderately dense superficial and deep lymphocytic infiltrate | May be confused with CTCL. Immunohistochemistry and T-cell rearrangement warranted |
| Phototesting | UVA (320–400 nm) UVB (290–320 nm) Visible light (400–700 nm) | Decreased MED Decreased MED May show decreased MED | Most common action spectrum for CAD is UVB + UVA. May also be seen with UVA or UVB alone, or with a combination of UVB + UVA + visible light |
| Laboratory | Lupus serologies Peripheral smear | ANA, anti-Ro/-La negative Sezary-like cells may be seen in erythrodermic CAD, but CD4:CD8 ratio will be low and T-cell clonality will be absent | Rule out other CTD Immunohistochemistry and gene rearrangement analysis can be conducted to further differentiate CTCL from CAD |
| | HIV | Negative | CAD may be a presenting sign of HIV in younger patients. Testing recommended in high risk patients |

*Abbreviations:* ANA, antinuclear antibody; CAD, chronic actinic dermatitis; CTCL, cutaneous T-cell lymphoma; CTD, connective tissue diseases; HIV, human immunodeficiency virus; MED, minimal erythema dose; UVA, ultraviolet A; UVB, ultraviolet B.

tacrolimus and pimecrolimus, although convincing evidence is lacking.

Systemic immunosuppressive therapy is frequently used for widespread or refractory disease. Oral corticosteroids (prednisone 0.5–1.0 mg/kg/d) can be given for several weeks at a time for flares. Chronic steroid use is not recommended because of its adverse side-effect profile, including, but not limited to, weight gain, high blood sugar, increased risk for infections, osteoporosis, and fractures, adrenal gland suppression, delayed wound healing, glaucoma or cataracts, and steroid psychosis. Other steroid-sparing agents with proven efficacy in the treatment of CAD include: cyclosporine (3.5–5 mg/kg/d),[49,50] azathioprine (1.0–2.5 mg/kg/d),[51,52] and mycophenolate mofetil (25–40 mg/kg/d or 1–2 g/d).[53] Patients should be counseled on the increased risk of infection with these medications. Additional potential side effects are noted in **Table 1**. Only single case reports exist to support the treatment of refractory CAD with low-dose thalidomide[54] and interferon-α.[55]

## PROGNOSIS

Spontaneous resolution of chronic actinic dermatitis has been reported to be 10% over 5 years, 20% over 10 years, and 50% over 15 years.[33] These findings were established from a historical cohort study of CAD patients in a Scottish tertiary referral center, and may underestimate the actual probability of remission. Patients may be counseled that their photosensitivity may eventually subside with photoprotection and avoidance of allergens.[56] In addition, a few case reports have suggested the possibility of malignant transformation of pseudolymphomatous CAD or association with other malignancies.[57–60] However, a chart review of 231 patients with CAD enrolled in the National Cancer Registry of the United Kingdom identified no significant increased risk of lymphoma and nonlymphoma cancers in a 20-year study period.[61] In addition, DNA flow cytometry of affected skin from patients with CAD did not demonstrate DNA aneuploidy.[62] Therefore, it does not appear that CAD is a premalignant condition, but patients should be aware of the increased risk of malignancy with immunosuppressant therapy.[63,64]

## SUMMARY

CAD is an immunologically mediated photodermatosis characterized by pruritic eczematous and lichenified plaques sharply demarcated to sun-exposed areas with notable sparing of eyelids, skin folds, submental chin, postauricular skin, and finger web spaces. It mostly affects men older than 50 years. The condition is thought to be due to secondary photosensitization of an endogenous antigen in the skin, resulting from either cross-reactivity with other contact allergens or photocontact allergens, or the lack of localized

**Table 2**
**Management of chronic actinic dermatitis**

| Therapy | Dosage | Comments |
| --- | --- | --- |
| Strict photoprotection | — | Long-sleeved clothing, wide-brimmed hats, sun avoidance during peak daylight hours (10 AM to 4 PM), UV filters or museum film for windows |
| Broad-spectrum (UVA/UVB-block) sunscreen | Minimum SPF 30 | ± inorganic filters |
| Topical tacrolimus (Protopic) ointment | 0.1% daily to BID | Black-box warning: increased risk of cutaneous malignancy and lymphoma |
| Prednisone | 0.5–1.0 mg/kg/d | For acute flares only<br>Potential side effects: weight gain, high blood sugar, high blood pressure, increased risk of infections, osteoporosis, and fractures, adrenal gland suppression, delayed wound healing, glaucoma or cataracts, steroid psychosis |
| Cyclosporine | 3.5–5 mg/kg/d | Side effects: gingival hyperplasia, hypertrichosis, headache, nausea, malaise, gout, hyperkalemia, hypomagnesemia, hypertension, nephrotoxicity, malignancy |
| Azathioprine | 1.0–2.5 mg/kg/d | Side effects: myelosuppression, hypersensitivity syndrome, GI symptoms, infection, lymphoproliferative malignancy |
| Mycophenolate mofetil (CellCept) | 25–40 mg/kg/d (1–2 g/d) | Side effects: GI upset, teratogenic, carcinogenic, neurologic symptoms (headache, tinnitus, weakness), increased risk of herpes zoster, risk of hepatotoxicity |

*Abbreviations:* BID, twice daily; CAD, chronic actinic dermatitis; GI, gastrointestinal; SPF, sun-protection factor; UV, ultraviolet; UVA, ultraviolet-A; UVB, ultraviolet-B.

photoimmunosuppression in such patients. Histology shows epidermal spongiosis with moderately dense superficial and deep lymphocytic infiltrate, which may be confused with CTCL. The most common action spectrum for CAD seen with phototesting is UVB plus UVA. As appropriate, patch testing and photopatch testing should also be performed. Laboratory workup should be aimed at excluding other potential diagnoses, such as CTCL and acute or subacute cutaneous lupus erythematosus. CAD may be a presenting sign of HIV in young patients with risk factors. **Table 2** outlines the therapeutic management of patients with CAD. Spontaneous resolution has been reported to be 10% over 5 years, 20% over 10 years, and 50% over 15 years. Therefore, patients should be counseled that their photosensitivity may eventually subside with avoidance of allergens and photoprotection. In addition, CAD does not appear to be a premalignant condition, but clinicians should provide counseling on the increased risk of malignancy with immunosuppressant therapy. Finally, CAD can have a moderate to large impact on quality of life, so proper diagnosis and management is essential.[65]

## REFERENCES

1. Hawk JL. Chronic actinic dermatitis. Photodermatol Photoimmunol Photomed 2004;20(6):312–4.
2. Gambichler T, Al-Muhammadi R, Boms S. Immunologically mediated photodermatoses: diagnosis and treatment. Am J Clin Dermatol 2009;10(3): 169–80.

3. Frain-Bell W, Lakshmipathi T, Rogers J, et al. The syndrome of chronic photosensitivity dermatitis and actinic reticuloid. Br J Dermatol 1974;91(6):617–34.

4. Ramsay CA, Black AK. Photosensitive eczema. Trans St Johns Hosp Dermatol Soc 1973;59(2):152–8.

5. Forsyth EL, Millard TP. Diagnosis and pharmacological treatment of chronic actinic dermatitis in the elderly: an update. Drugs Aging 2010;27(6):451–6.

6. Haxthausen H. Persistent hypersensitivity to light after intravenous injections of trypaflavine. Br J Dermatol 1933;45(1):16–8.

7. Ive FA, Magnus IA, Warin RP, et al. "Actinic reticuloid"; a chronic dermatosis associated with severe photosensitivity and the histological resemblance to lymphoma. Br J Dermatol 1969;81(7):469–85.

8. Epstein SS, Taylor FB. Photosensitizing compounds in extracts of drinking water. Science 1966;154(3746):261–3.

9. Hawk JL, Magnus IA. Chronic actinic dermatitis—an idiopathic photosensitivity syndrome including actinic reticuloid and photosensitive eczema [proceedings]. Br J Dermatol 1979;101(Suppl 17):24.

10. Lim HW, Buchness MR, Ashinoff R, et al. Chronic actinic dermatitis. Study of the spectrum of chronic photosensitivity in 12 patients. Arch Dermatol 1990;126(3):317–23.

11. Norris PG, Hawk JL. Chronic actinic dermatitis. A unifying concept. Arch Dermatol 1990;126(3):376–8.

12. Wong SN, Khoo LS. Analysis of photodermatoses seen in a predominantly Asian population at a photodermatology clinic in Singapore. Photodermatol Photoimmunol Photomed 2005;21(1):40–4.

13. Tan AW, Lim KS, Theng C, et al. Chronic actinic dermatitis in Asian skin: a Singaporean experience. Photodermatol Photoimmunol Photomed 2011;27(4):172–5.

14. Kyu-Won C, Chae-Young L, Yeong-Kyu L, et al. A Korean experience with chronic actinic dermatitis during an 18-year period: meteorological and photoimmunological aspects. Photodermatol Photoimmunol Photomed 2009;25(6):286–92.

15. Deng D, Hang Y, Chen H, et al. Prevalence of photodermatosis in four regions at different altitudes in Yunnan province, China. J Dermatol 2006;33(8):537–40.

16. Stratigos AJ, Antoniou C, Papathanakou E, et al. Spectrum of idiopathic photodermatoses in a Mediterranean country. Int J Dermatol 2003;42(6):449–54.

17. Que SK, Brauer JA, Soter NA, et al. Chronic actinic dermatitis: an analysis at a single institution over 25 years. Dermatitis 2011;22(3):147–54.

18. Lim HW, Morison WL, Kamide R, et al. Chronic actinic dermatitis. An analysis of 51 patients evaluated in the United States and Japan. Arch Dermatol 1994;130(10):1284–9.

19. Beach RA, Pratt MD. Chronic actinic dermatitis: clinical cases, diagnostic workup, and therapeutic management. J Cutan Med Surg 2009;13(3):121–8.

20. Kerr HA, Lim HW. Photodermatoses in African Americans: a retrospective analysis of 135 patients over a 7-year period. J Am Acad Dermatol 2007;57(4):638–43.

21. Lim HW, Cohen D, Soter NA. Chronic actinic dermatitis: results of patch and photopatch tests with Compositae, fragrances, and pesticides. J Am Acad Dermatol 1998;38(1):108–11.

22. Russell SC, Dawe RS, Collins P, et al. The photosensitivity dermatitis and actinic reticuloid syndrome (chronic actinic dermatitis) occurring in seven young atopic dermatitis patients. Br J Dermatol 1998;138(3):496–501.

23. Yones SS, Palmer RA, Hextall JM, et al. Exacerbation of presumed chronic actinic dermatitis by cockpit visible light in an airline pilot with atopic eczema. Photodermatol Photoimmunol Photomed 2005;21(3):152–3.

24. Creamer D, McGregor JM, Hawk JL. Chronic actinic dermatitis occurring in young patients with atopic dermatitis. Br J Dermatol 1998;139(6):1112–3.

25. Meola T, Sanchez M, Lim HW, et al. Chronic actinic dermatitis associated with human immunodeficiency virus infection. Br J Dermatol 1997;137(3):431–6.

26. Menage Hdu P, Sattar NK, Haskard DO, et al. A study of the kinetics and pattern of E-selectin, VCAM-1 and ICAM-1 expression in chronic actinic dermatitis. Br J Dermatol 1996;134(2):262–8.

27. van de Pas CB, Kelly DA, Seed PT, et al. Ultraviolet-radiation-induced erythema and suppression of contact hypersensitivity responses in patients with polymorphic light eruption. J Invest Dermatol 2004;122(2):295–9.

28. Freeman SE, Hacham H, Gange RW, et al. Wavelength dependence of pyrimidine dimer formation in DNA of human skin irradiated in situ with ultraviolet light. Proc Natl Acad Sci U S A 1989;86(14):5605–9.

29. Menage HD, Harrison GI, Potten CS, et al. The action spectrum for induction of chronic actinic dermatitis is similar to that for sunburn inflammation. Photochem Photobiol 1995;62(6):976–9.

30. Somani VK. Chronic actinic dermatitis—a study of clinical features. Indian J Dermatol Venereol Leprol 2005;71(6):409–13.

31. Heller P, Wieczorek R, Waldo E, et al. Chronic actinic dermatitis. An immunohistochemical study of its T-cell antigenic profile, with comparison to cutaneous T-cell lymphoma. Am J Dermatopathol 1994;16(5):510–6.

32. Pacheco D, Fraga A, Travassos AR, et al. Actinic reticuloid imitating Sezary syndrome. Acta Dermatovenerol Alp Panonica Adriat 2012;21(3):55–7.

33. Dawe RS, Crombie IK, Ferguson J. The natural history of chronic actinic dermatitis. Arch Dermatol 2000;136(10):1215–20.

34. Yap LM, Foley P, Crouch R, et al. Chronic actinic dermatitis: a retrospective analysis of 44 cases referred to an Australian photobiology clinic. Australas J Dermatol 2003;44(4):256–62.

35. Eadie E, Ferguson J, Moseley H. A preliminary investigation into the effect of exposure of photosensitive individuals to light from compact fluorescent lamps. Br J Dermatol 2009;160(3):659–64.

36. Bakels V, van Oostveen JW, Preesman AH, et al. Differentiation between actinic reticuloid and cutaneous T cell lymphoma by T cell receptor gamma gene rearrangement analysis and immunophenotyping. J Clin Pathol 1998;51(2):154–8.

37. Ferguson J. Diagnosis and treatment of the common idiopathic photodermatoses. Australas J Dermatol 2003;44(2):90–6.

38. Dawe R, Russell S, Ferguson J. Borrowing from museums and industry: two photoprotective devices. Br J Dermatol 1996;135(6):1016–7.

39. Uetsu N, Okamoto H, Fujii K, et al. Treatment of chronic actinic dermatitis with tacrolimus ointment. J Am Acad Dermatol 2002;47(6):881–4.

40. Grone D, Kunz M, Zimmermann R, et al. Successful treatment of nodular actinic reticuloid with tacrolimus ointment. Dermatology 2006;212(4):377–80.

41. Baldo A, Prizio E, Mansueto G, et al. A case of chronic actinic dermatitis treated with topical tacrolimus. J Dermatolog Treat 2005;16(4):245–8.

42. Schuster C, Zepter K, Kempf W, et al. Successful treatment of recalcitrant chronic actinic dermatitis with tacrolimus. Dermatology 2004;209(4):325–8.

43. Evans AV, Palmer RA, Hawk JL. Erythrodermic chronic actinic dermatitis responding only to topical tacrolimus. Photodermatol Photoimmunol Photomed 2004;20(1):59–61.

44. Suga Y, Hashimoto Y, Matsuba S, et al. Topical tacrolimus for chronic actinic dermatitis. J Am Acad Dermatol 2002;46(2):321–3.

45. Ogawa Y, Adachi A, Tomita Y. The successful use of topical tacrolimus treatment for a chronic actinic dermatitis patient with complications of idiopathic leukopenia. J Dermatol 2003;30(11):805–9.

46. Busaracome P, Wattanakrai P, Rajatanavin N. Chronic actinic dermatitis with leonine facies and iatrogenic adrenal insufficiency successfully treated with topical tacrolimus. Case Rep Dermatol 2011;3(1):49–54.

47. Ma Y, Lu Z. Treatment with topical tacrolimus favors chronic actinic dermatitis: a clinical and immunopathological study. J Dermatolog Treat 2010; 21(3):171–7.

48. Larangeira de Almeida H Jr. Successful treatment of chronic actinic dermatitis with topical pimecrolimus. Int J Dermatol 2005;44(4):343–4.

49. Norris PG, Camp RD, Hawk JL. Actinic reticuloid: response to cyclosporine. J Am Acad Dermatol 1989;21(2 Pt 1):307–9.

50. Gardeazabal J, Arregui MA, Gil N, et al. Successful treatment of musk ketone-induced chronic actinic dermatitis with cyclosporine and PUVA. J Am Acad Dermatol 1992;27(5 Pt 2):838–42.

51. Murphy GM, Maurice PD, Norris PG, et al. Azathioprine treatment in chronic actinic dermatitis: a double-blind controlled trial with monitoring of exposure to ultraviolet radiation. Br J Dermatol 1989;121(5):639–46.

52. Leigh IM, Hawk JL. Treatment of chronic actinic dermatitis with azathioprine. Br J Dermatol 1984; 110(6):691–5.

53. Thomson MA, Stewart DG, Lewis HM. Chronic actinic dermatitis treated with mycophenolate mofetil. Br J Dermatol 2005;152(4):784–6.

54. Safa G, Pieto-Le Corvaisier C, Hervagault B. Recalcitrant chronic actinic dermatitis treated with low-dose thalidomide. J Am Acad Dermatol 2005; 52(5):E6.

55. Parodi A, Gallo R, Guarrera M, et al. Natural alpha interferon in chronic actinic dermatitis. Report of a case. Acta Derm Venereol 1995;75(1):80.

56. Rose RF, Goulden V, Wilkinson SM. The spontaneous resolution of photosensitivity and contact allergy in a patient with chronic actinic dermatitis. Photodermatol Photoimmunol Photomed 2009; 25(2):114–6.

57. Sugita K, Shimauchi T, Tokura Y. Chronic actinic dermatitis associated with adult T-cell leukemia. J Am Acad Dermatol 2005;52(2 Suppl 1):38–40.

58. Thomsen K. The development of Hodgkin's disease in a patient with actinic reticuloid. Clin Exp Dermatol 1977;2(2):109–13.

59. De Silva BD, McLaren K, Kavanagh GM. Photosensitive mycosis fungoides or actinic reticuloid? Br J Dermatol 2000;142(6):1221–7.

60. Adachi Y, Horio T. Chronic actinic dermatitis in a patient with adult T-cell leukemia. Photodermatol Photoimmunol Photomed 2008;24(3):147–9.

61. Bilsland D, Crombie IK, Ferguson J. The photosensitivity dermatitis and actinic reticuloid syndrome: no association with lymphoreticular malignancy. Br J Dermatol 1994;131(2):209–14.

62. Norris PG, Newton JA, Camplejohn RS, et al. A flow cytometric study of actinic reticuloid. Clin Exp Dermatol 1989;14(2):128–31.

63. Ashinoff R, Buchness MR, Lim HW. Lymphoma in a black patient with actinic reticuloid treated with PUVA: possible etiologic considerations. J Am Acad Dermatol 1989;21(5 Pt 2):1134–7.

64. Thestrup-Pedersen K, Zachariae C, Kaltoft K, et al. Development of cutaneous pseudolymphoma following ciclosporin therapy of actinic reticuloid. Dermatologica 1988;177(6):376–81.

65. Jong CT, Finlay AY, Pearse AD, et al. The quality of life of 790 patients with photodermatoses. Br J Dermatol 2008;159(1):192–7.

# Drug-Induced Photosensitivity

Robert S. Dawe, MBChB, MD, FRCPE*, Sally H. Ibbotson, MBChB, MD, FRCPE

## KEYWORDS

• Drug • Xenobiotic • Photosensitivity • Phototoxicity • Photoallergy

## KEY POINTS

- Drug-induced photosensitivity is common.
- The principal mechanism of systemic drug photosensitivity is phototoxicity and the principal mechanism of topical drug photosensitivity is photoallergy.
- Photopatch testing is helpful to determine suspected topical agent photoallergies (eg, from ultraviolet filters in sunscreens) but generally not helpful in detecting systemic drug photosensitivity.
- Drug-induced photosensitivity is usually best managed by stopping the suspected drug.
- Other measures, including phototherapy using wavelengths that do not elicit the response, are sometimes necessary.

## INTRODUCTION

Drug-induced photosensitivity usually occurs through the mechanisms of phototoxicity and photoallergy.[1] Phototoxicity is non–immunologically mediated, whereas photoallergy requires immune sensitization. Most systemic drug photosensitivity is through a phototoxic mechanism, whereas photoallergy is more relevant to topical agent photosensitivity (such as from ultraviolet filters in sunscreens). Topical drugs, such as topically applied psoralens (whether therapeutically applied or from exposure to psoralen-containing plants), can also cause photosensitivity through a phototoxic mechanism.

Drug-induced photosensitivity can cause severe problems; therefore, diagnosis and management are important. Certain drugs that cause phototoxicity can also cause photocarcinogenesis[2–4]; this is best illustrated with the use of psoralens to cause phototoxicity as part of psoralen-ultraviolet A photochemotherapy (PUVA),[5,6] but may be an issue with some other drug groups.[7,8] It has recently become clear that increased risk of both melanoma and nonmelanoma skin cancers is an important issue with the photosensitizing antifungal voriconazole.[9] Vemurafenib, an inhibitor of mutated BRAF, shows promise as a treatment for metastatic malignant melanoma but is also associated with drug-induced phototoxicity and a greatly increased risk of squamous cell carcinoma of the skin.[10] It is plausible that the increased worldwide incidence of various skin cancers may be partly from the increased use of certain phototoxic drugs.

Phototoxicity will theoretically occur in any individual with exposure to enough phototoxin and appropriate irradiation, although idiosyncratic factors likely render some subjects more or less susceptible. Some drugs, such as psoralens and most fluoroquinolone antibiotics, can be expected to cause phototoxicity in anyone given a sufficiently high dose. However, the phototoxin is not always the parent drug: it may be a metabolite. It is likely that at least part of the reason why systemic drug phototoxicity can seem idiosyncratic, with only some individuals affected even if very high doses are administered, is because of individual differences in drug bioavailability and metabolism.

Disclosures: No conflicts of interest reported by either author.
Photobiology Unit, Department of Dermatology, Ninewells Hospital and Medical School, University of Dundee, Dundee DD1 9SY, Scotland, UK
* Corresponding author. Photobiology Unit, Level 8, Ninewells Hospital and Medical School, Dundee, Tayside DD1 9SY, Great Britain.
E-mail address: r.s.dawe@dundee.ac.uk

Dermatol Clin 32 (2014) 363–368
http://dx.doi.org/10.1016/j.det.2014.03.014

Even with drugs such as ciprofloxacin,[11] which frequently cause phototoxicity, marked variation is seen between individuals in the degree of photosensitivity produced by a given dose of drug (**Fig. 1**). Different patterns of phototoxic reactions occur in the skin, including an almost immediate prickling/burning sensation, urticaria, sunburn-like reactions, and skin fragility states (**Table 1**).

Photoallergy is usually associated with exposure to topical agents, such as ultraviolet filters and topical nonsteroidal anti-inflammatory drugs.[12] In some parts of the world, certain antiseptics may still be relevant.[13]

## EPIDEMIOLOGY

Although reported as the third most common cutaneous drug reaction in a recent Tunisian series,[14] drug-induced photosensitivity is frequently underdiagnosed. In tertiary referral populations seen at photodermatology centers, between 2% and 15% of patients were affected,[15–18] and 4% of those seen in the Dundee Photobiology Unit. Drug-induced phototoxicity is especially common in some populations, such as people with cystic fibrosis taking ciprofloxacin.[19] However, most who develop sunburn-like phototoxicity during a course of antibiotic therapy are likely to simply

stop the drug and not seek a formal diagnosis. The prevalence of different types of drug photosensitivity will vary geographically, not only because of differing patterns of exposure to causative drugs and patterns of ultraviolet and visible light exposure, but also because of variations in an individual's endogenous photoprotection and differences in drug metabolism between populations.

## PATHOGENESIS

The absorption of optical radiation by a photosensitizing drug or drug metabolite within the skin is an essential first step in both phototoxicity and photoallergy. Drug-induced photosensitivity can involve ultraviolet B (UVB) wavelengths, ultraviolet A (UVA) wavelengths, and visible wavelengths, depending on the absorption characteristics of the drug or drug metabolite. As a general rule, drug-induced photosensitivity is primarily a UVA phenomenon.

Once the energy is absorbed, photosensitizing radicals are produced through various mechanisms that can directly lead, again through a variety of mechanisms, to phototoxic effects. Alternatively, drug phototoxicity may be produced more indirectly by the altered chemicals, leading to alterations in endogenous porphyrin levels or triggering a lupus erythematosus–type reaction.

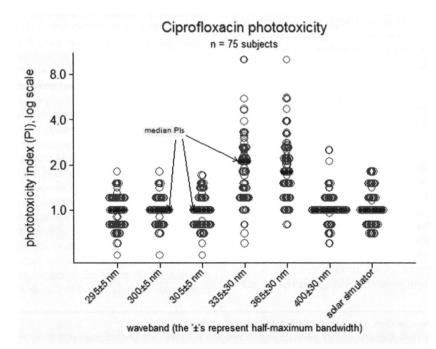

**Fig. 1.** Figure, taken from the results of several phototoxicity studies that included ciprofloxacin at a standard dose as a positive control drug, showing (1) the variability between individuals and (2) the wavelength dependency of phototoxicity with this particular drug. Note that at the 335 ± 30 nm waveband, the median phototoxic index (PI) is 2, indicating erythema with half the dose of this waveband that caused erythema without ciprofloxacin, but 2 individuals were severely photosensitive, with phototoxic indices greater than 8.

**Table 1**
**Major patterns of cutaneous phototoxicity**

| Skin Reactions | Photosensitizers |
| --- | --- |
| Prickling or burning during exposure; sometimes, but not always evident, immediate erythema; edema or urticaria with higher doses; sometimes delayed erythema or hyperpigmentation | Photofrin; amiodarone; chlorpromazine |
| Sunburn-type reactions | Fluoroquinolones; chlorpromazine; amiodarone; thiazide diuretics; quinine; demeclocycline; doxycycline; voriconazole |
| Dermatitis response | Thiazide diuretics |
| Late onset erythema; blisters with higher doses; hyperpigmentation | Psoralens |
| Increased skin fragility and blistering (pseudoporphyria) | Naproxen; nalidixic acid; demeclocycline; amiodarone; fluoroquinolone antibiotics; voriconazole |
| Telangiectasia on photoexposed site | Calcium channel antagonists |

In photoallergy, the altered chemical elicits a delayed type hypersensitization response, which on reexposure causes a reaction, typically of an allergic eczematous morphology and histopathology.

## CLINICAL MANIFESTATIONS

Systemic drug phototoxicity can display several different reaction patterns; the most frequent is a sunburn type reaction (see **Table 1**). Many different drugs cause photosensitivity through phototoxic mechanisms. The list in **Table 2** is not comprehensive but covers the most common photosensitizing drugs. Because the UVA wavelengths are often important (see **Table 2** for examples of wavelength dependency of common drugs that can cause phototoxicity), a history of sunburn-like reactions occurring when a normal, predominantly UVB sunburn would not be expected is a common finding. Some drugs cause sunburn-like reactions that occur within a different time course compared with normal sunburn. An example is systemic psoralen phototoxicity: the peak reaction is typically 72 to 96 hours after exposure to UVA.[20–22]

## LABORATORY FINDINGS

Laboratory testing is often not necessary, but if a type of cutaneous porphyria is in the differential (such as with early-onset prickling seen in erythropoietic protoporphyria or a skin fragility state akin to that seen in the bullous porphyrias), determination of plasma porphyrin levels and a porphyrin plasma scan (spectrofluorimetry) may be helpful. Unless a true porphyria is present or, rarely, the

mechanism of drug-induced photosensitivity involves an alteration in endogenous porphyrins, a porphyrin plasma scan will not show a peak typical of any of the porphyrias, although some drugs may themselves cause some abnormalities on spectrofluorimetry.

Lupus autoantibodies can be abnormal if a drug-induced lupus syndrome is the mechanism behind photosensitivity. Some drugs that cause a drug-induced lupus induce production of antihistone antibodies.

Various in vitro test systems can be used to assess the phototoxic potential of drugs. These systems are mostly used in drug development and are generally not useful in investigating patients with drug-induced photosensitivity.

## PHOTOBIOLOGICAL EVALUATION

For systemic drug phototoxicity, the key investigation is phototesting, ideally with a monochromator, to determine (1) the wavebands involved and degree of photosensitivity, and (2) the reaction to the suspected drug (sometimes for rechallenge). This testing also helps distinguish drug phototoxicity from other conditions, such as chronic actinic dermatitis.[23] Photopatch testing may or may not be positive (reflecting phototoxicity, not photoallergy),[24] presumably because it is not necessarily the parent drug, rather than a metabolite, that is the main cause of phototoxicity.

When investigating topical drug photoallergy, photopatch testing is the most important photobiological investigation. As with patch testing, use of the mid–upper back skin is recommended, avoiding the paravertebral groove area. The

**Table 2**
**Photosensitizing (phototoxic) drugs and predominant relevant wavelengths**

| | Photosensitizing Drugs | Predominant Wavelengths |
|---|---|---|
| Antibiotics | Fluoroquinolones | UVA/visible |
| | Nalidixic acid | UVA |
| | Tetracyclines (particularly demeclocycline and doxycycline) | UVA |
| | Sulphonamides | UVA |
| Antifungals | Griseofulvin | UVA |
| Diuretics and cardiovascular agents | Thiazides | UVB/UVA |
| | Furosemide (generally at high doses and/or in renal impairment) | UVA |
| | Amiodarone | UVA |
| | Quinidine | UVB/UVA |
| Nonsteroidal anti-inflammatory drugs | Naproxen | UVA |
| | Tiaprofenic acid | UVA |
| | Piroxicam | UVA |
| | Azapropazone | UVA |
| Calcium channel antagonists | Nifedipine | UVB/UVA |
| | Diltiazem | UVB/UVA |
| | Amlodipine | UVB/UVA |
| Psoralens | 8-Methoxypsoralen | UVA |
| | 5-Methoxypsoralen | UVA |
| Psychoactive drugs | Phenothiazines (chlorpromazine, thioridazine) | UVB/UVA |
| | Protriptyline | UVA |
| Retinoids | Isotretinoin | UVA |
| | Acitretin | UVA |
| Photodynamic therapy agents | Foscan | Visible |
| | Photofrin | Visible |

*Abbreviations:* UVA, ultraviolet A; UVB, ultraviolet B.

photoallergen series (eg, a standard European series),[12] are applied in duplicate. At 24 hours, both patch applications are removed and one set is irradiated, usually with a dose of 5 J/cm$^2$ UVA, followed by readings over the next 48 to 72 hours. Just as with patch testing, interpretation is critical. A reaction on an irradiated site, and not on unirradiated skin, to an unfamiliar substance during photopatch testing does not necessarily mean photoallergy.[25] Several reports of what has been labeled "photoallergy" to systemic drugs have based the diagnosis on a "positive" photopatch test, without reports on time course of reaction or on testing in controls to allow distinction between true photoallergy and phototoxicity.

Monochromator phototesting of volunteers on drug and on placebo in a blinded fashion can be used, particularly when assessing new potential drugs, to determine whether a particular drug has phototoxic effects.[26–28] However, even this testing cannot rule out rare idiosyncratic drug phototoxicity.

## MANAGEMENT

For many patients with suspected drug-induced photosensitivity, simply stopping the drug is all that is required. If the diagnosis of drug-induced photosensitivity is not clear (perhaps the main differential is between chronic actinic dermatitis and systemic drug phototoxicity, or between photoaggravated endogenous eczema and topical agent photoallergy), further investigations as detailed earlier are appropriate.

Drug-induced photosensitivity may be observed in patients undergoing phototherapy for various skin conditions. In general, drug-induced photosensitivity is less likely to be an issue with UVB therapy than phototherapy with longer wavelengths, although certain drugs that can cause phototoxicity with UVB wavelengths are associated with lower narrowband UVB minimal erythema doses (MEDs). Thus, if these drugs are initiated during a phototherapy course without assessment of pretreatment MED, they may potentially cause problems.[29]

With PUVA, the psoralen phototoxicity will usually be greater than with other photosensitizing drugs; therefore, the practical relevance of these other drugs would be anticipated to be low, although one study did show increased erythema reactions associated with other photosensitizing drugs.[30] The greatest concern is with ultraviolet A1 phototherapy, because this source is especially likely to cause drug-induced photosensitivity.[31–33] In practice, the action required regarding phototherapy in a patient on a potentially photosensitizing drug depends on a wide variety of factors (including the drug and its photosensitivity wavelength dependence, the form of phototherapy, and the ultraviolet dose), and should be decided on an individual basis. With a few exceptions (eg, phototherapy would seem unwise in a patient with voriconazole photosensitivity because of photocarcinogenesis concerns), photosensitizing drugs do not preclude phototherapy treatments. As a general rule, phototherapy should be stopped temporarily if a patient must be started on a short course of a drug that is known to cause photosensitivity at that particular wavelength. If a potentially problematic new drug is initiated during phototherapy and the drug course is expected to be prolonged, individual factors should be considered, such as the likelihood of causing phototoxicity (drug type and dose), type of phototherapy, ultraviolet dose reached during the course, potential interacting drugs, and patient's skin phototype. Lists of frequently used drugs unlikely to cause problems with the different phototherapies may be helpful.

Sometimes, stopping the drug is not appropriate. For example, a good antiarrhythmic alternative to amiodarone may not be available. In these instances, knowing the most relevant wavelengths can aid in advising the patient on appropriate photoprotection (behavioral, environmental, clothing, and sunscreen) measures. For some drugs with short half-lives, adjusting the time of dosing may avoid delivering the phototherapy during the time of peak plasma concentration of the drugs. Rarely, it is appropriate to use phototherapy, for example using narrowband UVB, to induce some protection against the effects of drug phototoxicity caused by longer wavelengths.[34]

## REFERENCES

1. Ferguson J. Photosensitivity due to drugs. Photodermatol Photoimmunol Photomed 2002;18:262–9.

2. Urbach F. Phototoxicity and possible enhancement of photocarcinogenesis by fluorinated quinolone antibiotics. J Photochem Photobiol B 1997;37:169–70.

3. O'Gorman SM, Murphy GM. Photosensitizing medications and photocarcinogenesis. Photodermatol Photoimmunol Photomed 2014;30:8–14.

4. Johnson BE, Gibbs NK, Ferguson J. Quinolone antibiotic with potential to photosensitize skin tumorigenesis. J Photochem Photobiol B 1997;37:171–3.

5. Lindelof B, Sigurgeirsson B, Tegner E, et al. PUVA and cancer risk: the Swedish follow-up study. Br J Dermatol 1999;141:108–12.

6. Stern RS, PUVA Follow-Up Study. The risk of squamous cell and basal cell cancer associated with psoralen and ultraviolet A therapy: a 30-year prospective study. J Am Acad Dermatol 2012;66:553–62.

7. Siiskonen SJ, Koomen ER, Visser LE, et al. Exposure to phototoxic NSAIDs and quinolones is associated with an increased risk of melanoma. Eur J Clin Pharmacol 2013;69:1437–44.

8. de Vries E, Trakatelli M, Kalabalikis D, et al. Known and potential new risk factors for skin cancer in European populations: a multicentre case-control study. Br J Dermatol 2012;167(Suppl 2):1–13.

9. Epaulard O, Leccia MT, Blanche S, et al. Phototoxicity and photocarcinogenesis associated with voriconazole. Med Mal Infect 2011;41:639–45.

10. Chapman PB, Hauschild A, Robert C, et al. Improved survival with vemurafenib in melanoma with BRAF V600E mutation. N Engl J Med 2011; 364:2507–16.

11. Ferguson J, Johnson BE. Ciprofloxacin-induced photosensitivity: in vitro and in vivo studies. Br J Dermatol 1990;123:9–20.

12. European Multicentre Photopatch Test Study (EMCPPTS) Taskforce. A European multicentre photopatch test study. Br J Dermatol 2012;166:1002–9.

13. Jindal N, Sharma NL, Mahajan VK, et al. Evaluation of photopatch test allergens for Indian patients of photodermatitis: preliminary results. Indian J Dermatol Venereol Leprol 2011;77:148–55.

14. Chaabane H, Masmoudi A, Amouri M, et al. Cutaneous adverse drug reaction: prospective study of 118 cases. Tunis Med 2013;91:514–20 [in French].

15. Fotiades J, Soter NA, Lim HW. Results of evaluation of 203 patients for photosensitivity in a 7.3-year period. J Am Acad Dermatol 1995;33:597–602.

16. Wong SN, Khoo LS. Analysis of photodermatoses seen in a predominantly Asian population at a photodermatology clinic in Singapore. Photodermatol Photoimmunol Photomed 2005;21:40–4.

17. Wadhwani AR, Sharma VK, Ramam M, et al. A clinical study of the spectrum of photodermatoses in dark-skinned populations. Clin Exp Dermatol 2013;38:823–9.

18. Frain-Bell W. Cutaneous photobiology. Oxford (United Kingdom): Oxford University Press; 1985. p. 125–52.

19. Tolland JP, Murphy BP, Boyle J, et al. Ciprofloxacin-induced phototoxicity in an adult cystic fibrosis

population. Photodermatol Photoimmunol Photomed 2012;28:258–60.

20. Ibbotson SH, Farr PM. The time-course of psoralen ultraviolet A (PUVA) erythema. J Invest Dermatol 1999;113:346–50.

21. Man I, Dawe RS, Ferguson J, et al. An intraindividual study of the characteristics of erythema induced by bath and oral methoxsalen photochemotherapy and narrowband ultraviolet B. Photochem Photobiol 2003;78:55–60.

22. Man I, McKinlay J, Dawe RS, et al. An intraindividual comparative study of psoralen-UVA erythema induced by bath 8-methoxypsoralen and 4, 5', 8-trimethylpsoralen. J Am Acad Dermatol 2003;49: 59–64.

23. O'Reilly FM, McKenna D, Murphy GM. Is monochromatic irradiation testing useful in the differentiation of drug-induced photosensitivity from chronic actinic dermatitis? Clin Exp Dermatol 1999;24:118–21.

24. Kerr A, Shareef M, Dawe R, et al. Photopatch testing negative in systemic quinine phototoxicity. Photodermatol Photoimmunol Photomed 2010;26:151–2.

25. Beattie PE, Traynor NJ, Woods JA, et al. Can a positive photopatch test be elicited by subclinical irritancy or allergy plus suberythemal UV exposure? Contact Dermatitis 2004;51:235–40.

26. Ferguson J, Dawe R. Phototoxicity in quinolones: comparison of ciprofloxacin and grepafloxacin. J Antimicrob Chemother 1997;40(Suppl A):93–8.

27. Dawe RS, Ibbotson SH, Sanderson JB, et al. A randomized controlled trial (volunteer study) of sitafloxacin, enoxacin, levofloxacin and sparfloxacin phototoxicity. Br J Dermatol 2003;149:1232–41.

28. Man I, Murphy J, Ferguson J. Fluoroquinolone phototoxicity: a comparison of moxifloxacin and lomefloxacin in normal volunteers. J Antimicrob Chemother 1999;43(Suppl B):77–82.

29. Cameron H, Dawe RS. Photosensitizing drugs may lower the narrow-band ultraviolet B (TL-01) minimal erythema dose. Br J Dermatol 2000;142:389–90.

30. Stern RS, Kleinerman RA, Parrish JA, et al. Phototoxic reactions to photoactive drugs in patients treated with PUVA. Arch Dermatol 1980;116: 1269–71.

31. Dawe RS. Ultraviolet A1 phototherapy. Br J Dermatol 2003;148:626–37.

32. Kerr AC, Ferguson J, Attili SK, et al. Ultraviolet A1 phototherapy: a British Photodermatology Group workshop report. Clin Exp Dermatol 2012;37: 219–26.

33. Beattie PE, Dawe RS, Traynor NJ, et al. Can St John's wort (hypericin) ingestion enhance the erythemal response during high-dose ultraviolet A1 therapy? Br J Dermatol 2005;153:1187–91.

34. Collins P, Ferguson J. Narrow-band UV (TL-01) phototherapy: an effective preventative treatment for the photodermatoses. Br J Dermatol 1995;132: 956–63.

# The Cutaneous Porphyrias

Danja Schulenburg-Brand, MBChB, MMed (Chem Path)[a],[*],
Ruwani Katugampola, BM, MRCP, MD[b], Alexander V. Anstey, MD, FRCP[c],[d],
Michael N. Badminton, BSc, MBChB, PhD, FRCPath[a],[e]

## KEYWORDS

- Cutaneous porphyria • Erythropoietic protoporphyria • Porphyria cutanea tarda
- Variegate porphyria • Congenital erythropoietic porphyria • Hereditary coproporphyria

## KEY POINTS

- Active cutaneous porphyria requires circulating porphyrins to reach the skin; therefore, a normal plasma porphyrin fluorescence emission screen excludes active cutaneous porphyria.
- The diagnosis of erythropoietic protoporphyria (EPP)/X-linked dominant protoporphyria (XLDPP) is suggested by the history of acute pain within minutes of sun exposure; physical signs are frequently absent but prolonged exposure can lead to erythema and edema, and an EDTA-preserved blood sample is essential to confirm the diagnosis.
- Lifelong effective photoprotection is key in the management of cutaneous porphyria.
- Porphyria cutanea tarda (PCT) can be treated with low-dose hydroxychloroquine or with phlebotomy in those patients with hemochromatosis and overt iron overload.
- All patients with variegate porphyria (VP) or hereditary coproporphyria (HCP) should be considered susceptible to acute attacks and advised on the known triggers, in particular, prescription medications and the requirement for lifelong vigilance.

## INTRODUCTION

The porphyrias are a group of mainly inherited disorders of heme biosynthesis where reduced activity of a pathway enzyme, or in 1 case a gain of function, results in accumulation of porphyrins and/or porphyrin precursors, giving rise to 2 types of clinical presentation: cutaneous photosensitivity and/or acute neurovisceral attacks (Table 1).[1] Skin problems related to circulating porphyrins are a feature of 6 of the 8 main types of porphyrias and fall into 2 categories. Acute painful photosensitivity due to the accumulation and circulation of excess protoporphyrin is associated with EPP and XLDPP, recently renamed X-linked EPP. Skin damage manifesting as fragility and blistering characterizes the bullous porphyrias, which comprise congenital erythropoietic porphyria (CEP) and PCT. Two of the acute porphyrias, HCP and VP, can also present with skin fragility, alone or in association with acute attacks.

## HISTORY

The earliest description of a cutaneous porphyria was in 1874,[2] and the link between photosensitive skin disease and hematoporphyrins excreted in the urine was made soon after in 1898.[3] The description of acute attacks appeared at approximately the time that sulfonal was introduced to clinical practice in the late 1800s,[4] and in 1911, Gunther[5] proposed a classification into "haematoporphyria

Funding Sources: None.
Conflict of Interest: None.
[a] Department of Medical Biochemistry and Immunology, University Hospital of Wales, Heath Park, Cardiff CF14 4XW, UK; [b] Department of Dermatology, University Hospital of Wales, Heath Park, Cardiff CF14 4XW, UK; [c] Department of Dermatology, Royal Gwent Hospital, Cardiff Road, Newport NP20 2UB, UK; [d] Institute of Medical Education, School of Medicine, Cardiff University, Heath Park, Cardiff, Wales CF14 4XN, UK; [e] Institute of Molecular and Experimental Medicine, School of Medicine, Cardiff University, Heath Park, Cardiff, Wales CF14 4XN, UK
* Corresponding author.
*E-mail address:* Danja.Schulenburg-Brand@wales.nhs.uk

Dermatol Clin 32 (2014) 369–384
http://dx.doi.org/10.1016/j.det.2014.03.001
0733-8635/14/$ – see front matter © 2014 Elsevier Inc. All rights reserved.

**Table 1**
**The porphyrias: inheritance, prevalence and clinical presentation**

| Porphyria | Gene | Inheritance Pattern | Estimated Prevalence[a] (per Million) | Acute Attacks | Fragile Skin/ Bullous Skin Lesions | Acute Photosensitivity |
|---|---|---|---|---|---|---|
| ADP | ALA-dehydratase (ALAD) | AR | Unknown | Yes | No | No |
| AIP | Hydroxymethylbilane synthase (HMBS) | AD | 7.2[34] | Yes | No | No |
| CEP | UROS | AR | 0.33[85] | No | Yes | No |
| PCT (HEP) | UROD | Complex (AR) | 40[47] (unknown) | No | Yes | No |
| HCP | Coproporphyrinogen oxidase (CPOX) | AD | 1[34] | Yes | Yes | No |
| VP | Protoporphyrinogen oxidase (PPOX) | AD | 3.2[34] | Yes | Yes | No |
| EPP | Ferrochelatase (FECH) | AD | 9.2[34] | No | No | Yes |
| XLDPP | ALA-synthase 2 (ALAS2) | XD | Unknown | No | No | Yes |

*Abbreviations:* ADP, ALA dehydratase deficiency porphyria; AR, autosomal recessive; XD, X-linked dominant.
[a] Symptomatic porphyria.

acuta" (acute attacks), "haematoporphyria conge-nita" (CEP), and "hematoporphyria chronica," a later-presenting cutaneous porphyria. In 1937, Waldenstrom proposed the term, *porphyria*, instead of haematoporphyria, and renamed hae-matoporphyria chronica as PCT.[5] As it became apparent, however, that some of these patients also experienced acute attacks and had similarly affected relatives, he proposed in 1957 the sub-group of PCT hereditaria, now known as VP. VP has been most extensively studied in South Africa,[6,7] where, due to a founder effect, an esti-mated 30,000 individuals who are descended from a Dutch couple who married in the Cape (now Cape Town) in 1688 are affected.[6,7] More recently, VP has been speculated to be the cause of King George III of Great Britain's mental illness,[8] although, on closer inspection of the evidence, this is now deemed implausible.[9] HCP was first described in 1949[10] and characterized as an auto-somal acute porphyria in 1955.[11] EPP was first recognized as a porphyria in 1961[12] and XLDPP was described for the first time in 2008.[13] EPP and XLDPP have identical clinical features, and it was the advent of molecular diagnostics that allowed the distinct pathogenetic mechanism in XLDPP to be elucidated.

## PATHOGENESIS OF SKIN LESIONS

In both categories of cutaneous porphyria, the skin problems are caused by the interaction be-tween porphyrins and visible light that occurs in the upper dermis. Due to their chemical ring struc-ture, porphyrins are photoreactive and absorb visible light strongly at approximately 400 to 410 nm (Soret peak), wavelengths that can pene-trate into the deep layers of the dermis. Absorption of energy creates an excited state porphyrin mole-cule that can either release energy as light (fluorescence, which is useful for laboratory mea-surement of porphyrins) or form reactive oxygen species through energy transfer. The creation of free radical species causes both direct damage to protein, lipids, and DNA as well as indirect tis-sue damage through degranulation of mast cells, complement activation, and metalloproteinase activation.[14–16] The distribution of porphyrins, which is determined by their differing physico-chemical properties, is thought to underlie the 2 different cutaneous presentations with hydrophobic protoporphyrin, with 2-carboxyl groups, having more affinity to lipid membranes, specifically endothelial cells, and the more water-soluble porphyrins (uroporphyrin and cop-roporphyrin with 8- and 4-carboxyl groups, respectively) diffusing into and accumulating in the lower dermis and basement membrane.[17] The histologic features in light-exposed skin are similar in all the cutaneous porphyrias and include thickening of papillary dermal blood vessel walls with hyalinization and periodic acid–Schiff–positive material, perivascular mucopolysaccha-ride material, and thickening of the dermis with hy-alinized collagen bundles.[18] In protoporphyria, the perivascular thickening may be more prominent, and in the bullous porphyrias, the epidermal atrophy and flattening of rete ridges predisposes to basement membrane splits and to the formation of subepidermal bullae.[19–22]

## DIAGNOSTIC APPROACH IN CUTANEOUS PORPHYRIA

Skin biopsy is not required to diagnose cutaneous porphyrias. Each porphyria has a unique porphyrin overproduction pattern that allows an accurate biochemical diagnosis, provided the correct samples are collected and protected from light degradation, accurately analyzed using sufficiently sensitive laboratory techniques, and interpreted by laboratory staff experienced in the diagnosis of porphyria.

Active skin lesions in cutaneous porphyria are always accompanied by excess circulating porphyrins produced in either the liver or bone marrow. The most informative initial test is, therefore, a plasma porphyrin fluorescence screen, which, if negative, excludes active cutaneous porphyria (**Fig. 1**). The preferred sample is EDTA-preserved whole blood, because erythrocytes are then available if further diagnostic testing is required. If the plasma emission scan[23] is abnormal, urine and/or feces and/or erythrocytes may be required to distinguish between the different types of porphyria (**Table 2**). A random urine sample, preferably early morning, is preferred to 24-hour urine collections, which unnecessarily delay diagnosis and risk sample degradation due to light exposure.

A plasma scan with an emission maximum wavelength greater than 623 nm is consistent with either VP or EPP/XLDPP; measurement of erythrocyte free and zinc-chelated protoporphyrin distinguishes these conditions (see **Fig. 1**, **Table 2**).[24] A plasma emission peak less than 623 nm is present in PCT, CEP, and HCP, which are differentiated by their characteristic urinary and fecal porphyrin patterns.[25–27] PCT is characterized by increased excretion of uroporphyrin and heptacarboxylic porphyrin in urine and isocoproporphyrin in feces. In HCP, the predominant porphyrin in urine and feces is coproporphyrin III in contrast to CEP, which is characterized by excess excretion of the isomer I series porphyrins, coproporphyrin I, and uroporphyrin I (see **Fig. 1**, **Table 2**).

DNA analysis is not required to confirm the biochemical diagnosis of porphyria except in XLDPP. It is, however, the preferred investigation for family screening, in particular, testing of asymptomatic family members for one of the autosomal dominant (AD) acute porphyrias (VP, HCP, or acute intermittent porphyria [AIP]). This requires knowledge of relevant family history and samples from an unequivocally affected relative for identification of the family-specific mutation. Family screening for familial PCT (PCT-F) is not recommended.[28] Confirming or disputing an alleged diagnosis of porphyria in an asymptomatic individual many years after the initial illness is a challenging clinical situation. Full analysis of blood, urine, and feces may not always result in a diagnosis, because porphyrin excretion may return to normal after long periods of remission. For family screening and testing of asymptomatic individuals, advice should be sought from a laboratory with specialist experience.

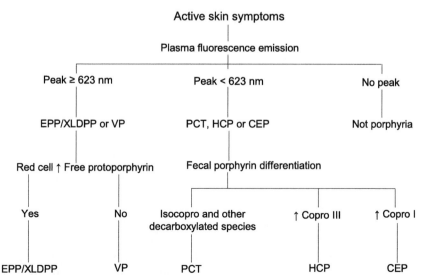

**Fig. 1.** Diagnostic algorithm for investigating cutaneous porphyria. Copro I, coproporphyrin I isomer; Copro III, coproporphyrin III isomer; nm, nanometer; ↑, increase.

**Table 2**
**Patterns of overproduction of heme precursors in clinical samples**

| Porphyria | Plasma Porphyrin Fluorescent Emission Peak | Urine Porphyrins and Precursors | Fecal Porphyrins | Erythrocyte Porphyrins |
|---|---|---|---|---|
| ADP | None | ALA > PBG Coproporphyrin | Not increased | Zinc protoporphyrin |
| AIP | 615–620 nm[a] | PBG > ALA Uroporphyrin[a] | Not increased | Normal |
| CEP | 615–620 nm | Normal ALA, PBG Uroporphyrin I > coproporphyrin I | Coproporphyrin I | Free and zinc protoporphyrin |
| PCT (HEP) | 615–620 nm | Normal ALA, PBG Uroporphyrin, 7-carboxyporphyrin | Isocoproporphyrin | Normal (free and zinc protoporphyrin) |
| HCP | 615–620 nm | PBG > ALA Coproporphyrin | Coproporphyrin III | Normal |
| VP | 624–627 nm | PBG > ALA Coproporphyrin | Protoporphyrin > coproporphyrin III | Normal |
| EPP | 626–634 nm | Normal ALA, PBG Normal porphyrin | ± Protoporphyrin | Free protoporphyrin |
| XLDPP | 626–634 nm | Normal ALA, PBG Normal porphyrin | ± Protoporphyrin | Free and zinc protoporphyrin |

Abbreviations: ADP, ALA dehydratase deficiency porphyria; nm, nanometer.
[a] Transient increased plasma porphyrin and urine uroporphyrin are believed to be from nonenzymatic metabolism of ALA and or PBG which may continue in vitro prior to analysis.

## GENERAL PHOTOPROTECTION

Patients with cutaneous porphyria require advice on how to adopt an effective strategy for photoprotection (**Box 1**). This should commence with an explanation that photosensitivity is mediated by visible light, not UV, light. Conventional sunscreens are not effective at blocking or absorbing visible light; visible light sunscreens are required. Furthermore, the photosensitivity can occur at any time of the day between sunrise and sunset and may also occur in the winter months. Unfortunately, these visible light sunscreens are opaque and are not dissimilar from wearing a makeup foundation cream. Some patients only use visible light sunscreens when playing sports.

Vitamin D monitoring and supplementation are required for all porphyria patients who adopt long-term photoprotection measures of this type.[29]

## PORPHYRIAS PRESENTING WITH ACUTE PHOTOSENSITIVITY
### Erythropoietic and X-Linked Dominant Protoporphyria

#### Epidemiology
The protoporphyrias are lifelong inherited metabolic disorders that usually present in early childhood with painful sun-induced photosensitivity resulting from dermal accumulation of the highly photosensitizing protoporphyrin IX.[30] EPP is an autosomal recessive condition caused by a

**Box 1**
**General photoprotection principles for patients with cutaneous porphyrias**

1. Clothing to cover skin: a broad-brimmed hat, clothing or fabric to cover the neck, long-sleeved top, gloves, long-sleeved trousers, closed shoes (not open sandals or lattice-style leather), and socks.

2. Sunglasses with side panels to protect the eyes and surrounding skin.

3. Restricted time outside on bright days between sunrise and sunset.

4. Reflectant sunscreen (containing zinc oxide or titanium oxide) to protect skin against visible light. In the United Kingdom, no commercial product is available; however, the Dundee reflectant sunscreen is available to the National Health Service via the Ninewells Pharmacy Production Unit, Ninewells Hospital, Dundee, Scotland. None is currently available in the United States.

reduction in ferrochelatase activity to below 30% of normal,[31] which in most patients is due to co-inheritance of a mutation that markedly decreases or abolishes enzyme activity with a common hypomorphic intronic polymorphism (IVS3-48C) that affects splicing efficiency.[32] The prevalence of EPP, therefore, varies in proportion to the prevalence of the hypomorphic allele in different populations, being highest in Japan, and lowest in sub-Saharan Africa.[33] The overall prevalence of EPP in Europe, which was calculated from prospective incidence data, was 1 in 108,000, with some variation between countries.[31,34] In contrast to EPP, XLDPP is transmitted in an X-linked dominant pattern[13,35] and is the consequence of gain-of-function mutations in the erythroid amino-levulinate synthase 2 (ALAS2) gene, resulting in increased flux through the heme pathway.[36] In the presence of normal ferrochelatase activity, limited iron availability results in accumulation of both free and zinc-chelated protoporphyrin.

## Clinical features

EPP typically presents in the first year of life, usually with distress within minutes of direct sun exposure. This reaction is so striking that although most parents of children with EPP suspect sunlight as the trigger for their child's distress, the absence of clinical signs means that the diagnosis may be delayed for many years.[30] Prolonged sun exposure occasionally occurs if a child is compelled to stay in direct sunlight and can lead to edema, erythema, and even purpura of the exposed skin, which may persist for several days. The photosensitivity reaction is mediated mainly by visible light, with a small contribution from UV-A. As a result, patients are symptomatic even in winter months when ambient UV levels are low. The typical onset of pain is usually within 5 to 15 minutes and subsides within minutes, provided patients remove themselves from ongoing sun exposure. Patients develop elaborate sun-avoidance strategies from an early age, preventing significant photo damage, and may, therefore, have subtle or no cutaneous signs (**Fig. 2**). Some patients show fine scarring on their noses, forehead, cheeks, or upper lip; others may develop waxy wrinkled appearance of the knuckles. Mild anemia is not uncommon in EPP and shows an apparent iron-deficiency pattern.[37] A minority of patients have changes in liver function tests, which may be an early sign of protoporphyric liver damage. Less than 2% of these progress to fulminant liver failure,[38] which usually requires liver transplantation.

## Differential diagnosis

The differential diagnosis of photosensitivity occurring within minutes of sun exposure includes solar urticaria and Smith-Lemli-Opitz syndrome. Both of these conditions are easily distinguished from EPP due to the rapid onset of a rash of the sun-exposed skin. In contrast, redness and swelling occur only after prolonged sun exposure in EPP and arises a few hours later.

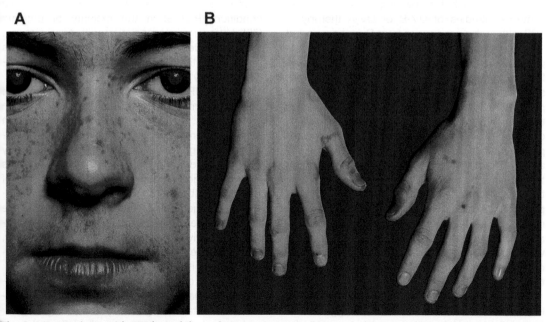

**A**     **B**

**Fig. 2.** Most patients with EPP have (*A*) no obvious cutaneous signs, as is the case in this patient; some have (*B*) scarring on the dorsum of the hands.

## Laboratory findings

Analysis of blood (plasma and erythrocyte) porphyrins is essential for the diagnosis of protoporphyria, because protoporphyrin is hydrophobic and not excreted in the urine. Increased circulating plasma protoporphyrin usually gives rise to a distinct fluorescence emission peak at 630 to 634 nm and is accompanied by increased erythrocyte free protoporphyrin in EPP and both free and zinc-chelated protoporphyrin in XLDPP (see **Table 2**).[13] The diagnosis of XLDPP should be confirmed by mutation analysis of the ALAS2 gene, because knowledge and experience of this condition is still evolving.

## Management

General principles of photoprotection should be followed (see **Box 1**). Visible light sunscreens help some patients with protoporphyria but may be cosmetically unacceptable.[30] In contrast to the bullous cutaneous porphyrias, because of symptoms associated with sun exposure, patients with protoporphyria have a strong motivating factor for adherence to rigorous photo protection strategies.

Several different treatments have been used for EPP (and XLDPP). Some patients derive therapeutic benefit from antihistamines, with diminished discomfort during photosensitivity reactions. β-Carotene (Lumitene, Tishcon Corporation, Westbury, NY, USA), containing Roche beadlets, has been assessed by clinical trials with conflicting results.[39,40] Both UV-A and UV-B therapy cause the skin to undergo photo adaptation, which includes tanning. There are no controlled studies of UV-B or UV-A therapy in EPP, although a case series from Dundee reported increased sun tolerance after narrowband UV-B phototherapy in all 6 patients treated.[41] The Dundee group has recently updated their retrospective case series, which now includes 12 EPP patients (9 female and 3 male) who have been treated with 80 courses of narrowband UV-B over the past 20 years. This treatment was reported to have been beneficial and well tolerated.[42] There are, however, no clinical reports of the therapeutic use of UV-A for EPP other than the self-reported use of sun beds by 34 patients.[30] A subcutaneous implant of an α–melanocyte-stimulating hormone analog, which promotes melanocyte-mediated skin pigmentation without UV exposure, is under investigation. Initial open studies reported apparent efficacy for this treatment.[43]

Although patients with protoporphyria have lower hemoglobin with iron indices suggestive of iron deficiency,[37] iron therapy tends not to be effective unless the anemia is profound and may even exacerbate the photosensitivity.[44] The risk of severe liver disease in EPP and XLDPP is low but can be rapidly progressive and require urgent liver transplantation.[45] Intraoperative protection with specific light filters to prevent intra-abdominal phototoxic tissue injury by theater lights is required during transplant surgery.[46] Patients should be advised to report an increase in photosensitivity, and both liver function and erythrocyte porphyrins should be monitored annually. If problems arise, patients should be referred urgently to a liver center with expertise in treating protoporphyric liver disease.[38]

Although genetic testing is not essential to confirm the diagnosis in EPP, patients and their families may request referral to clinical genetics for family counseling. Analysis for the hypomorphic allele (IVS3-48C) in the unaffected partner may be all that is required to advise on the likelihood of having an affected child.

# PORPHYRIAS PRESENTING WITH FRAGILE SKIN

## Porphyria Cutanea Tarda

### Epidemiology and pathogenesis

PCT is the most common of the cutaneous porphyrias in most populations and results from inhibition of the fifth enzyme in the heme synthesis pathway, uroporphyrinogen decarboxylase (UROD). It is predominantly a disease of adulthood with an estimated prevalence of approximately 40 per 1,000,000.[47] PCT differs from the other porphyrias in that it occurs as an acquired sporadic condition (PCT-S) in the majority of patients (75%), usually in association with liver disease. The remainder (25%) of patients inherit PCT as an AD condition (PCT-F)[48,49] although these proportions may vary in different populations.[50,51]

Hepatic UROD inhibition results in release of porphyrins into the plasma with accumulation in the dermis. The sunlight-induced reaction (described previously) results in the typical symptoms and signs of PCT, which are skin fragility and bullae formation where the epidermis splits from damaged basal lamina. The process of UROD inhibition is complex, with both environmental and genetic risk factors playing a role. The consequence at the cellular level is reduced hepatic UROD activity due to production of an inhibitor, uroporphomethene, from iron-dependent oxidation of uroporphyrinogen.[52,53]

PCT-F is characterized by low clinical penetrance, so that a family history is not always present. Presentation is generally at a younger age,[50] males and females are equally affected, and UROD is deficient in all tissues. Genetically determined half-normal enzyme activity is further reduced by the same risk factors that cause PCT-S.

PCT-S is usually associated with liver disease and is seen more commonly in males. Many patients have abnormal liver function, and a majority have hepatic iron overload with increased transferrin saturation and ferritin concentrations. Risk factors associated with UROD inhibition include hepatitis C infection, excessive alcohol intake, prescribed estrogen, and HIV infection.[50,54–57] The hereditary hemochromatosis HFE genotypes C282Y and H63D confer an increased risk of developing PCT, the highest risk associated with C282Y homozygotes.[50,58] A recent study showed that the hepcidin antimicrobial peptide (HAMP) gene expression of hepcidin (preventing iron overload) may be down-regulated in PCT, independent of the HFE phenotype,[51] hence increasing the risk of iron overload.

## Clinical features

Chronic bullous skin lesions, worse in summer, occur in sun-exposed areas, such as the dorsal aspect of the hands (Fig. 3A), arms, feet, and face. Skin fragility is the dominant feature; daily minor trauma results in skin erosions and blisters (see Fig. 3B), which can become secondarily infected, forming crusts and scarring. Hypertrichosis (see Fig. 3C), hyper- or hypopigmentation, and milia (see Fig. 3B) (typically on the dorsum of the digits) occur commonly.

## Differential diagnosis

The cutaneous symptoms of PCT, VP, HCP, and CEP are identical, although CEP tends to be a more severe disease, usually presenting in childhood. Unlike VP and HCP, PCT patients do not suffer from acute neurovisceral attacks. Similar skin lesions due to drug reactions or associated with hemodialysis can occur with normal porphyrin metabolism (termed *pseudoporphyria*). Other bullous dermatoses that should be considered include bullous pemphigoid, pemphigus, epidermolysis bullosa, and dermatitis herpetiformis.

## Laboratory findings

Active PCT is always associated with an abnormal plasma porphyrin screen, and analysis of urine and feces showing increased excretion of specific porphyrins (see Table 1) distinguishes PCT from the other bullous porphyrias. Particularly useful is the presence of the pathognomonic porphyrin in PCT, isocoproporphyrin, in feces (see Fig. 1,

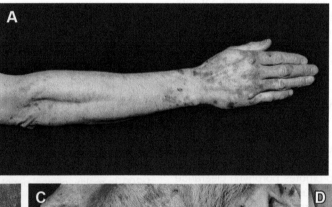

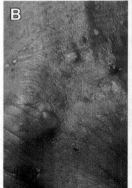 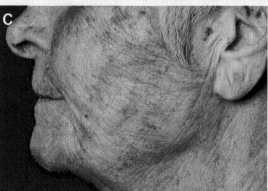 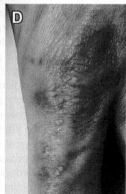

Fig. 3. Cutaneous manifestations of the AD porphyrias. (A) Note the demarcation of cutaneous manifestations on photoexposed skin on the dorsum of the hands and sparing of the photoprotected skin of the forearm. (B) Blisters and milia on the dorsum of the hand of a patient with porphyria cutanea tarda. (C) Hypertrichosis on the face of a patient with porphyria cutanea tarda. (D) Milia on the dorsum of the hands of a patient with VP.

Table 1). The different forms of PCT can be distinguished by measuring erythrocyte UROD activity, which is reduced in PCT-F but not PCT-S, or genotyping the UROD gene. Distinguishing between these different forms of PCT, however, is not essential because management of the 2 conditions is identical.

## Management

Once a diagnosis of PCT has been made, causative risk factors should be investigated. Alcohol consumption and prescribed estrogen intake should be evaluated. Liver function testing, transferrin saturation, ferritin, and genotyping (if indicated) for hereditary hemochromatosis should be performed. Viral serology for hepatitis B and C should be done and testing for HIV should be considered where appropriate.

General measures of adequate visible light photoprotection should be followed (see Box 1). Limiting alcohol intake until biochemical remission is achieved is desirable. Specific treatment options available in PCT are phlebotomy and/or oral chloroquine. The 2 treatments seem equally effective in achieving remission[59]; however, phlebotomy is required for those patients with hemochromatosis and iron overload. A unit of blood is removed weekly or every 2 weeks until patients are borderline iron deficient (transferrin saturation <16%; ferritin <15 ug/L) but without making them anemic.

When phlebotomy is not required to treat concomitant iron overload or is medically contraindicated, oral treatment with low-dose chloroquine (125 mg) (Avloclor, Alliance Pharmaceuticals, Chippenham, Wiltshire, UK or Aralen, Sanofi-Aventis, Paris, France)[60] or hydroxychloroquine (100–200 mg) (Plaquenil, Sanofi-Aventis) twice a week is preferred.[59] Chloroquine complexes with uroporphyrin[61] and promotes porphyrin clearance and excretion in the urine. Treatment should continue until urinary porphyrin excretion normalizes. Higher doses should not be given because this can precipitate acute photosensitivity and hepatotoxicity.[62] In a study[60] of 53 patients treated with chloroquine, the median time to relapse after biochemical remission was 2 years. Relapse was earlier in patients who were more severely affected when treatment was started. Clinical remission is usually achieved several months before biochemical remission. For patients who cannot tolerate phlebotomy or chloroquine, alternative methods of reducing iron stores are effective.

## Complications

Once in remission, patients should be followed-up for relapse and liver function should be monitored annually because there is an increased risk of developing cirrhosis or hepatocellular carcinoma. The incidence of hepatocellular carcinoma seems to be 3.5 times higher in PCT compared with matched chronic liver disease controls.[63]

## The Autosomal Dominant Acute Porphyrias

### Epidemiology

The AD acute porphyrias affect all populations worldwide, and in most countries, AIP, with no cutaneous manifestations, is the most common (see Table 1). As noted previously, the exception is in South Africa, where, due to a founder effect, VP is the most common. First acute attacks generally present in a patient's mid-20s, although in VP this is usually slightly later. Estimation of the clinical prevalence of overt porphyria varies, probably not only because in some series overt and latent porphyria have been included but also because the definition of symptomatic porphyria is observer dependent and can be biased by knowledge of an individual's mutation status. A 3-year prospective incidence study in Europe was used to calculate the prevalence of overt AIP (6 per million) and VP (3 per million).[34] Not surprisingly, clinical penetrance has also been difficult to estimate accurately. Family studies, which report penetrance between 10% and 50%, are not the answer, because there may be co-inheritance of additional genetic factors affecting disease expression. For example, overall clinical penetrance of VP (acute and cutaneous) was 40% in adult members of a large South African family.[64] There is also increasing evidence from population screening studies[65] and the Exome Sequencing Project (University of Washington, Seattle, WA, USA) that heterozygote frequency for hydroxymethylbilane synthase (HMBS) variants may be as high as 1:200. In reality, clinical penetrance may, therefore, be as low as 0.1%.

### Pathogenesis of acute attacks

Acute attacks manifest when hepatic heme synthesis is induced in the presence of partial hydroxymethylbilane synthase deficiency, which becomes rate limiting with consequent overproduction of aminolevulinic acid (ALA) and porphobilinogen (PBG). In AIP, this deficiency is the primary defect, but in HCP and VP it is believed secondary to porphyrin metabolites.[66] Factors that can induce the pathway include menstrual hormonal changes, certain prescribed and illicit drugs, stress, infection, and excess alcohol consumption. Evidence from liver transplantation indicates that hepatic porphyrin precursor production alone, probably ALA, is sufficient to cause the axonal degeneration and patchy demyelination that characterizes the neurologic lesions.[67,68] This neuronal damage results in rapidly progressive autonomic, motor and central neurologic system changes, and consequent clinical features (described later).

## Clinical manifestations

Although in AIP the only clinical manifestation is acute neurovisceral attacks, fragile skin with blisters (see Fig. 3B, D) indistinguishable from those that occur in PCT can affect patients with VP and HCP. In VP, 60% to 80% of patients with overt porphyria have skin symptoms only, 10% to 20% acute attacks only, and 10% to 20% both. Skin symptoms are much less common in HCP, with less than 10% presenting with skin lesions alone, often provoked by hepatobiliary disease. Approximately one-quarter of those who present with an acute attack are noted to have skin lesions at the time.[69]

Acute neurovisceral attacks affect mainly women (male-to-female ratio 1:3) and are rare before puberty and unusual after menopause. They almost invariably start with abdominal pain, which becomes increasingly severe but with no localizing features or evidence of peritonism.[70] Pain may also affect lower back and inner thighs and usually requires high-dose parenteral opiates for effective analgesia. The autonomic neuropathy also causes nausea, vomiting, constipation, hypertension, and tachycardia in a proportion of patients.[71] Features of central nervous system involvement, such as agitation, confusion, and unusual behavior, are common and can progress to psychosis with hallucinations. Other neurologic manifestations that may be seen include transient acute mental changes, such as anxiety, confusion, insomnia, and occasionally hallucinations. Convulsions, which may be secondary to hyponatremia, also can occur. Undiagnosed and severe attacks can result in a peripheral motor neuropathy, which initially involves distal muscles but can progress to a flaccid paraparesis that requires ventilatory support. There is no evidence that porphyria results in chronic mental illness.[72] Other less common neurologic features include sensory changes in a similar distribution to the motor neuropathy, cerebellar syndrome, and transient cortical blindness.[73]

## Laboratory findings

Acute attacks are always accompanied by an increased urinary excretion of ALA and PBG.[74] Screening tests for PBG are sufficient in the first instance but should always be confirmed by quantitation. When a patient is stable, further biochemical investigation to determine the type of acute porphyria usually requires analysis of plasma and fecal porphyrins. A positive plasma porphyrin fluorescence emission screen with a maximum emission greater than 623 nm is diagnostic of VP. If a plasma porphyrin screen is negative or has a wavelength maximum less than 623 nm, then fecal porphyrin analysis is required to distinguish between AIP and HCP.[75]

## Management

At present, it is not possible to predict which patients will go on to develop an acute attack and when; therefore, all are treated as equally at risk. Family studies to identify those who have inherited the condition are advised, and those affected can then be counseled as to how to minimize their risk of an attack.[28] Newly diagnosed patients should be provided with patient information leaflets and information on drug safety and how to keep this up to date.[76]

Acute attacks are managed in identical fashion, independent of the type of acute porphyria.[76,77] The first step is a careful assessment of likely precipitating causes. Symptomatic relief usually requires high-dose opiates, antiemetics, and anxiolytics. Where intravenous fluid therapy is required, dextrose in saline is preferred to avoid hyponatremia, which may precipitate convulsions. Complications (hypertension, tachycardia, and convulsions) should be treated with drugs known to be safe (see the Welsh Medicines Information Centre Web site). Patients with severe acute attacks, or where the attack is accompanied by neurologic complications, such as weakness, convulsions, and/or hyponatremia, should be treated with intravenous human hemin, available either as heme arginate (Normosang, Orphan Europe; not available in the United States) or hematin (Panhematin, Recordati Rare Diseases, Lebanon, NJ, USA).

A small proportion of patients, mainly female, develop severe, recurrent acute attacks, which may be related to the luteal phase of the menstrual cycle. Gonadorelin analogs administered to induce a chemical menopause can be effective, although duration of treatment is limited by side effects.[77,78] Noncyclic attacks can be prevented by prophylactic hemin administration, usually administered biweekly or weekly via an indwelling intravenous infusion device. Orthotopic liver transplantation is curative but generally reserved for patients in whom medical therapy is no longer effective, who suffer repeated life-threatening attacks, or in whom quality of life is poor.[68] Late complications of acute porphyria include chronic hypertension,[78] renal impairment,[79] and hepatocellular carcinoma.[80,81]

### Congenital Erythropoietic Porphyria

CEP is an extremely rare autosomal recessive cutaneous porphyria caused by deficient uroporphyrinogen-III synthase (UROS) activity, the fourth enzyme of the heme biosynthetic pathway. There is wide allelic heterogeneity resulting in homozygosity or compound heterozygosity for mutations throughout the UROS gene.[82–85]

#### Epidemiology

CEP affects both genders and is panethnic. The prevalence of less than 1 per million quoted in the literature has not been verified by references.[86] The estimated crude minimum prevalence in the United Kingdom is 1 per 3 million population.[85]

#### Clinical manifestations

CEP is a multisystem disease. Clinical manifestations are summarized in (**Fig. 4, Table 3**). It typically presents shortly after birth with passage of red urine and discoloration of diapers that fluoresce under Wood light. Its predominant characteristic, lifelong bullous cutaneous photosensitivity to visible light and skin fragility, starts in

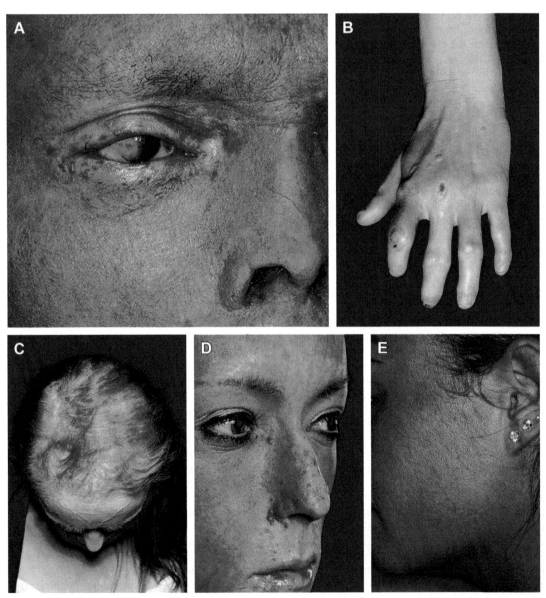

**Fig. 4.** Cutaneous manifestations of CEP include (*A*) photomutilation due to scarring of photoexposed skin of the face, including distortion of the nasal structure, loss of eyelashes, ectropion, and conjunctival scarring; (*B*) resorption of fingertips and flexion deformities of the hands; (*C*) scarring alopecia; (*D*) pink-erythematous facial papules; and (*E*) hypertrichosis.

**Table 3**
**Clinical manifestations and complications of congenital erythropoietic porphyria**

| Affected Site | Manifestations |
|---|---|
| Skin | Skin fragility, blistering, scarring leading to photomutilation, pink-erythematous facial papules |
| Nails | Longitudinal ridging, subungual blisters, hyperkeratosis and hematomas, onycholysis/shedding, rudimentary nails, anonychia; fingernails more severely affected than toe nails |
| Hair | Facial hypertrichosis and/or scarring alopecia |
| Hematology | Mild to severe, transfusion-dependant hemolytic anemia or pancytopenia; hemolysis, ineffective erythropoiesis, and sequestration of red blood cells with hemolysis in the spleen |
| Skeletal system | Scarring of fingers, fixed flexion deformities, resorption of finger tips, osteomyelitis due to recurrent infection of nonhealing ulcers of overlying skin, osteoporosis secondary to bone marrow hyperplasia, vitamin D deficiency or insufficiency |
| Eye | Photophobia, blepharitis, loss of eyelashes, ectropion, lagophthalmos, sclerokeratitis, lipid keratopathy, scleromalacia, conjunctivitis, conjunctival and corneal ulcers and scarring, leading to blindness |
| Mouth | Erythrodontia, microstomia |
| Liver | Neonatal jaundice ± hemolytic anemia, mild to massive hepatomegaly resulting in increased intra-abdominal pressure |
| Spleen | Splenomegaly and secondary pancytopenia |

early infancy, leading to scarring and progressive photomutilation. Some, however, may experience acute-onset of cutaneous and noncutaneous symptoms and signs immediately after visible light exposure.[85] CEP is genetically and phenotypically heterogeneous; disease severity can range from fetal hydrops in utero to adult-onset mild cutaneous photosensitivity.[85,87,88] Genotype-phenotype correlation in CEP can predict disease prognosis in some but not all cases.[85,89,90] Photoprotective behavior and environmental and epigenetic factors are likely to contribute to the lack of consistent genotype-phenotype correlation in CEP.[85] The main poor prognostic factors are early age of onset and hematological complications.[85]

### Laboratory findings
The diagnosis of CEP is based on elevated fecal and urinary porphyrins with a predominance (approximately 80%) of isomer series I porphyrins, mainly uroporphyrin I and coproporphyrin I, which is a consequence of nonenzymatic cyclization of the linear tetrapyrrole hydroxymethylbilane (see Table 2). Identification of UROS gene mutations may support the diagnosis but is not required routinely.

### Differential diagnosis
In addition to the other porphyrias, diseases to consider in the differential diagnosis of cutaneous

photosensitivity in early infancy include xeroderma pigmentosum, Bloom syndrome, Cockayne syndrome, Kindler syndrome, and Smith-Lemli-Opitz syndrome, all of which are inherited in an autosomal recessive manner.[91]

### Management
Due to the lack of consistent genotype-phenotype correlation, the management challenge in CEP is weighing the risks and benefits of treatment interventions against predicted disease prognosis.[92] Despite minimal intervention, some individuals with CEP have a good prognosis with no impact on their health-related quality of life (HRQOL), although others develop progressive severe disease with treatment-associated complications (such as iron overload and blood-borne infections). Other conservative treatments, such as β-carotene, oral cholestyramine, and/or oral charcoal, are of no benefit.[92] The only curative treatment option for CEP at present is hematopoietic stem cell transplantation, with 21 published cases in children treated with either bone marrow or umbilical cord stem cell transplantation.[78,92–107] All resulted in symptomatic and biochemical cure apart from 3 transplant related deaths and 1 transplant failure.

A multidisciplinary management algorithm has been proposed to aid management decisions in CEP.[92] The initial assessment of patients should include a detailed clinical history and examination, including a detailed dental, ophthalmology, and psychological assessment with baseline laboratory and radiologic investigations.[92] Regular follow-up and monitoring every 6 or 12 months depending on disease severity are recommended.[92] Assessment of the spleen volume by ultrasound and bone health by dual energy x-ray absorptiometry scan every 2 to 3 years are recommended.

All patients need repeated counseling regarding rigorous lifelong general photoprotection (see **Box 1**). The exact cause and impact of suboptimal serum vitamin D concentration on the severity of bone disease in CEP is unclear. In those with vitamin D insufficiency or deficiency, dietary review and vitamin D replacement are essential. If radiologic investigations demonstrate progressive bone loss, treatment with bisphosphonates should be initiated. Progressive hemolytic anemia and/or thrombocytopenia should be investigated by bone marrow aspirate. Those with evidence of ineffective erythropoiesis should be considered for bone marrow transplant where a suitable HLA-matched donor is available.

Parents and family members also require support and advice. This should include genetic counseling about their risk of having an affected child. Parents of affected children should be offered the option of prenatal diagnosis for subsequent pregnancies (see European Porphyria Network and British Association of Dermatologists Web sites).

### Complications

The complications of CEP are summarized in **Table 3**. Disease- and treatment-related complications can have an impact on the psychological well-being and HRQOL of affected individuals and their families.[85] For example, leisure activities may be restricted due to severe photosensitivity, skin fragility, and risk of osteoporotic fractures.

## RARE PORPHYRIA VARIANTS

Mutations in the genes responsible for all of the AD porphyrias are frequent enough in the general population to give rise to rare homozygous variants of VP[108] and HCP[109] in which at least 1 allele must have sufficient residual activity to sustain heme synthesis essential for intrauterine development. Dual porphyrias, in which patients inherit more than 1 form, have also been described, most frequently PCT in combination with VP, HCP, or AIP.[110]

Hepatoerythropoietic porphyria (HEP), resulting from homozygosity or compound heterozygosity for mutations in the *UROD* gene, is rare, with 31

families reported to date.[47] It manifests as severe bullous photosensitivity before the age of 2 years in most cases. Photomutilation can be as severe as in CEP but hematological problems are usually minimal. Treatment is focused on photoprotection, because neither phlebotomy nor oral chloroquine therapy has been shown effective. Excess porphyrin production is mainly hepatic in origin, and bone marrow transplantation is, therefore, not an option.[111]

## REFERENCES

1. Puy H, Gouya L, Deybach JC. Porphyrias. Lancet 2010;375:924–37.
2. Schultz JH. Ein Fall von Pemphigus leprosus complicirt durch Lepra visceralis. Inaugural Dissertation. University of Griefswald; 1874.
3. Anderson TM. Hydroea aestivale in two brothers complicated with the presence of haematoporphyrin in the urine. Br J Dermatol 1898;10:1.
4. Stokvis BJ. Zur pathgenese der hamatoporphyrinurie. Z Klin Med 1895;28:1–21.
5. Goldberg A. Historical perspective. Clin Dermatol 1998;16:189–93.
6. Barnes HD. Further South African cases of porphyrinuria. S Afr J Clin Sci 1951;2:117–69.
7. Dean G. Porphyria variegata: a new disease. In: The porphyrias: a story of inheritance and environment. London: Pitman Medical; 1971. p. 4–13.
8. Macalpine I, Hunter R, Rimington C. Porphyria in the royal houses of Stuart, Hanover, and Prussia. A follow-up study of George 3d's illness. Br Med J 1968;1:7–18.
9. Hift RJ, Peters TJ, Meissner PN. A review of the clinical presentation, natural history and inheritance of variegate porphyria: its implausibility as the source of the 'Royal Malady'. J Clin Pathol 2012;65:200–5.
10. Watson CJ, Schwartz S, Schulze W, et al. Studies of coproporphyrin III. Idiopathic coproporphyrinuria; a hitherto unrecognized form characterized by lack of symptoms in spite of the excretion of large amounts of coproporphyrin. J Clin Invest 1949;28:465–8.
11. Berger H, Goldberg A. Hereditary coproporphyria. Br Med J 1955;2:85–8.
12. Magnus IA, Jarrett A, Pranker TA, et al. Erythropoietic protoporphyria. A new porphyria syndrome with solar urticaria due to protoporphyrinaemia. Lancet 1961;278:448–51.
13. Whatley SD, Ducamp S, Gouya L, et al. C-terminal deletions in the ALAS2 gene lead to gain of function and cause X-linked dominant protoporphyria without anemia or iron overload. Am J Hum Genet 2008;83:408–14.
14. Lim HW, Poh-Fitzpatrick MB, Gigli I. Activation of the complement system in patients with porphyrias

after irradiation in vivo. J Clin Invest 1984;74:1961–5.

15. Poh-Fitzpatrick MB. Molecular and cellular mechanisms of porphyrin photosensitization. Photodermatol 1986;3:148–57.

16. Poh-Fitzpatrick MB. Porphyrin-sensitized cutaneous photosensitivity: pathogenesis and treatment. Clin Dermatol 1985;3:41–82.

17. Brun A, Sandberg S. Mechanisms of photosensitivity in porphyric patients with special emphasis on erythropoietic protoporphyria. J Photochem Photobiol B 1991;10:285–302.

18. Epstein JH, Tuffanelli DL, Epstein WL. Cutaneous changes in the porphyrias. A microscopic study. Arch Dermatol 1973;107:689–98.

19. Sneddon IB. Congenital porphyria. Proc R Soc Med 1974;67:593–4.

20. Bhutani LK, Sood SK, Das PK, et al. Congenital erythropoietic porphyria. An autopsy report. Arch Dermatol 1974;110:427–31.

21. Bhutani LK, Deshpande SG, Bedi TR, et al. Cyclophosphamide and congenital erythropoietic porphyria. Photodermatol 1985;2:394–8.

22. Jacobo A, Almeida HL Jr, Jorge VM. Congenital erythropoietic porphyria in two siblings. Dermatol Online J 2005;11:15.

23. Poh-Fitzpatrick MB. A plasma pophyrin fluorescence marker for variegate porphyria. Arch Dermatol 1980;116:543–7.

24. Piomelli S. A micromethod for free erythrocyte porphyrins: the FEP test. J Lab Clin Med 1973;81:932–40.

25. Blake D, Poulos V. Diagnosis of porphyria- recommended methods for peripheral laboratories. Clin Biochem Rev 1992;13:S1–24.

26. Lockwood WH, Poulos V, Rossi E, et al. Rapid procedure for fecal porphyrin assay. Clin Chem 1985;31:1163–7.

27. Lim CK, Peters TJ. Urine and faecal porphyrin profiles by reversed-phase high-performance liquid chromatography in the porphyrias. Clin Chim Acta 1984;139:55–63.

28. Whatley SD, Badminton MN. Role of genetic testing in the management of patients with inherited porphyria and their families. Ann Clin Biochem 2013;50:204–16.

29. Holme SA, Anstey AV, Badminton MN, et al. Serum 25-hydroxyvitamin D in erythropoietic protoporphyria. Br J Dermatol 2008;159:211–3.

30. Holme SA, Anstey AV, Finlay AY, et al. Erythropoietic protoporphyria in the U.K.: clinical features and effect on quality of life. Br J Dermatol 2006;155:574–81.

31. Lecha M, Puy H, Deybach JC. Erythropoietic protoporphyria. Orphanet J Rare Dis 2009;4:19.

32. Gouya L, Puy H, Robreau AM, et al. The penetrance of dominant erythropoietic protoporphyria is modulated by expression of wildtype FECH. Nat Genet 2002;30:27–8.

33. Gouya L, Martin-Schmitt C, Robreau AM, et al. Contribution of a common single-nucleotide polymorphism to the genetic predisposition for erythropoietic protoporphyria. Am J Hum Genet 2006;78:2–14.

34. Elder G, Harper P, Badminton M, et al. The incidence of inherited porphyrias in Europe. J Inherit Metab Dis 2013;36:849–57.

35. Elder GH, Gouya L, Whatley SD, et al. The molecular genetics of erythropoietic protoporphyria. Cell Mol Biol (Noisy-le-grand) 2009;55:118–26.

36. Balwani M, Doheny D, Bishop DF, et al. Loss-of-function ferrochelatase and gain-of-function erythroid-specific 5-aminolevulinate synthase mutations causing erythropoietic protoporphyria and x-linked protoporphyria in North American patients reveal novel mutations and a high prevalence of X-linked protoporphyria. Mol Med 2013;19:26–35.

37. Holme SA, Worwood M, Anstey AV, et al. Erythropoiesis and iron metabolism in dominant erythropoietic protoporphyria. Blood 2007;110:4108–10.

38. Anstey AV, Hift RJ. Liver disease in erythropoietic protoporphyria: insights and implications for management. Gut 2007;56:1009–18.

39. Mathews-Roth MM, Pathak UA, Fitzpatrick TB, et al. Beta-carotene as an oral photoprotective agent in erythropoietic protoporphyria. JAMA 1974;228:1004–8.

40. Corbett MF, Herxheimer A, Magnus IA, et al. The long term treatment with beta-carotene in erythropoietic protoporphyria: a controlled trial. Br J Dermatol 1977;97:655–62.

41. Collins P, Ferguson J. Narrow-band UVB (TL-01) phototherapy: an effective preventative treatment for the photodermatoses. Br J Dermatol 1995;132:956–63.

42. Sivaramakrishnan M, Woods J, Dawe R. Narrowband UVB phototherapy in erythropoietic protoporphyria: case series. Br J Dermatol 2014, in press.

43. Harms J, Lautenschlager S, Minder CE, et al. An alpha-melanocyte-stimulating hormone analogue in erythropoietic protoporphyria. N Engl J Med 2009;60:306–7.

44. Milligan A, Graham-Brown RA, Sarkany I, et al. Erythropoietic protoporphyria exacerbated by oral iron therapy. Br J Dermatol 1988;119:63–6.

45. McGuire BM, Bonkovsky HL, Carithers RL Jr, et al. Liver transplantation for erythropoietic protoporphyria liver disease. Liver Transpl 2005;11:1590–6.

46. Wahlin S, Srikanthan N, Hamre B, et al. Protection from phototoxic injury during surgery and endoscopy in erythropoietic protoporphyria. Liver Transpl 2008;14:1340–6.

47. Badminton MN, Elder GH, Whatley SD. Clinical and molecular epidemiology of the porphyrias. In: Fereira GC, Kadish KM, Smith KM, et al, editors. Handbook of porphyrin science. New Jersey: World Scientific; 2013. p. 119–50.

48. Mendez M, Poblete-Gutierrez P, Garcia-Bravo M, et al. Molecular heterogeneity of familial porphyria cutanea tarda in Spain: characterization of 10 novel mutations in the UROD gene. Br J Dermatol 2007; 157:501–7.

49. Bygum A, Christiansen L, Petersen NE, et al. Familial and sporadic porphyria cutanea tarda: clinical, biochemical and genetic features with emphasis on iron status. Acta Derm Venereol 2003;83: 115–20.

50. Aarsand AK, Boman H, Sandberg S. Familial and sporadic porphyria cutanea tarda: characterization and diagnostic strategies. Clin Chem 2009;55: 795–803.

51. Ajioka RS, Phillips JD, Weiss RB, et al. Down-regulation of hepcidin in porphyria cutanea tarda. Blood 2008;112:4723–8.

52. Phillips JD, Kushner JP, Bergonia HA, et al. Uroporphyria in the Cyp1a2-/- mouse. Blood Cells Mol Dis 2011;47:249–54.

53. Phillips JD, Bergonia HA, Reilly CA, et al. A porphomethene inhibitor of uroporphyrinogen decarboxylase causes porphyria cutanea tarda. Proc Natl Acad Sci U S A 2007;104:5079–84.

54. Jalil S, Grady JJ, Lee C, et al. Associations among behavior-related susceptibility factors in porphyria cutanea tarda. Clin Gastroenterol Hepatol 2010;8: 297–302.

55. Gisbert JP, Garcia-Buey L, Pajares JM, et al. Prevalence of hepatitis C virus infection in porphyria cutanea tarda: systematic review and meta-analysis. J Hepatol 2003;39:620–7.

56. Munoz-Santos C, Guilabert A, Moreno N, et al. Familial and sporadic porphyria cutanea tarda: clinical and biochemical features and risk factors in 152 patients. Medicine 2010;89:69–74.

57. Bulaj ZJ, Phillips JD, Ajioka RS, et al. Hemochromatosis genes and other factors contributing to the pathogenesis of porphyria cutanea tarda. Blood 2000;95:1565–71.

58. Ellervik C, Birgens H, Tybjaerg-Hansen A, et al. Hemochromatosis genotypes and risk of 31 disease endpoints: meta-analysis including 66000 cases and 226000 controls. Hepatology 2007;46: 1071–80.

59. Singal AK, Kormos-Hallberg C, Lee C, et al. Low-dose hydroxychloroquine is as effective as phlebotomy in treatment of patients with porphyria cutanea tarda. Clin Gastroenterol Hepatol 2012; 10:1402–9.

60. Valls V, Ena J, Enriquez-De-Salamanca R. Low-dose oral chloroquine in patients with porphyria

cutanea tarda and low-moderate iron overload. J Dermatol Sci 1994;7:169–75.

61. Chinarro S, de Salamanca RE, Perpina J, et al. Studies on in vitro formation of complexes between porphyrins and chloroquine. Biochem Int 1983;6: 565–8.

62. Rossmann-Ringdahl I, Olsson R. Porphyria cutanea tarda: effects and risk factors for hepatotoxicity from high-dose chloroquine treatment. Acta Derm Venereol 2007;87:401–5.

63. Francanzani AL, Taioli E, Sampietro M, et al. Liver cancer risk is increased in patients with porphyria cutanea tarda in comparison to matched control patients with chronic liver disease. J Hepatol 2001;35:498–503.

64. Hift RJ, Meissner D, Meissner PN. A systematic study of the clinical and biochemical expression of variegate porphyria in a large South African family. Br J Dermatol 2004;151:465–71.

65. Nordmann Y, Puy H, Da Silva V, et al. Acute intermittent porphyria: prevalence of mutations in the porphobilinogen deaminase gene in blood donors in France. J Intern Med 1997;242:213–7.

66. Meissner PN, Adams P, Kirsh R. Allosteric inhibition of human lymphoblast and purified porphobilinogen deaminase by protoporphyrinogen and coproporphyrinogen. J Clin Invest 1993;91:1436–44.

67. Meyer UA, Schuurmans MM, Lindberg RL. Acute porphyrias: pathogenesis of neurological manifestations. Semin Liver Dis 1998;18:43–52.

68. Dowman JK, Gunson BK, Bramhall S, et al. Liver transplantation from donors with acute intermittent porphyria. Ann Intern Med 2011;154:571–2.

69. Brodie MJ, Thompson GG, Moore MR, et al. Hereditary coproporphyria. Demonstration of the abnormalities in haem biosynthesis in peripheral blood. Q J Med 1977;46:229–41.

70. Hift RJ, Meissner PN. An analysis of 112 acute porphyric attacks in Cape Town, South Africa: evidence that acute intermittent porphyria and variegate porphyria differ in susceptibility and severity. Medicine (Baltimore) 2005;84:48–60.

71. Mustajoki P, Nordmann Y. Early administration of heme arginate for acute porphyric attacks. Arch Intern Med 1993;153:2004–8.

72. Millward LM, Kelly P, King A, et al. Anxiety and depression in the acute porphyrias. J Inherit Metab Dis 2005;28:1099–107.

73. Pischik E, Kauppinen R. Neurological manifestations of acute intermittent porphyria. Cell Mol Biol (Noisy-le-grand) 2009;55:72–83.

74. Deacon AC, Elder GH. ACP best practice no 165: front line tests for the investigation of suspected porphyria. J Clin Pathol 2001;54:500–7.

75. Whatley SD, Mason NG, Woolf JR, et al. Diagnostic strategies for autosomal dominant acute porphyrias: retrospective analysis of 467 unrelated

patients referred for mutational analysis of the HMBS, CPOX, or PPOX gene. Clin Chem 2009;55: 1406–14.

76. Stein P, Badminton M, Barth J, et al. Best practice guidelines on clinical management of acute attacks of porphyria and their complications. Ann Clin Biochem 2013;50:217–23.

77. Anderson KE, Bloomer JR, Bonkovsky HL, et al. Recommendations for the diagnosis and treatment of the acute porphyrias. Ann Intern Med 2005;142: 439–50.

78. Andersson C, Lithner F. Hypertension and renal disease in patients with acute intermittent porphyria. J Intern Med 1994;236:169–75.

79. Andersson C, Wikberg A, Stegmayr B, et al. Renal symptomatology in patients with acute intermittent porphyria. A population-based study. J Intern Med 2000;248:319–25.

80. Lithner F, Wetterberg L. Hepatocellular carcinoma in patients with acute intermittent porphyria. Acta Med Scand 1984;215:271–4.

81. Andant C, Puy H, Bogard C, et al. Hepatocellular carcinoma in patients with acute hepatic porphyria: frequency of occurrence and related factors. J Hepatol 2000;32:933–9.

82. Astrin KH, Warner CA, Yoo HW, et al. Regional assignment of the human uroporphyrinogen III synthase (UROS) gene to chromosome 10q25.2->q26.3. Hum Genet 1991;87:18–22.

83. Aizencang G, Solis C, Bishop DF, et al. Human uroporphyrinogen-III synthase: genomic organization, alternative promoters, and erythroid-specific expression. Genomics 2000;70:223–31.

84. Ged C, Moreau-Gaudry F, Richard E, et al. Congenital erythropoietic porphyria: mutation update and correlations between genotype and phenotype. Cell Mol Biol (Noisy-le-grand) 2009; 55:53–60.

85. Katugampola RP, Badminton MN, Finlay AY, et al. Congenital erythropoietic porphyria: a single-observer clinical study of 29 cases. Br J Dermatol 2012;167:901–13.

86. Anderson K, Sassa S, Bishop D, et al. Disorders of heme biosynthesis: X-linked sideroblastic anemia and the porphyrias. In: Scriver CR, Beaudet AL, Sly WS, et al, editors. The metabolic and molecular basis of inherited disease. 8th edition. New York: McGraw-Hill Publishing; 2001. p. 2991–3062.

87. Verstraeten L, Van Regemorter N, Pardou A, et al. Biochemical diagnosis of a fatal case of Gunther's disease in a newborn with hydrops foetalis. Eur J Clin Chem Clin Biochem 1993;31:121–8.

88. Daikha-Dahmane F, Dommergues M, Narcy F, et al. Congenital erythropoietic porphyria: prenatal diagnosis and autopsy findings in two sibling fetuses. Pediatr Dev Pathol 2001;4:180–4.

89. Desnick RJ, Astrin KH. Congenital erythropoietic porphyria: advances in pathogenesis and treatment. Br J Haematol 2002;117:779–95.

90. De Verneuil H, Ged C, Moreau-Gaudry F. Congenital erythropoietic porphyria. In: Kadish KM, Smith KM, Guilard R, editors. The porphyrin handbook. 2nd edition. New York: Elsevier Science (USA); 2003. p. 43–63.

91. Anstey A. School in photodermatology: Smith-Lemli-Opitz syndrome. Photodermatol Photoimmunol Photomed 2006;22:200–4.

92. Katugampola RP, Anstey AV, Finlay AY, et al. A management algorithm for congenital erythropoietic porphyria derived from a study of 29 cases. Br J Dermatol 2012;167:888–900.

93. Kaufman L, Evans D, Stevens R, et al. Bone-marrow transplantation for congenital erythropoietic porphyria. Lancet 1991;337:1510–1.

94. Zix-Kieffer I, Langer B, Eyer D, et al. Successful cord blood stem cell transplantation for congenital erythropoietic porphyria (Gunther's disease). Bone Marrow Transplant 1996;18:217–20.

95. Thomas C, Ged C, Nordmann Y, et al. Correction of congenital erythropoietic porphyria by bone marrow transplantation. J Pediatr 1996; 129:453–6.

96. Lagarde C, Hamel-Teillac D, De Prost Y, et al. Allogeneic bone marrow transplantation in congenital erythropoietic porphyria. Gunther's disease. Ann Dermatol Venereol 1998;125:114–7.

97. Tezcan I, Xu W, Gurgey A, et al. Congenital erythropoietic porphyria successfully treated by allogeneic bone marrow transplantation. Blood 1998;92: 4053–8.

98. Shaw PH, Mancini AJ, McConnell JP, et al. Treatment of congenital erythropoietic porphyria in children by allogeneic stem cell transplantation: a case report and review of the literature. Bone Marrow Transplant 2001;27:101–5.

99. Harada FA, Shwayder TA, Desnick RJ, et al. Treatment of severe congenital erythropoietic porphyria by bone marrow transplantation. J Am Acad Dermatol 2001;45:279–82.

100. Dupuis-Girod S, Akkari V, Ged C, et al. Successful match-unrelated donor bone marrow transplantation for congenital erythropoietic porphyria (Gunther disease). Eur J Pediatr 2005;164:104–7.

101. Phillips JD, Steensma DP, Pulsipher MA, et al. Congenital erythropoietic porphyria due to a mutation in GATA1: the first trans-acting mutation causative for a human porphyria. Blood 2007;109: 2618–21.

102. Taibjee SM, Stevenson OE, Abdullah A, et al. Allogeneic bone marrow transplantation in a 7-year-old girl with congenital erythropoietic porphyria: a treatment dilemma. Br J Dermatol 2007;156: 567–71.

103. Faraci M, Morreale G, Boeri E, et al. Unrelated HSCT in an adolescent affected by congenital erythropoietic porphyria. Pediatr Transplant 2008; 12:117–20.

104. Lebreuilly-Sohyer I, Morice A, Acher A, et al. Congenital erythropoeietic porphyria treated by haematopoietic stem cell allograft. Ann Dermatol Venereol 2010;137:635–9.

105. Hogeling M, Nakano T, Dvorak CC, et al. Severe neonatal congenital erythropoietic porphyria. Pediatr Dermatol 2011;28:416–20.

106. Singh S, Khanna N, Kumar L. Bone marrow transplantation improves symptoms of congenital erythropoietic porphyria even when done post puberty. Indian J Dermatol Venereol Leprol 2012;78:108–11.

107. Fritsch C, Lang K, Bolsen K, et al. Congenital erythropoietic porphyria. Skin Pharmacol Appl Skin Physiol 1998;11:347–57.

108. Korda V, Deybach JC, Martasek P, et al. Homozygous variegate porphyria. Lancet 1984;1:851.

109. Grandchamp B, Phung N, Nordmann Y. Homozygous case of hereditary coproporphyria. Lancet 1977;2:1348–9.

110. Poblete-Gutierrez P, Badeloe S, Wiederholt T, et al. Dual porphyrias revisited. Exp Dermatol 2006;15: 685–91.

111. Elder GH. Porphyria cutanea tarda and related disorders. In: Kadish KM, Smith KM, Guilard R, editors. The porphyrin handbook. 1st edition. San Diego (CA): Elsevier Science (USA); 2003. p. 67–92.

# Photoaggravated Disorders

Susan M. O'Gorman, MB BCh[a,]*, Gillian M. Murphy, MB BCh[a,b]

## KEYWORDS

• Photoaggravated • Photodermatoses • Photosensitivity • Ultraviolet radiation

## KEY POINTS

- Photoaggravated skin disorders are diseases that occur as entities without UV radiation (UVR).
- They can be subdivided into conditions that are frequently exacerbated by UVR and conditions that are sometimes exacerbated by UVR.
- Conditions frequently exacerbated by UVR include cutaneous lupus erythematosus (LE), Darier disease (DD), dermatomyositis (DM), lichen planus (LP) actinicus, pellagra, rosacea, and Smith-Lemli-Opitz syndrome.
- Conditions sometimes exacerabated by UVR include acne, atopic dermatitis (AD), carcinoid syndrome, cutaneous T-cell lymphoma, erythema multiforme, pemphigus, pityriasis rubra pilaris, psoriasis, reticulate erythematous mucinosis syndrome, seborrheic dermatitis, transient acantholytic dermatosis (Grover disease), and viral infections.
- Polymorphous light eruption (PMLE) is a common photodermatosis, making it important to differentiate photoaggravation of an underlying disorder from superimposed PMLE.

## INTRODUCTION

Photoaggravated skin disorders are diseases that occur as entities without UV radiation (UVR) but are sometimes or frequently exacerbated by UVR. The specific UV wavelengths most capable of causing a flare in the disease are referred to as the action spectrum, and many photoaggravated diseases have distinct action spectra. In conditions, such as lupus erythematosus (LE), photoaggravation occurs in a majority of patients, and photoprotection is an essential component of management. In conditions, such as psoriasis and atopic dermatitis (AD), exposure to UVR results in improvement in a majority of patients but may exacerbate a subset. Photoaggravated conditions affect both fair-skinned and dark-skinned individuals. A recent study from India of 362 patients with Fitzpatrick types IV or V skin who were

suspected of having a photodermatosis documented a range of photoaggravated conditions: AD in 6.1%, systemic LE (SLE) in 3.6%, discoid LE (DLE) in 3%, rosacea in 3.3% (topical steroid–related in 2.2%), actinic lichen planus (LP) in 2.2%, dermatomyositis (DM) in 1.2%, and photoaggravated psoriasis in 0.6%.[1]

PMLE is a common photodermatosis in all skin types; therefore, it is important to differentiate photoaggravation of an underlying disorder from superimposed PMLE.[2] Among patients with suspected PMLE, up to 10% are subsequently diagnosed with LE, making this an important differential.[3] True photoaggravation causes exacerbation of the primary disease-specific lesions, and histology reflects the underlying dermatosis.

Disease-specific treatments should be instituted where possible. A key component of management of these photoaggravated conditions is

Author Disclosures: None declared.

[a] Dermatology Department, Beaumont Hospital, Beaumont Road, Beaumont, Dublin 9, Ireland; [b] National Photodermatology Unit, Dermatology Department, Mater Misericordiae University Hospital, Eccles Street, Dublin 7, Ireland
* Corresponding author.
E-mail address: ogormansm@hotmail.com

Dermatol Clin 32 (2014) 385–398
http://dx.doi.org/10.1016/j.det.2014.03.008

derm.theclinics.com

photoprotection in the form of sun avoidance between 10:00 AM and 4:00 PM in temperate zones and use of long-sleeved clothing, wide-brimmed hats, and broad-spectrum sunscreen. When photoprotection is advised, consideration should be given to vitamin D supplementation.[4]

Counterintuitively, in photoaggravated conditions, if photoprotection and disease-specific measures prove insufficient, low-dose phototherapy may be indicated. The study of this group of disorders is hampered by inconsistent terminology; for example, the terms, *photosensitive psoriasis, photoaggravated psoriasis*, and *photoexacerbated psoriasis*, describe the same subset of patients.

This article covers the conditions usually exacerbated by UVR and briefly covers a selection of conditions sometimes exacerbated by UVR (**Box 1**).

## DISEASES USUALLY EXACERBATED BY UVR
### Cutaneous Lupus Erythematosus

#### Introduction
LE encompasses several related conditions (**Box 2**), sharing the common feature of autoimmunity against nuclear constituents.

---

**Box 1**
Diseases exacerbated by UVR

Diseases usually exacerbated by UVR

  Cutaneous lupus erythematosus

  Darier disease (keratosis follicularis)

  Dermatomyositis

  Lichen planus actinicus

  Pellagra

  Rosacea

  Smith-Lemli-Opitz syndrome

Diseases sometimes exacerbated by UVR

  Acne

  *Atopic dermatitis*

  Carcinoid syndrome (**Fig. 1**)

  Cutaneous T-cell lymphoma

  Erythema multiforme

  *Pemphigus*

  Pityriasis rupra pilaris

  *Psoriasis*

  Reticulate erythematous mucinosis syndrome

  Seborrhoeic dermatitis

  Viral infections

---

**Box 2**
Subtypes of lupus erythematosus

Systemic lupus erythematosus

• Rowell syndrome

Subacute cutaneous lupus erythematosus

Chronic cutaneous lupus erythematosus

• Discoid lupus erythematosus

• Lupus tumidus

• Lupus profundus

---

#### History
Cazenave[5] first coined the term, *lupus erythematosus*, in the mid-nineteenth century and helped differentiate it from lupus vulgaris, a cutaneous form of tuberculosis. In the mid-twentieth century, Dubois[6] described the spectrum of disease seen with LE, ranging from cutaneous to multisystem disease.

#### Epidemiology
The epidemiology of LE varies by subtype. SLE is more common in women than men (6:1), with a higher prevalence in African American populations compared with white populations.[7] The early cutaneous manifestations of SLE may be overlooked in dark-skinned individuals. Subacute cutaneous LE (SCLE) and DLE also occur more commonly in women, but the ratio at 3:1 is not as marked as for SLE.[8] The mean age at presentation for SCLE

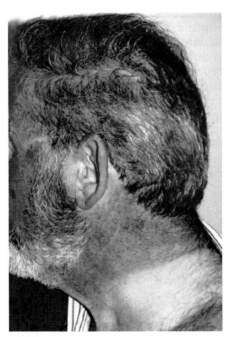

Fig. 1. Photoaggravation in carcinoid syndrome.

is in the sixth decade.[9] Although DLE can be seen in any age group, it most commonly presents in the fifth decade.[9]

The association between photosensitivity and LE varies worldwide, with a higher prevalence of photosensitivity in lupus in Asia compared with Africa.[10]

## Pathogenesis

In LE, a patient's immune system loses its tolerance to self, resulting in immune-mediated injury to organs, including the skin. The underlying pathogenesis, although not fully understood, reflects an interaction between host factors, such as susceptibility genes, sex hormones, and environmental factors, including viruses, drugs, and UVR.

Photosensitivity has long been recognized in LE,[11,12] with UVR playing a significant role in the induction and exacerbation of cutaneous LE.[13] UVR results in the aggravation of lupus through a variety of established mechanisms. UV-generated reactive oxygen species render DNA antigenic. The resultant autoantibodies recognize both this altered DNA and also native DNA.[14,15] UV-B displaces the typically intracellular antigens, Ro/SS-A and La/SS-B, to the surface of the keratinocyte,[16–18] resulting in antibody-mediated cytotoxic keratinocyte damage.[19] UV-induced destruction of keratinocytes through apoptosis occurs even in a normal setting; however, in lupus, slow clearance of apoptotic cells leads to prolonged exposure of DNA and extractable nuclear antigen (ENA) to the immune system, generating anti-DNA and anti-ENA antibodies.[20,21] The mechanisms underlying this process have been reviewed recently.[22,23] UV light also upregulates adhesion molecules, such as intercellular adhesion molecule 1,[24] in patients with LE. Nitric oxide synthase, capable of inducing cytokines, is released from keratinocytes after UV irradiation. In patients with lupus, this release is delayed but prolonged.[25] The promoter polymorphism 308A of tumor necrosis factor (TNF)-$\alpha$ is seen with increased frequency in SCLE,[26] and transcription is photoregulated.[27]

It may be difficult to elicit a history of photosensitivity, because the delay between UV exposure and exacerbation (sometimes 1–3 weeks) means patients may not make this association. UV-A and UV-B radiation are both implicated in the pathogenesis of LE, as shown by in vitro[28] and in vivo[29] studies. One study documented that photosensitivity in cutaneous LE was UV-B induced in 33% of cases, was UV-A induced in 14%, and in a majority of cases (53%) was mediated by a combination of UV-B and UV-A.[13] Nonsolar sources of UV-A, such as photocopiers,[30] and UV-B, such

as fluorescent lighting,[31] can aggravate LE. Although UV-B consistently aggravates LE, studies document reduction in LE disease activity with low-dose UV-A1 (340–400 nm) irradiation.[32–34] Subtypes of LE have varying degrees of photoaggravation, with lupus tumidus[35] and SCLE seeming the most photosensitive of the LE subtypes[2,36]; however, one study of phototesting with UV-A, UV-B, and visible light in 100 patients (24 with SLE, 30 with SCLE, and 46 with DLE) found no association between photosensitivity and LE subtype.[37] Phototesting is not routinely required in clinical practice to make a diagnosis of LE, because clinical history, examination, serologic studies, and skin biopsy for histology and direct immunofluorescence (DIF) suffice.

PMLE is seen with increased frequency in patients with underlying LE (49%), and the onset of PMLE precedes the onset of LE by more than 7 years in half of patients. This suggests that there may be features of pathogenesis common to both entities and that PMLE may predispose to LE in a subset of patients.[38]

## Clinical manifestations

Although the underlying disease process is similar across LE subtypes, the clinical presentation is diverse. Patients with SLE can present acutely with end-organ damage secondary to circulating autoantibodies (**Fig. 2**). No organ is protected from immune-mediated destruction, and SLE can present with nephritis, arthralgia, pleuritis, vasculitis, and central nervous system involvement. These patients can die from their disease manifestations. At the other end of the spectrum, patients may develop cutaneous lesions and never progress to systemic involvement.

Cutaneous manifestations of LE can be divided into LE nonspecific and LE specific. LE-nonspecific mucocutaneous manifestations include mouth ulcers, scarring alopecia, Raynaud's syndrome, and vasculitis. The characteristic cutaneous manifestation of SLE is a confluent, edematous erythema in a malar distribution; in a majority of cases,

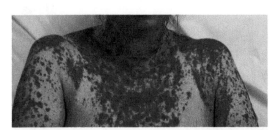

**Fig. 2.** Acute cutaneous lupus presenting in a patient with SLE. (*Courtesy of* Dr Aoife Lally, Saint Vincent's University Hospital, Dublin, Ireland.)

this malar rash is associated with underlying visceral involvement. SLE may present with erythema multiforme–like lesions, a condition termed, *Rowell syndrome*. Cutaneous lesions of SCLE include sharply demarcated psoriasiform plaques with fine scale and erosions and annular lesions with an erythematous border and a collarette of scale (**Fig. 3**). The cutaneous lesions of DLE are characteristically coin-shaped plaques on the face and neck, with fine adherent scale and follicular plugging. There may be appreciable scarring and hypo- or hyperpigmentation. After a diagnosis of DLE, the probability of receiving a diagnosis of SLE is 9.8% in the first year and 16.7% after 3 years. The corresponding figures are higher for SCLE, at 22% in the first year and 24.7% after 3 years.[8] Classification criteria for SLE have been defined by the American College of Rheumatology.[39,40]

The cutaneous lesions of DLE heal with central atrophy resulting in scarring. The cutaneous lesions associated with SCLE and SLE are non-scarring, although lesions of SCLE may result in hypo- and hyperpigmentation. Lupus tumidus is typified by violaceous, nonscaling papules and plaques on sun-exposed and non–sun-exposed sites.

There is a seasonal variation in manifestations of LE, with skin and joint symptoms flaring during summer months but an apparent increase in renal involvement in winter months.[41,42]

### Histology

Histologic features are central to the diagnosis of cutaneous LE. There is a lymphocytic infiltrate in the dermis that is both perivascular and periadnexal. At the dermoepidermal junction, the lymphocytic infiltrate is lichenoid with liquefactive degeneration of the basal keratinocytes and presence of epidermal cytoid bodies. Typically in DLE, follicular plugging and basement membrane thickening are marked, although occasionally epidermal changes are not prominent and dermal changes predominate. In SCLE, the epidermal features are minimal, and the findings are dermal vacuolar change with lymphocytic infiltration. In lupus tumidus, mucin is abundant, with positive DIF, in addition to the previously described dermal features.

### Laboratory findings

SLE is the LE subtype most strongly associated with positive antinuclear antibody (ANA) and double-stranded DNA.[9] Given the propensity of SLE to affect internal organs, a comprehensive systemic work-up, including complete blood cell count, complement levels, and parameters of renal function, including urinalysis, should be undertaken. The presence of anti-Ro (SS-A) and anti-La (SS-B) is associated with a pathologic photoprovocation reaction.[2] Anti-Ro (SS-A) is found in 72% of patients with SCLE, 47% of patients with acute cutaneous LE, and 22% of patients with chronic cutaneous LE (CCLE). Anti-La antibodies are found in 36% of patients with SCLE, 27% of patients with acute cutaneous LE, and 7% of patients with CCLE.[9] These antibodies are also strongly associated with Sjögren syndrome, which may overlap with SCLE. Additionally, Sjögren syndrome may be photoaggravated.[43] Drug-induced lupus is associated with antihistone antibodies and may demonstrate features identical to SLE, SCLE, and CCLE (as noted previously).

### Management

Essential lifestyle changes for patients with cutaneous LE are photoprotection[44] and smoking cessation. Given the implication of both UV-A and UV-B in the action spectrum of LE, broad-spectrum sunscreen is recommended.[45] Patients with cutaneous LE who practice rigorous photoprotection have suboptimal levels of vitamin D, which may be treated with oral supplementation.[4] Topical corticosteroids, antimalarials, and topical retinoids[46] are first-line treatment options for cutaneous LE. Second-line treatment options include dapsone,[47] thalidomide,[48] oral retinoids,[49] and immunosuppressive medications, such as mycophenylate mofetil,[50,51] azathioprine, and methotrexate. Every patient with cutaneous and systemic LE should be evaluated to ensure no causative drug is implicated. SCLE rarely is a paraneoplastic disease.[52]

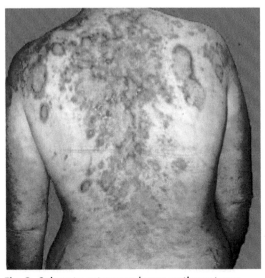

**Fig. 3.** Subacute cutaneous lupus erythematosus.

## Darier Disease

### Introduction

This uncommon autosomal dominant, late-onset genodermatosis, Darier disease (DD), is a disorder of keratinization. It is also known as keratosis follicularis or Darier-White disease.

### History

Jean Darier,[53] at the Hospital Saint-Louis in Paris, and James C. White,[54] Professor of Dermatology at Harvard University, independently described cases of DD in 1889. The eponym, Darier-White disease, is sometimes used. Darier recognized a striking number of epidermal round bodies (grains and corps ronds) on histology but mistakenly believed these to be parasitic elements. These are now known to represent abnormally keratinized keratinocytes. White recognized DD as a genetically inherited condition when the daughter of his index case also developed the disease.[55]

### Epidemiology

DD affects both genders and all ethnicities equally. Its prevalence is estimated at 1 in 36,000 in the United Kingdom[56] and 1 in 100,000 in Denmark.[57]

### Pathogenesis

DD is a genodermatosis inherited in an autosomal dominant manner, with complete penetrance and variable expression. It results from a mutation in the ATP2A2 gene on chromosome band 12q23-24, coding for SERCA2, a calcium pump protein of the sarco/endoplasmic reticulum, demonstrating the importance of calcium in maintaining normal epidermal function.[58,59]

DD is photoaggravated by UV-B but not UV-A irradiation.[60] Similarly, Hailey-Hailey disease, a genetically distinct but mechanistically related disorder of keratinization, may be induced by UV-B.[61]

### Clinical manifestations

DD manifests most commonly in puberty.[62] Follicular plugs result in brown papules in a seborrheic distribution, coalescing into papillomatous plaques with overlying yellow, greasy scale. Hypopigmented macules (guttate leukoderma) may be noted, particularly in darker skin types. Patients may have bullous, erosive, or vegetating lesions with associated distressing malodor. Although vesicles may be a feature of DD, it is essential to put rule herpetic infection.[63] Affected areas are typically the face, ears, and scalp (in particular the hairline), upper chest, inframammary area, back, sides of the neck, groin, and axillae. Additional features include papules resembling planar warts on the dorsum of hands and feet, small white papules on the oral mucosa, and palmoplantar pits

(identification of which may be facilitated by obtaining finger or palm prints).[62,64] Nail abnormalities with longitudinal ridging, red or white streaks, V-shaped notching at the distal margin, nail fragility, and subungal hyperkeratosis are highly consistent and specific features of the disease. A postzygotic ATP2A2 mutation can result in cutaneous features of DD following Blaschko lines, a condition known as acantholyic dyskeratotic epidermal nevus. A further subtype affects acral skin only and may be difficult to distinguish from acrokeratosis verruciformis. DD runs a relapsing-remitting course. Exacerbating factors include sunlight or artificial UV irradiation,[65] heat, friction, sweating, and infections, with increased susceptibility to pyogenic infections and herpes. The clinical severity of DD can vary greatly between different families and also between individuals affected within the same family. Cutaneous involvement can range from limited to extensive.

### Histology

A skin biopsy is essential for diagnosis. The presence of individually keratinized apoptotic cells (dyskeratosis) is pathognomonic of DD. These are seen as pink condensed cells. These dyskeratotic keratinocytes are called grains in the upper epidermis and corps ronds in the statum spinosum. A further feature is suprabasal loss of adhesion between keratinocytes (acantholysis), resulting in suprabasal clefting.

### Management

Patients should be advised on photoprotection, minimization of exacerbating factors, and wearing lightweight loose clothing. Urea or lactic acid–containing emollients may reduce crusting. Topical retinoids[66] can also be effective but irritation may limit their use. Emollient use and alternate-day application may be helpful to reduce irritation. Newer formulations of retinoids, such as tazarotene, may be better tolerated than older forms of retinoids.[67] Topical corticosteroids, although less effective as monotherapy than retinoids, may be useful in combination, because they calm the irritation associated with retinoid use. Reports testify to the efficacy of 5-fluorouracil.[68] Topical tacrolimus may be effective, even in extensive disease. Patients with DD tend to develop secondary infections that require disinfectants, antibiotics, antivirals, or antifungals. Treatment with oral retinoids, although characterized by relapse after cessation and limited by teratogenicity and side effects, is required for more extensive disease.[69,70] It may be possible to interrupt treatment in winter months. Many patients have prolonged remissions.

## Dermatomyositis

### Introduction

DM is an autoimmune disease of the skin and striated muscle. It is associated with an increased risk of malignancy, which is highest in the first 3 years after diagnosis of myositis but is increased for up to 5 years.[71]

### History

Although DM has been recognized since the late nineteenth century, Bohan and Peter compiled generally accepted diagnostic criteria in 1975.[72,73] Recent revisions of the classification no longer require muscle involvement for diagnosis.[74]

### Epidemiology

The incidence is 9 per million with a female predominance (3:1)[75] but no ethnic predilection. In Europe, an increasing prevalence of DM relative to polymyositis is seen with decreasing latitude,[76] and an association has been identified between surface UVR intensity and expression of anti-Mi2 autoantbodies.[77] Although DM may occur at any age, 2 peaks are seen: between the age of 5 and 10 years in children and in adults in the sixth decade.

### Pathogenesis

Antigen mimicry is theorized to be the pathogenic trigger for DM. It is driven by CD8+ T cells and is associated with other autoimmune diseases and viral infections. The primary target seems to be capillaries, with immunologic attack resulting in the development of foci of ischemic myocyte necrosis.

DM is frequently photoaggravated.[78,79] The pathogenesis of photosensitivity in DM and LE may overlap, because polymorphisms of TNF-$\alpha$[80] and increased keratinocyte apoptosis occur in both conditions.[81]

### Clinical manifestations

The skin and striated muscle may be affected to varying degrees, but both are typically involved. Cutaneous findings accompany muscle involvement in 60% of cases and precede it in 30%. In approximately 10% of cases, there is no muscle involvement, and this is described as DM sine myositis or amyopathic DM. Cutaneous findings include edematous, erythematous, or bluish-purple plaques and patches affecting the face and the V of the neck (**Fig. 4**). The characteristic heliotrope rash refers to a lilac discoloration of the eyelids with periorbital edema. Examination of the dorsum of the hands may demonstrate mauve linear plaques along the back of the fingers and dusky erythematous papules with atrophy,

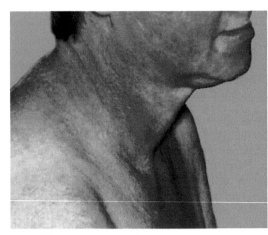

**Fig. 4.** Photoaggravation in dermatomyositis.

termed *Gottron papules*, over the joints. These Gottron papules represent a hyperkeratotic response to inflammation. The nail folds are hyperkeratotic with hemorrhage. Seen with capillary microscopy, the vessels in the nail folds are coiled and enlarged. Photosensitivity is seen with poikilodermatous change (telangiectasia, atrophy, and hyper- and hypopigmentation) of sun-exposed sites.

Proximal muscles tend to be most affected; the triceps and the quadriceps are symmetrically involved with slow onset of weakness and myalgia. Patients may have difficulty brushing their hair or getting up from a seated position. Only in advanced disease are distal muscles affected. Involvement of the pharyngeal muscles may occur and manifests as difficulty breathing or swallowing. Complications include pulmonary fibrosis, vasculitis, and myocarditis.

DM may be chronic or spontaneously remit in 2 to 3 years. If an underlying malignancy is present, removal can result in rapid resolution.

### Histology

A muscle biopsy demonstrates CD8+ T cells surrounding and infiltrating the muscle fibers with associated apoptosis, atrophy, regeneration, and hypertrophy. The primary target of immunologic attack seems to be capillaries resulting in the development of foci of ischemic myocyte necrosis. Deposition of antibodies and complement in the microvasculature precedes inflammation; the perifascicular atrophy of muscle fibers and inflammation support a microvascular pathology. Epidermal atrophy, a sparse lymphocytic infiltrate, and vacuolar interface change are seen. Findings on histology can be difficult to differentiate from LE. Examination of Gottron papules may demonstrate acanthosis and a dense, lichenoid infiltrate.

## Laboratory findings

A positive ANA is present in more than 90% of cases with specific antibodies against mRNP, PM-Scl, Mi2, and Jo1 found in approximately 30% of cases. Elevation of creatine kinase (also known as creatine phosphokinase) and aldolase indicates muscle involvement, and these enzyme levels can be monitored to track response to treatment. A muscle biopsy and electromyography confirm the diagnosis.

## Photobiologic evaluation

Routine photobiologic evaluation is not usually undertaken. Studies have indicated, however, that approximately 50% of patients with DM have a reduced UV-B minimal erythema dose (MED).[79] The action spectrum remains unknown.

## Management

Drug-induced DM, such as that seen with hydroxyurea, should be excluded. Photoprotection, including broad-spectrum sunscreen use, is advisable. First-line therapies for cutaneous disease include topical corticosteroids and antimalarials, such as hydroxychloroquine[82] or chloroquine. Muscle involvement requires prednisone, 1 mg/kg per day, with options for steroid-sparing agents, including methotrexate or azathioprine. High-dose intravenous immunoglobulin[83] may be warranted if there is failure to respond or significant muscle involvement.

## Lichen Planus Actinicus

### Introduction

Lichen planus (LP) actinicus is a variant of classical LP. It is triggered by UVR, resulting in skin lesions in a photodistributed pattern.

### Epidemiology

LP actinicus is seen more often in dark-skinned individuals in subtropical climates[84–89]; thus, this condition has also been termed LP subtropicus.[90]

### Pathogenesis

The exact pathogenesis is unknown, but UV seems to be a trigger in most cases, with artificial UV-B exposure sufficient to induce new lesions.[91] The relationship to UVR is further supported by the seasonal variation with exacerbation in summer and resolution in winter months.[85,89] Sun protection may suffice to induce remission.[86] Drug-induced LP and allergic contact dermatitis, which can also present as a photosensitive lichenoid eruption,[92] should be excluded. Photosensitive LP has also been described in association with human immunodeficiency virus (HIV).[93–95]

### Clinical manifestations

Lesions may resemble the violaceous, polygonal papules of classical LP, but morphologic variants described include melasma-like patches, dyschromic papules, and annular hyperpigmented plaques.[84,85,96,97] Areas affected include the forehead, face, neck, and dorsal hands. The lesions are usually pruritic. An earlier age at onset, ethnic predilection, and seasonal variation help distinguish LP actinicus from classical LP,[84,85,89] as does the absence of nail changes and Koebner phenomenon.

### Histology

Histology is identical to classical LP, the hallmark being lichenoid or interface dermatitis with a linear band of T cells along the basement membrane zone. Epidermal damage results in the normally smoothly undulating rete ridges becoming jagged or sawtooth-shaped. Anucleate, apoptotic basal keratinocytes, termed Civatte bodies, are seen. The histologic findings of LP may mimic erythema multiforme in these regards, but a distinguishing feature is the evidence of chronicity with epidermal hyperplasia, hypergranulosis, and hyperkeratosis seen in LP.

### Management

In addition to photoprotection, treatments with reported efficacy include hydroxychloroquine, acitretin, and topical corticosteroids.[88,90,98]

## Pellagra

### Introduction

Pellagra, meaning rough skin, refers to a triad of dermatitis, dementia, and diarrhea seen with niacin (vitamin $B_3$) deficiency.

### Epidemiology

Niacin deficiency is the result of nutritional deficiency and is seen with increased frequency among economically deprived communities where maize is the staple diet. In the setting of excess maize (corn) consumption, leucine, present in maize, interferes with the metabolism of niacin. In developed countries, it is seen among alcoholics and patients with chronic illnesses, such as HIV or protracted diarrheal illness, including carcinoid syndrome.

### Pathogenesis

Pellagra results from niacin deficiency. Niacin refers to both nicotinic acid and its active metabolites (eg, nicotinamide). In the form of nicotinamide, a coenzyme for both nicotinamide adenine dinucleotide (NAD) and NAD phosphate (NADP), it is essential for cellular metabolism. Niacin is present in grains, seed oils, and legumes and a small amount in meat. In some grains, such as corn, niacin is present but is in a bound, non-absorbable form. Due to tissue stores, there is a delay of months from the onset of dietary deficiency to the onset of symptoms. The pathogenic mechanisms underlying photosensitivity in pellagra remain to be understood. Theories include alterations in porphyrin metabolism, deficiency in NAD/NADP, cutaneous deficiency in urocanic acid, and an accumulation in kynurenic acid.[99]

### Clinical manifestations
The characteristic features of pellagra are dermatitis, dementia, and diarrhea, and the condition can be fatal if untreated. Dermatitis, the sole manifestation in 3% of patients, presents as bilaterally symmetric erythema and scaling on sun-exposed sites and on areas exposed to friction, pressure, or heat, such as the scrotum. At onset, erythema and roughening of the skin may predominate, replaced in later stages by thick scaling and desquamation. A well-demarcated erythema with thick scaling can be seen on the dorsum of the hands, and when present on the neck, is termed, *Casal necklace*. Painful fissures may be present on the palms and soles. Additional features include anorexia, nausea and vomiting, glossitis, muscle weakness, depression, and psychosis. It is important to consider pellagra in the context of an ill, malnourished patient in a hospital setting.

### Laboratory findings
The measurement of urinary excretion of niacin metabolites is the most reliable test. Serologic assays are neither sensitive nor specific.

### Management
Nicotinic acid can be replaced orally in mild cases and intravenously or intramuscularly in more advanced cases. When treatment is instituted, improvement is noted in days.

## Rosacea

### Introduction
Rosacea is a common skin condition in fair-skinned white populations, particularly in northern latitudes. The prevalence of rosacea in Ireland is in the range of 3% to 4%.[100,101]

### History
Papulopustular rosacea was the first subtype to be described by Robert Willan, a British physician, in the late eighteenth century.[102]

### Epidemiology
Rosacea, although it may occur at any age, typically occurs over the age of 40. Although rosacea is seen more frequently in women,[103] it manifests more severely in men. It is seen with increased frequency in patients with fair skin, Fitzpatrick types I and II, such as patients of Celtic origin.

### Pathogenesis
Pathologic factors include dysregulation of blood flow to the affected areas, *Demodex* colonization, induction of innate antimicrobial peptides, and chronic UV light exposure.

### Clinical manifestations
Papules and pustules are seen on a background of erythema and telangiectasia in a midfacial distribution involving the forehead, nose, cheeks, and chin. Unlike acne, comedones are not a feature. Papulopustular, erythematotelangiectatic, ocular, and phymatous subtypes exist, with rhinophyma a typical example of the latter. Lymphedema may also be a feature. Among those with rosacea, 60% report photoaggravation, although photo-testing on the back and face shows no abnormality, unless a patient is taking photosensitizing medications, such as doxycycline.[104] Hot drinks, spicy foods, alcohol, and emotional stress may trigger flushing that is initially sporadic but later persistent.

### Histology
The diagnosis is usually made clinically without the need for a skin biopsy; however, in cases where the diagnosis is uncertain, a skin biopsy may be useful to distinguish it from conditions, such as LE. Histologic findings in rosacea are nonspecific and only mild edema and vascular ectasia may be seen. A perivascular and perifollicular lymphohistiocytic infiltrate may be seen in the inflammatory papulopustular form.

### Management
Photoprotection and avoidance of triggers should be advised. Topical treatment options include metronidazole 1% cream or 0.75% gel[105–107] or azelaic acid 20% cream[108] and should be prescribed long term. Antibiotics are the mainstay of management and options include lymecycline (not available in the United States), erythromycin, and minocycline. Low-dose doxycycline (40 mg daily) may be effective and is prescribed frequently in the United States. Severe or refractory rosacea may respond to isotretinoin. If fulminant, a short course of oral steroids may be indicated in addition to isotretinoin. Laser ablation can be used for telangiectasias, and clonidine may be given to treat flushing, although the risk of rebound hypertension limits its use. Patients with ocular rosacea, present in 30%, need ophthalmologic referral due to the remote risk of blindness. Effective

treatment of rosacea usually abolishes the aggravation by UVR, although the fair skin of the individual still requires photoprotection.

## Smith-Lemli-Opitz Syndrome

Smith-Lemli-Opitz syndrome is a rare autosomal recessive disorder of cholesterol metabolism, resulting from an inborn deficiency of 7-dehydrocholesterol reductase. Excess metabolite results in intellectual disability and a range of physical and behavioral characteristics. Severe UV-A–mediated photosensitivity (peak at 350 nm) is a feature seen in more than 50% of patients with Smith-Lemli-Opitz syndrome.[109,110] The lack of a correlation between levels of 7-dehydrocholesterol and severity of photosensitivity suggests that the observed photosensitivity is not a direct phototoxic effect. A high cholesterol diet may reduce photosensitivity.[110]

## DISEASES SOMETIMES EXACERBATED BY UVR

### Atopic Dermatitis

Eczema presenting in a photosensitive distribution can represent photoaggravated atopic dermatitis (AD), drug-induced photosensitivity, or chronic actinic dermatitis. Positive monochromator light tests and photoprovocation testing using a solar simulator are useful to identify chronic actinic dermatitis. There is a subset of young adults with AD who have acquired photoaggravation and abnormal phototesting,[111,112] making it difficult in some cases to draw a clear distinction between photoaggravated AD and chronic actinic dermatitis.

In a retrospective study in the Netherlands of 3804 patients with eczema, 145 patients underwent phototesting due to a clinical suspicion of photosensitivity. Photoprovoked reactions occurred in 108 of these 145 patients (prevalence of 3% [ie, 108/3804]) with a reduced MED for UV-B in 8 patients (7%) and for UV-A in 5 patients (5%). Sensitivity to UV-A and UV-B was noted in 72 patients (67%) of the 108 patients who had a photoprovoked reaction, sensitivity to UV-B solely in 18 patients (17%), and sensitivity to UV-A solely in 18 patients (17%). In 51 patients (47%), this photoprovoked reaction consisted of an erthythematous, papular, pruritic reaction, developing within hours and resolving in days, resembling PMLE. These patients were diagnosed with AD and coexisting PMLE; 44 patients (41%) developed an eczematous photoprovoked reaction, which took days to develop and was more persistent, and 11 (10%) patients had a combination of both types of reactions.[113]

## Pemphigus

Pemphigus erythematosus (PE), also known as Sinear-Usher syndrome, is one of the 6 subtypes of pemphigus. PE affects all races and both genders. Although children can be affected, it most typically affects adults ages 50 to 60 years. PE is a rare condition in which pemphigus foliaceus (PF) occurs with a positive ANA, and it may represent an overlap of pemphigus and LE due to epitope spread. Blisters that tend to ooze, crust, and scale develop on chronically sun-exposed skin, such as the face and scalp. They can result in scarring and infection. There is an absence of blisters on mucous membranes, helping to differentiate this from other subtypes of pemphigus vulgaris. Similar to other forms of PF, the pathogenesis results from antibodies that attack desmosomes, which are the bridges that connect epidermal cells. Destruction of these connections results in the formations of blisters, which are superficial and, therefore, rupture easily (**Fig. 5**). PF can be photoaggravated,[114,115] as can pemphigus vulgaris.[116] Photoprotection should be advised to prevent exacerbation by UVR.

## Psoriasis

In the majority of patients with psoriasis, UV exposure improves disease control; however, a defined subset of patients, in the range of 5% to 20%, experiences exacerbation of psoriasis with UV

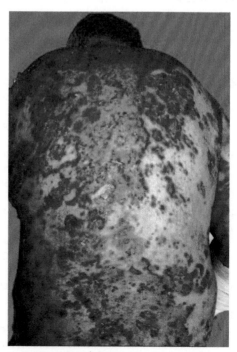

**Fig. 5.** Pemphigus foliaceus.

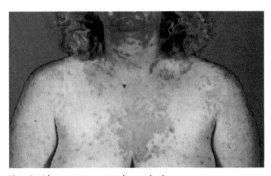

Fig. 6. Photoaggravated psoriasis.

exposure (Fig. 6).[117–119] This patient subset tends to be female of advanced age with a positive family history of psoriasis, with early age at onset of psoriasis, and with psoriasis affecting the dorsal surface of the hands.[118–120] There is a strong association with HLA-Cw*0602.[119] Approximately 50% develop PMLE after sun exposure with subsequent development of psoriasis within PMLE lesions, whereas the other 50% have photoaggravated psoriasis with no associated PMLE.[118] In the former group, PMLE preceding psoriasis is more easily provoked by UV-A, whereas UV-B is more effective in provoking photoaggravated psoriasis without PMLE.[121] Patients considered to have photoaggravated psoriasis should undergo confirmatory phototesting, and photoprotection is advisable.

## REFERENCES

1. Wadhwani AR, Sharma VK, Ramam M, et al. A clinical study of the spectrum of photodermatoses in dark-skinned populations. Clin Exp Dermatol 2013;38(8):823–9.
2. Hasan T, Nyberg F, Stephansson E, et al. Photosensitivity in lupus erythematosus, UV photoprovocation results compared with history of photosensitivity and clinical findings. Br J Dermatol 1997;136(5):699–705.
3. Murphy GM, Hawk JL. The prevalence of antinuclear antibodies in patients with apparent polymorphic light eruption. Br J Dermatol 1991;125(5): 448–51.
4. Cusack C, Danby C, Fallon JC, et al. Photoprotective behaviour and sunscreen use: impact on vitamin D levels in cutaneous lupus erythematosus. Photodermatol Photoimmunol Photomed 2008; 24(5):260–7.
5. Cazenave PL. Lupus erythemateux (erytheme centrifuge). Ann Mal Peau Syph 1851;3:297–9.
6. Dubois EL. Lupus erythematosus: a review of the current status of discoid and systematic lupus erythematosus and their variants. New York: McGraw-Hill, Blakiston Division; 1966.
7. Feldman CH, Hiraki LT, Liu J, et al. Epidemiology and sociodemographics of systemic lupus erythematosus and lupus nephritis among US adults with Medicaid coverage, 2000-2004. Arthritis Rheum 2013;65(3):753–63.
8. Gronhagen CM, Fored CM, Granath F, et al. Cutaneous lupus erythematosus and the association with systemic lupus erythematosus: a population-based cohort of 1088 patients in Sweden. Br J Dermatol 2011;164(6):1335–41.
9. Biazar C, Sigges J, Patsinakidis N, et al. Cutaneous lupus erythematosus: first multicenter database analysis of 1002 patients from the European Society of Cutaneous Lupus Erythematosus (EUSCLE). Autoimmun Rev 2013;12(3):444–54.
10. Scheinfeld N, Deleo VA. Photosensitivity in lupus erythematosus. Photodermatol Photoimmunol Photomed 2004;20(5):272–9.
11. Baer RL, Harber LC. Photobiology of lupus erythematosus. Arch Dermatol 1965;92:124–8.
12. Everett MA, Olson RL. Response of cutaneous lupus erythematosus to ultraviolet light. J Invest Dermatol 1965;44:133–8.
13. Lehmann P, Holzle E, Kind P, et al. Experimental reproduction of skin lesions in lupus erythematosus by UVA and UVB radiation. J Am Acad Dermatol 1990;22(2 Pt 1):181–7.
14. Ashok BT, Ali R. Antigen binding characteristics of experimentally-induced antibodies against hydroxyl radical modified native DNA. Autoimmunity 1999; 29(1):11–9.
15. Davis P, Russell AS, Percy JS. Antibodies to UV light denatured DNA in systemic lupus erythematosus: detection by filter radioimmunoassay and clinical correlations. J Rheumatol 1976;3(4):375–9.
16. Jones SK. Ultraviolet radiation (UVR) induces cell-surface Ro/SSA antigen expression by human keratinocytes in vitro: a possible mechanism for the UVR induction of cutaneous lupus lesions. Br J Dermatol 1992;126(6):546–53.
17. Golan TD, Elkon KB, Gharavi AE, et al. Enhanced membrane binding of autoantibodies to cultured keratinocytes of systemic lupus erythematosus patients after ultraviolet B/ultraviolet A irradiation. J Clin Invest 1992;90(3):1067–76.
18. Furukawa F, Kashihara-Sawami M, Lyons MB, et al. Binding of antibodies to the extractable nuclear antigens SS-A/Ro and SS-B/La is induced on the surface of human keratinocytes by ultraviolet light (UVL): implications for the pathogenesis of photosensitive cutaneous lupus. J Invest Dermatol 1990;94(1):77–85.
19. Bennion SD, Ferris C, Lieu TS, et al. IgG subclasses in the serum and skin in subacute cutaneous lupus erythematosus and neonatal lupus erythematosus. J Invest Dermatol 1990;95(6): 643–6.

20. Caricchio R, McPhie L, Cohen PL. Ultraviolet B radiation-induced cell death: critical role of ultraviolet dose in inflammation and lupus autoantigen redistribution. J Immunol 2003;171(11):5778–86.

21. Majai G, Kiss E, Tarr T, et al. Decreased apoptophagocytic gene expression in the macrophages of systemic lupus erythematosus patients. Lupus 2014;23:133–45.

22. Janko C, Schorn C, Grossmayer GE, et al. Inflammatory clearance of apoptotic remnants in systemic lupus erythematosus (SLE). Autoimmun Rev 2008;8(1):9–12.

23. Yu C, Chang C, Zhang J. Immunologic and genetic considerations of cutaneous lupus erythematosus: a comprehensive review. J Autoimmun 2013;41: 34–45.

24. Norris DA, Lyons MB, Middleton MH, et al. Ultraviolet radiation can either suppress or induce expression of intercellular adhesion molecule 1 (ICAM-1) on the surface of cultured human keratinocytes. J Invest Dermatol 1990;95(2):132–8.

25. Kuhn A, Fehsel K, Lehmann P, et al. Aberrant timing in epidermal expression of inducible nitric oxide synthase after UV irradiation in cutaneous lupus erythematosus. J Invest Dermatol 1998;111(1):149–53.

26. Millard TP, Kondeatis E, Cox A, et al. A candidate gene analysis of three related photosensitivity disorders: cutaneous lupus erythematosus, polymorphic light eruption and actinic prurigo. Br J Dermatol 2001;145(2):229–36.

27. Werth VP, Zhang W, Dortzbach K, et al. Association of a promoter polymorphism of tumor necrosis factor-alpha with subacute cutaneous lupus erythematosus and distinct photoregulation of transcription. J Invest Dermatol 2000;115(4):726–30.

28. Golan TD, Foltyn V, Roueff A. Increased susceptibility to in vitro ultraviolet B radiation in fibroblasts and lymphocytes cultured from systemic lupus erythematosus patients. Clin Immunol Immunopathol 1991;58(2):289–304.

29. Nived O, Johansen PB, Sturfelt G. Standardized ultraviolet-A exposure provokes skin reaction in systemic lupus erythematosus. Lupus 1993;2(4): 247–50.

30. Klein LR, Elmets CA, Callen JP. Photoexacerbation of cutaneous lupus erythematosus due to ultraviolet A emissions from a photocopier. Arthritis Rheum 1995;38(8):1152–6.

31. Rihner M, McGrath H Jr. Fluorescent light photosensitivity in patients with systemic lupus erythematosus. Arthritis Rheum 1992;35(8):949–52.

32. McGrath H Jr. Ultraviolet A1 (340-400 nm) irradiation and systemic lupus erythematosus. J Investig Dermatol Symp Proc 1999;4(1):79–84.

33. Molina JF, McGrath H Jr. Longterm ultraviolet-A1 irradiation therapy in systemic lupus erythematosus. J Rheumatol 1997;24(6):1072–4.

34. McGrath H, Martinez-Osuna P, Lee FA. Ultraviolet-A1 (340-400 nm) irradiation therapy in systemic lupus erythematosus. Lupus 1996;5(4):269–74.

35. Kuhn A, Sonntag M, Richter-Hintz D, et al. Phototesting in lupus erythematosus tumidus–review of 60 patients. Photochem Photobiol 2001;73(5):532–6.

36. Chlebus E, Wolska H, Blaszczyk M, et al. Subacute cutaneous lupus erythematosus versus systemic lupus erythematosus: diagnostic criteria and therapeutic implications. J Am Acad Dermatol 1998; 38(3):405–12.

37. Sanders CJ, Van Weelden H, Kazzaz GA, et al. Photosensitivity in patients with lupus erythematosus: a clinical and photobiological study of 100 patients using a prolonged phototest protocol. Br J Dermatol 2003;149(1):131–7.

38. Nyberg F, Hasan T, Puska P, et al. Occurrence of polymorphous light eruption in lupus erythematosus. Br J Dermatol 1997;136(2):217–21.

39. Tan EM, Cohen AS, Fries JF, et al. The 1982 revised criteria for the classification of systemic lupus erythematosus. Arthritis Rheum 1982; 25(11):1271–7.

40. Hochberg MC. Updating the American College of Rheumatology revised criteria for the classification of systemic lupus erythematosus. Arthritis Rheum 1997;40(9):1725.

41. Duarte-Garcia A, Fang H, To CH, et al. Seasonal variation in the activity of systemic lupus erythematosus. J Rheumatol 2012;39(7):1392–8.

42. Szeto CC, Mok HY, Chow KM, et al. Climatic influence on the prevalence of noncutaneous disease flare in systemic lupus erythematosus in Hong Kong. J Rheumatol 2008;35(6):1031–7.

43. Tsukazaki N, Watanabe M, Shimizu K, et al. Photoprovocation test and immunohistochemical analysis of inducible nitric oxide synthase expression in patients with Sjogren's syndrome associated with photosensitivity. Br J Dermatol 2002;147(6): 1102–8.

44. Stege H, Budde MA, Grether-Beck S, et al. Evaluation of the capacity of sunscreens to photoprotect lupus erythematosus patients by employing the photoprovocation test. Photodermatol Photoimmunol Photomed 2000;16(6):256–9.

45. Kuhn A, Gensch K, Haust M, et al. Photoprotective effects of a broad-spectrum sunscreen in ultraviolet-induced cutaneous lupus erythematosus: a randomized, vehicle-controlled, double-blind study. J Am Acad Dermatol 2011;64(1):37–48.

46. Seiger E, Roland S, Goldman S. Cutaneous lupus treated with topical tretinoin: a case report. Cutis 1991;47(5):351–5.

47. Neri R, Mosca M, Bernacchi E, et al. A case of SLE with acute, subacute and chronic cutaneous lesions successfully treated with Dapsone. Lupus 1999;8(3):240–3.

48. Duong DJ, Spigel GT, Moxley RT 3rd, et al. American experience with low-dose thalidomide therapy for severe cutaneous lupus erythematosus. Arch Dermatol 1999;135(9):1079–87.

49. Newton RC, Jorizzo JL, Solomon AR Jr, et al. Mechanism-oriented assessment of isotretinoin in chronic or subacute cutaneous lupus erythematosus. Arch Dermatol 1986;122(2):170–6.

50. Schanz S, Ulmer A, Rassner G, et al. Successful treatment of subacute cutaneous lupus erythematosus with mycophenolate mofetil. Br J Dermatol 2002;147(1):174–8.

51. Kreuter A, Tomi NS, Weiner SM, et al. Mycophenolate sodium for subacute cutaneous lupus erythematosus resistant to standard therapy. Br J Dermatol 2007;156(6):1321–7.

52. Torchia D, Caproni M, Massi D, et al. Paraneoplastic toxic epidermal necrolysis-like subacute cutaneous lupus erythematosus. Clin Exp Dermatol 2010;35(4):455–6.

53. Darier J. De la psorospermose folliculaire vegetante. Ann Dermatol Syphiligr 1889;10:597–612.

54. White J. A case of keratosis (ichthyosis) follicularis. J Cutan Genito-Urin Dis 1889;7:201–9.

55. White J. Keratosis follicularis (psorospermose folliculaire vegetante). A second case. J Cutan Genito-Urin Dis 1890;8:13–20.

56. Munro CS. The phenotype of Darier's disease: penetrance and expressivity in adults and children. Br J Dermatol 1992;127(2):126–30.

57. Svendsen IB, Albrectsen B. The prevalence of dyskeratosis follicularis (Darier's disease) in Denmark: an investigation of the heredity in 22 families. Acta Derm Venereol 1959;39:256–69.

58. Hovnanian A. Darier's disease: from dyskeratosis to endoplasmic reticulum calcium ATPase deficiency. Biochem Biophys Res Commun 2004; 322(4):1237–44.

59. Dhitavat J, Dode L, Leslie N, et al. Mutations in the sarcoplasmic/endoplasmic reticulum Ca2+ ATPase isoform cause Darier's disease. J Invest Dermatol 2003;121(3):486–9.

60. Baba T, Yaoita H. UV radiation and keratosis follicularis. Arch Dermatol 1984;120(11):1484–7.

61. Mayuzumi N, Ikeda S, Kawada H, et al. Effects of ultraviolet B irradiation, proinflammatory cytokines and raised extracellular calcium concentration on the expression of ATP2A2 and ATP2C1. Br J Dermatol 2005;152(4):697–701.

62. Burge SM, Wilkinson JD. Darier-White disease: a review of the clinical features in 163 patients. J Am Acad Dermatol 1992;27(1):40–50.

63. Telfer NR, Burge SM, Ryan TJ. Vesiculo-bullous Darier's disease. Br J Dermatol 1990;122(6):831–4.

64. Macleod RI, Munro CS. The incidence and distribution of oral lesions in patients with Darier's disease. Br Dent J 1991;171(5):133–6.

65. Hedblad MA, Nakatani T, Beitner H. Ultrastructural changes in Darier's disease induced by ultraviolet irradiation. Acta Derm Venereol 1991;71(2):108–12.

66. Burge SM, Buxton PK. Topical isotretinoin in Darier's disease. Br J Dermatol 1995;133(6):924–8.

67. Burkhart CG, Burkhart CN. Tazarotene gel for Darier's disease. J Am Acad Dermatol 1998; 38(6 Pt 1):1001–2.

68. Schmidt H, Ochsendorf FR, Wolter M, et al. Topical 5-fluorouracil in Darier disease. Br J Dermatol 2008;158(6):1393–6.

69. Burge S. Darier's disease–the clinical features and pathogenesis. Clin Exp Dermatol 1994; 19(3):193–205.

70. Christophersen J, Geiger JM, Danneskiold-Samsoe P, et al. A double-blind comparison of acitretin and etretinate in the treatment of Darier's disease. Acta Derm Venereol 1992;72(2):150–2.

71. Buchbinder R, Forbes A, Hall S, et al. Incidence of malignant disease in biopsy-proven inflammatory myopathy. A population-based cohort study. Ann Intern Med 2001;134(12):1087–95.

72. Bohan A, Peter JB. Polymyositis and dermatomyositis (first of two parts). N Engl J Med 1975;292(7): 344–7.

73. Bohan A, Peter JB. Polymyositis and dermatomyositis (second of two parts). N Engl J Med 1975; 292(8):403–7.

74. Sontheimer RD. Cutaneous features of classic dermatomyositis and amyopathic dermatomyositis. Curr Opin Rheumatol 1999;11(6):475–82.

75. Bendewald MJ, Wetter DA, Li X, et al. Incidence of dermatomyositis and clinically amyopathic dermatomyositis: a population-based study in Olmsted County, Minnesota. Arch Dermatol 2010;146(1):26–30.

76. Hengstman GJ, van Venrooij WJ, Vencovsky J, et al. The relative prevalence of dermatomyositis and polymyositis in Europe exhibits a latitudinal gradient. Ann Rheum Dis 2000;59(2):141–2.

77. Okada S, Weatherhead E, Targoff IN, et al. Global surface ultraviolet radiation intensity may modulate the clinical and immunologic expression of autoimmune muscle disease. Arthritis Rheum 2003;48(8): 2285–93.

78. Cheong WK, Hughes GR, Norris PG, et al. Cutaneous photosensitivity in dermatomyositis. Br J Dermatol 1994;131(2):205–8.

79. Dourmishev L, Meffert H, Piazena H. Dermatomyositis: comparative studies of cutaneous photosensitivity in lupus erythematosus and normal subjects. Photodermatol Photoimmunol Photomed 2004; 20(5):230–4.

80. Werth VP, Callen JP, Ang G, et al. Associations of tumor necrosis factor alpha and HLA polymorphisms with adult dermatomyositis: implications for a unique pathogenesis. J Invest Dermatol 2002;119(3):617–20.

81. Pablos JL, Santiago B, Galindo M, et al. Keratinocyte apoptosis and p53 expression in cutaneous lupus and dermatomyositis. J Pathol 1999;188(1): 63–8.

82. Woo TY, Callen JP, Voorhees JJ, et al. Cutaneous lesions of dermatomyositis are improved by hydroxychloroquine. J Am Acad Dermatol 1984; 10(4):592–600.

83. Dalakas MC, Illa I, Dambrosia JM, et al. A controlled trial of high-dose intravenous immune globulin infusions as treatment for dermatomyositis. N Engl J Med 1993;329(27):1993–2000.

84. Isaacson D, Turner ML, Elgart ML. Summertime actinic lichenoid eruption (lichen planus actinicus). J Am Acad Dermatol 1981;4(4):404–11.

85. Katzenellenbogen I. Lichen planus actinicus (lichen planus in subtropical countries). Dermatologica 1962;124:10–20.

86. Bedi TR. Summertime actinic lichenoid eruption. Dermatologica 1978;157(2):115–25.

87. Verhagen AR, Koten JW. Lichenoid melanodermatitis. A clinicopathological study of fifty-one Kenyan patients with so-called tropical lichen planus. Br J Dermatol 1979;101(6):651–8.

88. Zanca A. Lichen planus actinicus. Int J Dermatol 1978;17(6):506–8.

89. Dostrovsky A, Sagher F. Lichen planus in subtropical countries; study of an annular type with inverse localization (uncovered surfaces of the skin). Arch Derm Syphilol 1949;59(3):308–28.

90. Kilaimy M. Lichen planus subtropicus. Arch Dermatol 1976;112(9):1251–3.

91. van der Schroeff JG, Schothorst AA, Kanaar P. Induction of actinic lichen planus with artificial UV sources. Arch Dermatol 1983;119(6):498–500.

92. Verma KK, Sirka CS, Ramam M, et al. Parthenium dermatitis presenting as photosensitive lichenoid eruption. A new clinical variant. Contact Derm 2002;46(5):286–9.

93. Fitzgerald E, Purcell SM, Goldman HM. Photodistributed hypertrophic lichen planus in association with acquired immunodeficiency syndrome: a distinct entity. Cutis 1995;55(2):109–11.

94. Berger TG, Dhar A. Lichenoid photoeruptions in human immunodeficiency virus infection. Arch Dermatol 1994;130(5):609–13.

95. Bilu D, Mamelak AJ, Nguyen RH, et al. Clinical and epidemiologic characterization of photosensitivity in HIV-positive individuals. Photodermatol Photoimmunol Photomed 2004;20(4):175–83.

96. Salman SM, Kibbi AG, Zaynoun S. Actinic lichen planus. A clinicopathologic study of 16 patients. J Am Acad Dermatol 1989;20(2 Pt 1):226–31.

97. Salman SM, Khallouf R, Zaynoun S. Actinic lichen planus mimicking melasma. A clinical and histopathologic study of three cases. J Am Acad Dermatol 1988;18(2 Pt 1):275–8.

98. Jansen T, Gambichler T, von Kobyletzki L, et al. Lichen planus actinicus treated with acitretin and topical corticosteroids. J Eur Acad Dermatol Venereol 2002;16(2):174–5.

99. Wan P, Moat S, Anstey A. Pellagra: a review with emphasis on photosensitivity. Br J Dermatol 2011; 164(6):1188–200.

100. Gibson GE, Codd MB, Murphy GM. Skin type distribution and skin disease in Ireland. Ir J Med Sci 1997;166(2):72–4.

101. McAleer MA, Fitzpatrick P, Powell FC. Papulopustular rosacea: prevalence and relationship to photodamage. J Am Acad Dermatol 2010;63(1):33–9.

102. Robert Willan. On cutaneous diseases. Vol. 1. London: Printed for J.Johnson, 180

103. Berg M, Liden S. An epidemiological study of rosacea. Acta Derm Venereol 1989;69(5):419–23.

104. Murphy G. Ultraviolet light and rosacea. Cutis 2004;74(3 Suppl):13–6, 32–4.

105. Nielsen PG. A double-blind study of I% metronidazole cream versus systemic oxytetracycline therapy for rosacea. Br J Dermatol 1983;109(1):63–5.

106. Jorizzo JL, Lebwohl M, Tobey RE. The efficacy of metronidazole 1% cream once daily compared with metronidazole 1% cream twice daily and their vehicles in rosacea: a double-blind clinical trial. J Am Acad Dermatol 1998;39(3):502–4.

107. Dahl MV, Katz HI, Krueger GG, et al. Topical metronidazole maintains remissions of rosacea. Arch Dermatol 1998;134(6):679–83.

108. Bjerke R, Fyrand O, Graupe K. Double-blind comparison of azelaic acid 20% cream and its vehicle in treatment of papulo-pustular rosacea. Acta Derm Venereol 1999;79(6):456–9.

109. Anstey AV, Ryan A, Rhodes LE, et al. Characterization of photosensitivity in the Smith-Lemli-Opitz syndrome: a new congenital photosensitivity syndrome. Br J Dermatol 1999;141(3):406–14.

110. Anstey AV, Taylor CR. Photosensitivity in the Smith-Lemli-Opitz syndrome: the US experience of a new congenital photosensitivity syndrome. J Am Acad Dermatol 1999;41(1):121–3.

111. Ogboli MI, Rhodes LE. Chronic actinic dermatitis in young atopic dermatitis sufferers. Br J Dermatol 2000;142(3):845.

112. Russell SC, Dawe RS, Collins P, et al. The photosensitivity dermatitis and actinic reticuloid syndrome (chronic actinic dermatitis) occurring in seven young atopic dermatitis patients. Br J Dermatol 1998;138(3):496–501.

113. ten Berge O, van Weelden H, Bruijnzeel-Koomen CA, et al. Throwing a light on photosensitivity in atopic dermatitis: a retrospective study. Am J Clin Dermatol 2009;10(2):119–23.

114. Igawa K, Matsunaga T, Nishioka K. Involvement of UV-irradiation in pemphigus foliaceus. J Eur Acad Dermatol Venereol 2004;18(2):216–7.

115. Kano Y, Shimosegawa M, Mizukawa Y, et al. Pemphigus foliaceus induced by exposure to sunlight. Report of a case and analysis of photochallenge-induced lesions. Dermatology 2000;201(2):132–8.

116. Reis VM, Toledo RP, Lopez A, et al. UVB-induced acantholysis in endemic pemphigus foliaceus (fogo selvagem) and pemphigus vulgaris. J Am Acad Dermatol 2000;42(4):571–6.

117. Farber EM, Bright RD, Nall ML. Psoriasis. A questionnaire survey of 2,144 patients. Arch Dermatol 1968;98(3):248–59.

118. Ros AM, Eklund G. Photosensitive psoriasis. An epidemiologic study. J Am Acad Dermatol 1987; 17(5 Pt 1):752–8.

119. Rutter KJ, Watson RE, Cotterell LF, et al. Severely photosensitive psoriasis: a phenotypically defined patient subset. J Invest Dermatol 2009;129(12):2861–7.

120. Nalluri R, Arun B, Rhodes LE. Photoaggravated hand and foot psoriasis. Photodermatol Photoimmunol Photomed 2010;26(5):261–2.

121. Ros AM, Wennersten G. Photosensitive psoriasis—clinical findings and phototest results. Photodermatol 1986;3(6):317–26.

# UV-Based Therapy

Mariam B. Totonchy, MD[a], Melvin W. Chiu, MD, MPH[b],*

## KEYWORDS

- Phototherapy - Narrowband UVB - PUVA - UV-A1 - Excimer - Psoralen - Psoriasis - UV therapy

## KEY POINTS

- UV phototherapy is a useful tool in several common and rare dermatoses.
- Because of its more favorable side-effect profile, narrowband UV-B has supplanted psoralen and UV-A light (PUVA) as the first-line treatment in photo-responsive dermatoses; although for some, PUVA may have superior efficacy.
- Excimer phototherapy has proven to be an excellent option in the treatment of localized photo-responsive dermatoses.
- UV-A1 has emerged as a useful therapeutic option, especially for sclerotic skin disorders, with an improved side-effect profile over PUVA.

## INTRODUCTION

UV phototherapy has become increasingly influential as a therapeutic modality in dermatology. UV radiation is divided into UV-C (200–290 nm), UV-B (290–320 nm), and UV-A (320–400 nm). UV-A is further divided into UV-A1 (340–400 nm) and UV-A2 (320–340 nm) (**Table 1**). The authors specifically focus on the main types of UV therapy used for the treatment of dermatologic conditions: narrowband UV-B (NB–U-VB), excimer laser, psoralen and UV-A light (PUVA) photochemotherapy, and finally UV-A1.

## HISTORY

Although targeted UV therapies have emerged more recently, the use of sunlight for the treatment of skin disease dates back as far as 2000 to 1400 BC in India and Egypt, where psoralen and the plant *Ammi majus*, in combination with sun exposure, were used to treat vitiligo.[1,2] In 1947, Fahmy and collaborators[3-5] isolated 8-methoxypsoralen (8-MOP) from *Ammi majus* and used it along with sunlight to treat vitiligo. In the 1960s, topical and oral 8-MOP were used with UV radiation for the

treatment of psoriasis.[6] Shortly after, UV-A tubes were used for total body irradiation in combination with topical 8-MOP. Although topical 8-MOP was shown to be effective with UV-A tubes, the output of these tubes was still ineffective with orally administered 8-MOP. In the landmark trial performed by Parrish and colleagues[7] in 1974, a novel type of high-intensity UV-A tube was used for the treatment of psoriasis with oral 8-MOP. This development marked the beginning of PUVA for the treatment of psoriasis.

In 1925, Goeckerman[8] found that UV radiation from mercury quartz lamps in combination with crude tar oil was more effective for the treatment of psoriasis than either treatment alone. This finding formed the basis for UV therapy for psoriasis, commonly used worldwide, for many subsequent decades.[8] In 1953, Ingram[9] described the standard treatment of psoriasis in England with tar, UV radiation, and dithranol. In the 1960s, Wiskemann[10] introduced broadband (BB) UV-B using a filtered wavelength of UV-B light as opposed to the unfiltered UV radiation from the mercury quartz lamp. In 1978, Wiskemann[10] used BB–UV-B to treat psoriasis, and Gilchrest and colleagues[11]

Funding Sources: None.

Conflicts of Interest: None.

[a] Department of Dermatology, Yale School of Medicine, New Haven, CT, USA; [b] Division of Dermatology, Department of Medicine, David Geffen School of Medicine at UCLA, 52-121 Center for the Health Sciences, 10833 Le Conte Avenue, Los Angeles, CA 90095, USA

* Corresponding author.

*E-mail address:* mchiu@mednet.ucla.edu

Dermatol Clin 32 (2014) 399–413

http://dx.doi.org/10.1016/j.det.2014.03.003

derm.theclinics.com

**Table 1**
**UV spectrum (10–400 nm)**

| Abbreviation | Wavelength (nm) |
|---|---|
| UV-A | 320–400 |
| UV-A1 | 340–400 |
| UV-A2 | 320–340 |
| UV-B | 290–320 |
| UV-C | 200–290 |

began using BB–UV-B for the treatment of uremic pruritus. However, BB–UV-B was not as effective as PUVA for psoriasis therapy. In the early 1980s, the most effective UV-B wavelengths for the treatment of psoriasis were examined under closer scrutiny, showing a peak action spectrum at 313 nm.[12–14] NB–UV-B (311–313 nm) lamps were ultimately developed and were proven to be more effective than conventional BB–UV-B in treating psoriasis.[15,16] NB–UV-B has subsequently replaced BB–UV-B as the first-line therapy for psoriasis treatment.

UV-A1 was introduced in the early 1990s for treatment of atopic dermatitis.[17] Because UV-A1 has a longer wavelength, 340 to 400 nm, it is able to penetrate deeper than UV-B, reaching the deep dermal components of the skin. It has been shown to effectively upregulate matrix metalloproteinases. It has, therefore, been targeted for use in skin conditions with a predominantly dermal component, with particular emphasis placed on sclerotic diseases of the skin.[18]

## UV-B
### Mechanism of Action

UV-B alters cytokines within the skin, induces apoptosis, promotes immunosuppression, causes DNA damage, and decreases the proliferation of dendritic cells and other cells of the innate immune system. The skin contains 3 main types of helper T cells: Th1, Th2, and Th17. In psoriasis, there is thought to be an overactivity of Th1 and Th17 cells, increasing cytokines produced by these helper T cells, which in turn increase inflammation in the skin and hyperproliferation of keratinocytes.[19,20] In contrast, Th2-related cytokines, such as interleukin (IL)-10, are relatively decreased, whereas Th1 cytokines IL-12 and tumor necrosis factor (TNF)-alpha are elevated as compared with normal skin.[19,20] UV-B is thought to counterbalance this by upregulating IL-10 and downregulating IL-12.[21,22] NB–UV-B has been found to suppress the Th1/Th17 cytokines IL-12, IL-17, and interferon (IFN)-gamma while increasing Th2 cytokine IL-4 in psoriatic lesions.[23–26] IL-4 suppresses pathways activated by Th1/Th17 cells, thus, contributing to the therapeutic effects of NB–UV-B. NB–UV-B has also been shown to isomerize urocanic acid (UCA) from the *trans* to the *cis* form; it not only acts to change the skin from a Th1 to a Th2 environment but also causes generalized UV-induced immunosuppression.[27–29]

Another way NB–UV-B therapy exerts its action is by promoting apoptosis in T cells and keratinocytes in psoriatic lesions.[30–32] Although Langerhans cells decrease in number following NB–UV-B therapy, the mechanism of their depletion remains unclear; a possible explanation is thought to relate to their migration away from the epidermis into the lymph nodes rather than through apoptotic mechanisms.[33–35] NB–UV-B has also been shown to induce DNA damage and disrupt lipid membranes, cellular content, and cellular cytoskeleton, which can lead to cell cycle arrest and cell death at high enough doses. UV-B not only decreases the number of Langerhans cells in the epidermis but also decreases their functionality,[33,34,36–38] depletes T cells,[30] decreases inflammatory dendritic cells,[23] and suppresses the contact hypersensitivity reaction, which is thought to be a measure of T-cell activity.[39–42] Long-term, low-dose UV-B therapy has been shown to suppress the mixed epidermal cell lymphocyte reaction used to measure immune responsiveness.[36,43] UV-B phototherapy has also been implicated in increasing regulatory T cells that can prevent immune system activation.[44] The excimer laser at 308 nm also induces T-cell apoptosis and does so more efficiently than NB–UV-B.[45]

### Modes of Delivery

#### BB–UV-B phototherapy
BB–UV-B phototherapy (280–320 nm) was the first type of restricted UV wavelength phototherapy used to treat psoriasis. In one study, 18 out of 20 patients with psoriasis achieved clearance with BB–UV-B 3 times weekly for a total of 10 to 38 treatments.[46] A similar study using erythemogenic doses of home-based UV-B achieved resolution of psoriasis in 20 out of 28 patients.[47]

#### NB–UV-B phototherapy
Beginning in the late 1990s, BB–UV-B has been gradually replaced by NB–UV-B (311–313 nm), which has proven to be safer and more efficacious, with faster clearance rates and longer remission than BB–UV-B for the treatment of psoriasis.[48–52] NB–UV-B causes a greater degree of T-cell depletion in psoriatic lesions as compared with BB–UV-B, likely because of deeper penetration of NB–UV-B into the dermis. With NB–UV-B,

a greater amount of energy can be delivered with less potential for burning.[31] In fact, Schindl and colleagues[53] compared apoptosis of epidermal cells following varying doses of UV radiation and found that about 5 to 10 times higher doses of BB–UV-B were required to cause comparable amounts of cell death compared with NB–UV-B. Because NB–UV-B is more efficient in clearing psoriasis, it requires a lower minimal erythema dose (MED) equivalent of fluence to clear psoriasis as compared with BB–UV-B.[54] Depletion of Langerhans cells and apoptosis of epidermal T cells as well as mast cells seem to be less following exposure to BB–UV-B as compared with NB–UV-B.[30,31,48,55] Lastly, NB–UV-B also has been shown to be more effective at isomerization of UCA from *trans* to *cis* isomer and overall is more immunosuppressive of innate immune cells as well as cytokine responses when compared with BB–UV-B.[55,56] Therefore, treatment with NB–UV-B is emphasized in this issue, given that BB–UV-B is almost no longer used in practice.

## Targeted Phototherapy: Excimer Lasers and Lamps

The excimer (308 nm) lasers and lamps have become increasingly popular in the last decade, as they allow for targeted phototherapy treatment with high doses of 308 nm light. Although excimer lamps, emitting incoherent output with a peak at 308 nm, are used in Europe and Asia, they are not available in the United States. Therefore, this section focuses on excimer laser only.

With NB–UV-B, both diseased and normal skin is irradiated; however, the excimer laser is able to target only the involved skin. The excimer laser is, therefore, more selective and delivers short impulses with higher intensity than NB–UV-B, giving a more rapid response. However, when treating large body surface areas, the excimer laser can be quite labor intensive and time consuming.

## Indications

Common indications for NB–UV-B phototherapy are psoriasis, vitiligo,[57,58] atopic dermatitis, mycosis fungoides, and pruritus (**Table 2**).

## Contraindications

NB–UV-B is contraindicated in those with lupus erythematous, basal cell nevus syndrome, or xeroderma pigmentosum. Patients with Fitzpatrick skin types I and II should undergo UV-B therapy with greater caution given their tendency to burn.

**Table 2**
**Phototherapy indications**

| NB–UV-B | PUVA | UV-A1 |
|---|---|---|
| Common | Common | Common |
| Psoriasis | Psoriasis | Morphea |
| Vitiligo | Vitiligo | Lichen sclerosis |
| Atopic dermatitis | Atopic dermatitis | Atopic dermatitis |
| Mycosis fungoides | Mycosis fungoides | Less common |
| Pruritus (associated with renal disease, polycythemia vera) | Less common | Cutaneous graft-versus-host disease |
| Less common | Alopecia areata | Cutaneous mastocytosis |
| Acquired perforating dermatosis | Cutaneous graft-versus-host disease | Granuloma annulare |
| Chronic urticarial | Cutaneous mastocytosis | Lichen planus |
| Cutaneous graft-versus-host disease | Polymorphous light eruption | Mycosis fungoides |
| Polymorphous light eruption | Dermatitis herpetiformis | Necrobiosis lipoidica |
| Cutaneous mastocytosis | Dyshidrotic eczema | Pityriasis lichenoides |
| Granuloma annulare | Granuloma annulare | Sarcoidosis |
| Lichen planus | Histiocytosis | Systemic lupus erythematosus |
| Lichen simplex chronicus | Lichen planus | |
| Lymphomatoid papulosis | Lichen sclerosis | |
| Parapsoriasis | Morphea | |
| Pityriasis lichenoides | Pityriasis rosea | |
| Pityriasis rosea | Urticaria | |
| Pityriasis rubra pilaris | | |
| Seborrheic dermatitis | | |

*Adapted from* Walker D, Jacobe H. Phototherapy in the age of biologics. Semin Cutan Med Surg 2011;30(4):190–8; with permission.

Patients with a history of arsenic ingestion, radiation exposure, melanoma or nonmelanoma skin cancers, or anyone with a medical condition that makes standing for long periods of time or in an enclosed space difficult should exercise caution.[54] Although phototherapy is considered a safe treatment option for those with a personal history of nonmelanoma skin cancer, patients with multiple nonmelanoma skin cancers or with a personal history of melanoma should consider other treatment options.

### Treatment Protocol

Table 3 lists a general protocol for treatment with NB–UV-B. When receiving treatment, patients should be instructed to use goggles and use genital shields in male patients. MED to NB–UV-B (MED-B) can vary widely depending on skin type, so MED-B testing is recommended before beginning treatment. UV-B therapy can be initiated 24 hours after MED testing. However, MED testing can be time consuming and labor intensive; approval for insurance coverage can be quite laborious, so the initial dose can be based on skin type. The

frequency of treatment with NB–UV-B should be 3 times a week, as no statistical difference in efficacy was seen between 3 and 5 times per week.[59–61] Treatment 3 times a week, with low incremental increases in dose, helps minimize toxicities and the total UV-B exposure dose. The initial UV-B dose should be between 50% and 70% of MED, which has been found to have maximum efficacy and safety in both dark- and light-skinned patients.[29,62] In a randomized, double-blind comparison, Kleinpenning and colleagues[63] tested high-dose NB–UV-B (0.7 MED, 40% incremental increases) against low-dose NB–UV-B (0.35 MED, 20% incremental increases) and found that there was no statistically significant difference in the number of patients who achieved clearance or in cumulative doses of UV-B. They did find, however, that on average the high-dose patients required fewer treatments than the low-dose patients at 20.6 versus 24.1 total treatments, respectively.

The goal of NB–UV-B treatment is to maintain a mild amount of erythema for optimal results.[64] Although some studies suggest 40% MED

---

**Table 3**
**NB–UV-B treatment protocols[a,b]**

| | | Treatment by Skin Type | | |
| Skin Type | Initial Dose (mJ/cm$^2$) | Subsequent Increase in Dose (mJ/cm$^2$) | Estimated Goal (mJ/cm$^2$) | Maximum Dose (mJ/cm$^2$) |
| --- | --- | --- | --- | --- |
| I | 50–120 | 15–50 | 520 | 2000 |
| II | 100–220 | 25–50 | 880 | 2000 |
| III | 200–260 | 30–50 | 1040 | 3000 |
| IV | 250–330 | 45–75 | 1320 | 3000 |
| V | 300–350 | 50–100 | 1400 | 5000 |
| VI | 350–400 | 50–100 | 1600 | 5000 |
| Vitiligo | Treat as skin type I | | | |

Treatment by MED
  Initial dose: 50% MED
  Treatments 1–20 increase dose by 10% of initial MED
  Treatments 21+ increase dose per discretion of ordering physician
Next treatment if treatments are missed for
  <7 d: keep same dose per protocol
  1–2 wk: decrease dose by 25%
  2–3 wk: decrease dose by 50% or start over
  >3 wk: start over
Maintenance regimen after satisfactory clearance
  2 times per wk for 4 wk: same dose
  1 time per wk for 4 wk: same dose
  1 time per 2 wk for 4 wk: decrease dose by 25%
  1 time per 4 wk: decrease dose by 50%

[a] This protocol is a representative protocol for psoriasis and vitiligo. Although no consensus exists, NB–UV-B phototherapy protocols for other indications are generally similar to those used in psoriasis.

*Adapted from* Menter A, Korman NJ, Elmets CA, et al. Guidelines of care for the management of psoriasis and psoriatic arthritis: section 5. Guidelines of care for the treatment of psoriasis with phototherapy and photochemotherapy. J Am Acad Dermatol 2010;62(1):118; with permission.

increases, others have found incremental increases of 5% to 10% are equally effective as high-dose incremental increases.[61,63,65]

If combined with acitretin, this medication should be started about 2 weeks before the initiation of phototherapy. The standard dosage is 25 to 50 mg/d for patients that are 70 kg or more. For those that are less than 70 kg, 10 mg/d is the suggested dosage. The initial dose of phototherapy should be reduced to 25% the normal dose with NB–UV-B monotherapy.[54] If acitretin is started while patients are receiving NB–UV-B, the NB–UV-B dose should be decreased by 33%, and then increased at 5% to 15% per treatment as tolerated.

Although some suggest maintenance therapy with NB–UV-B may allow for a longer length of remission,[66] there are no agreed-on guidelines for the use of long-term NB–UV-B maintenance therapy.[67] Therefore, maintenance therapy tends to be left to the discretion of the clinician, taking into account the patients' response to treatment, severity of the disease, and access/ease of undergoing additional treatments. Generally, once satisfactory clearance is achieved, the treatment frequency is decreased with concordant decreases in dosing (see **Table 3**).[68]

Lastly, it is important to calibrate the NB–UV-B phototherapy booth at least once weekly. The output of the lamps can slowly decay; so if output is not measured regularly, undertreatment of patients may occur.[54] However, all the currently marketed units, with the notable exception of home phototherapy units, have internal meters that measure the output as the dose is being delivered and, hence, will internally adjust the treatment time as the output decreases.

For the excimer laser, treatment sessions are typically performed 2 to 3 times per week, with a minimum of 48 hours between treatments, for a period of 3 to 6 weeks for psoriasis.[69] Maintenance therapy with excimer may also be valuable depending on the extent of the disease burden, willingness or availability of patients to undergo further treatments, and insurance approval. A maintenance protocol was tested in a study of 5 patients with psoriasis achieving 75% improvement in Psoriasis Area and Severity Index (PASI) score after 15 treatments of biweekly excimer laser therapy. The maintenance therapy consisted of one treatment per week for 4 weeks, then one treatment every other week for 4 weeks, and finally one treatment 4 weeks later, for a total of 7 maintenance treatments. No flares (defined as 25% worsening over baseline) were noted after the first month of taper; during the taper period, all patients maintained a 50% improvement in PASI score.[70] **Table 4** describes the recommended treatment regimens for excimer laser.

**Table 4**
**Excimer laser treatment protocol[a,b]**

| | Initial Dose for Psoriasis | |
|---|---|---|
| Plaque Thickness | Fitzpatrick Skin Type I–III (Dose in mJ/cm$^2$) | Fitzpatrick Skin Type IV–VI (Dose in mJ/cm$^2$) |
| Mild | 500 | 400 |
| Moderate | 500 | 600 |
| Severe | 700 | 900 |
| | Dose for Subsequent Treatments | | | | |
| Effect | No Effect with No Erythema | Minimal Effect with Mild Erythema | Good Effect with Mild to Moderate Erythema | Considerable Improvement | Moderate to Severe Erythema (±Blistering) |
| Dosing recommendation | Increase dose by 25% | Increase dose by 15% | Maintain dose | Maintain dose or reduce dose by 15% | Skip treatment or treat nonblistered area with reduced dose by 25% |

[a] Excimer treatment protocol for vitiligo is similar to that for psoriasis, with treatments occurring 2 to 3 times per week, with a minimum of 48 hours between treatments, for a period of 4 to 36 weeks.

*Adapted from* Menter A, Korman NJ, Elmets CA, et al. Guidelines of care for the management of psoriasis and psoriatic arthritis: section 5. Guidelines of care for the treatment of psoriasis with phototherapy and photochemotherapy. J Am Acad Dermatol 2010;62(1):124; with permission.

## Expected Outcome

It typically takes 20 to 36 treatments to see significant improvement for moderate to severe psoriasis treatment with NB–UV-B.[71] Psoriasis treatment with NB–UV-B typically achieves clearance rates in the 60% to 70% range.[49,72–76] With excimer laser, one can expect clearance after 8 to 10 treatments.[77–79] Photocarcinogenicity is directly related to cumulative UV dose,[80] suggesting that treatment with excimer laser may have less photocarcinogenic potential than treatment with NB–UV-B; however, it should be emphasized that currently there are no data on this topic.

## Side Effects

Acute side effects may include itching, burning, blistering, stinging, dryness, and erythema. Maximal erythema occurs around 8 to 24 hours after phototherapy.[64] Protective eyewear is important to reduce the risk of UV-B–related cataract formation. However, it has been demonstrated that UV does not penetrate the eyelids[81]; therefore, for patients who require periocular treatment, it can be safely done by having patients close their eyelids during the irradiation period. Photoaging, reactivation of herpes simplex virus, and anxiety in children have also been reported with UV-B therapy. Lesional blister formation following NB–UV-B has also been rarely reported.[82] No significant increased risk of basal cell carcinoma (BCC), squamous cell carcinoma (SCC), or melanoma has been seen in association with NB–UV-B phototherapy.[83–86] NB–UV-B and excimer laser are safe for use in pregnancy.[87,88] There have been conflicting reports of folic acid depletion during NB–UV-B treatment. Because of the adverse effects of folic acid deficiency in the fetus, practitioners should discuss folic acid supplementation with female patients of childbearing potential before starting NB–UV-B phototherapy.[87,88]

Excimer laser has similar side effects as nontargeted UV-B therapies. The most common adverse effects include blistering, erythema, hyperpigmentation, mild burning, itching, and erosions; but all side effects are generally well tolerated.[69]

## PUVA AND UV-A1
### Mechanism of Action

PUVA therapy combines UV-A light with photosensitizing compounds called *psoralens*, such as 8-MOP, which are used in the clinical treatment of psoriasis. Psoralens are furocoumarins that are found naturally in some plants and are also synthetically produced. Psoralens allow cells in the skin to become sensitized to UV-A light (320–400 nm). PUVA creates both oxygen-independent type 1 reactions and oxygen-dependent type 2 reactions.[29] Oxygen-independent reactions occur when psoralen intercalates between DNA base pairs. When the skin is subsequently exposed to UV-A, psoralen-DNA cross-links are formed, creating pyrimidine dimers that prevent DNA replication and result in T lymphocyte and keratinocyte cell cycle arrest. The DNA cross-links in the epidermis can predispose patients to develop SCC with long-term PUVA treatment (discussed later). Lymphocytes and antigen-presenting cells are much more sensitive than keratinocytes to apoptosis from PUVA therapy. Clinical response to PUVA correlates with depletion of lymphocytes in the epidermis, which may account for response of cutaneous T-cell lymphomas (CTCL) and inflammatory skin disease, such as psoriasis and atopic dermatitis, to PUVA therapy.[89]

Reactive oxygen species are also induced from PUVA therapy in type 2 oxygen-dependent reactions. Reactive oxygen species are formed when excited psoralens react with molecular oxygen, leading to cell and mitochondrial membrane damage from lipid peroxidation, which can result in cell death. Singlet oxygen-mediated reactions and free radicals also act to alter proteins and lipids within the cell. The 8-MOP photooxidized product inhibits C5a, an anaphylatoxin. The 8-MOP photooxidized product inhibits the anaphylatoxin C5a, resulting in the inhibition of polymorphonuclear neutrophils' chemotactic activity to C5a.[90]

PUVA therapy also alters cytokines and cytokine receptors, causing a decline in keratinocyte epidermal growth factor receptor activity as well as decreased expression of Th1/Th17-mediated cytokines IFN-gamma and IL-23 in the epidermis and dermis of psoriatic lesions.[91] In studies using a mouse model of psoriasis,[92] PUVA led to the suppression of Th1/Th17, with significantly depressed levels of IL-17, IL-12, IFN-gamma, and IL-23. Th2 cytokines, such as IL-10, were upregulated, similar to what occurs after UV-B therapy, as discussed earlier. In addition to local changes in the skin, studies have also found decreased levels of these cytokines in the serum of patients treated with PUVA therapy.[93,94]

UV-A1 is proposed to work by inducing T- and B-cell apoptosis, decreasing Langerhans cells and mast cells, decreasing inflammatory cytokines, upregulating matrix metalloproteinases, and decreasing collagen production. UV-A1 has been shown to activate apoptosis cascades, leading to apoptosis of both T and B lymphocytes.[95] UV-A1 also decreases inflammatory cytokines TNF-alpha, IFN-gamma and IL-12.[22,96] Like UV-B, UV-A1 causes photoisomerization of cis to trans UCA, which also has immunomodulatory functions.[22] Intercellular adhesion molecule 1 (ICAM-1), an ICAM that mediates leukocyte and keratinocyte adhesion, is upregulated through cytokines induced by UV-A1.[97] In vitro, cultures of fibroblasts from samples of patients with morphea, unaffected patients, and in mouse models of scleroderma treated with UV-A1 were shown to produce increased collagenase mRNA and protein.[98] Other in vitro studies on normal human fibroblast cultures and in cultures of fibroblasts from mouse models of scleroderma have shown decreased hydroxyproline and collagen levels with UV-A1 exposure.[99] Studies have also shown that proinflammatory cytokines IL-6 and IL-8, interleukins shown to be active in localized scleroderma, are significantly reduced following UV-A1 therapy.[100]

## Modes of Delivery

### PUVA

As previously discussed in relation to NB–UV-B treatment, PUVA therapy remains the most effective UV-based therapy for extensive psoriasis. PUVA has been found to be particularly successful in the treatment of thick plaque and palmoplantar psoriasis.[101] Yet with the advent of NB–UV-B, biologic therapies, and excimer laser, and given the adverse effects and inconvenience of psoralen administration, as well as the increased risk of skin cancer with PUVA as compared with other phototherapy treatment modalities, its use has declined in recent years.

Oral psoralen is listed as pregnancy category C. A few studies have evaluated the rate of congenital malformations in infants born to mothers treated with PUVA and have not found an increased risk when compared with the general population.[102–104] In a study of 504 infants born to mothers treated with PUVA during conception or pregnancy, researchers found no increased risk of malformations, although there was an increase in low birth weight infants.[103] However, there was no control group of infants born to mothers with moderate to severe psoriasis without phototherapy treatment. PUVA is generally not recommended for use in children with psoriasis because of the increased risk of skin cancer. It is recommended that oral PUVA be used with caution only in those children who are at least 12 years old or at least 100 lb.[105]

In addition to orally administered psoralen, PUVA can be administered topically. Topical, soak (usually hands and/or feet) or bath PUVA was developed to deliver the efficacy of oral PUVA without the associated toxicity.

### UV-A1

It was in the early 1990s that UV-A1 began to emerge as a potentially effective form of phototherapy with the study of Krutmann and Schopf[106] who used UV-A1 to successfully treat patients with acute exacerbations of atopic dermatitis. When compared with UV-A2, UV-A1 is less erythemogenic and penetrates deeper into the skin and possibly the subcutis. UV-A1 has been found to be effective for treating atopic dermatitis and localized scleroderma as is discussed further later.[18]

### Indications

Indications for PUVA and UV-A1 are similar to those for NB–UV-B; but because of the deeper penetration of UV-A, it is more frequently used for dermal conditions, such as sclerotic skin disorders (see **Table 2**).

### Contraindications

PUVA and UV-A1 are contraindicated in those with xeroderma pigmentosum, photosensitivity, or in patients with long-term immunosuppression. However, it should be noted that PUVA has been used successfully for desensitization therapy in polymorphous light eruption.

Patients with prior radiation exposure, those who have ingested arsenic, as well as those with Fitzpatrick skin type I or II should undergo PUVA treatment with caution. Caution should also be exercised in those with a history of melanoma or nonmelanoma skin cancer, those who are pregnant or nursing, those with liver disease that could lead to elevated levels of psoralens on PUVA, anyone with past or current exposure to methotrexate or cyclosporine, or anyone with medical issues that make prolonged exposure to heat or standing for an increased length of time difficult. PUVA is not contraindicated in patients with cataracts or aphakia, as most lens implants block UV light. Cataracts are actually protective of the retina, but patients with cataracts or aphakia should practice caution and make sure to wear protective eyewear during all treatments.

### Expected Outcome

Psoriasis clearance rates with oral PUVA therapy are typically in the range of 75% to 88%, with median numbers of treatments needed for clearance at about 16 to 17.[72,73,75,76] According to studies by Gordon and colleagues[72] and Yones and colleagues,[76] 41% to 68% of those who cleared after oral PUVA therapy remained clear of psoriasis at 6 months. Patients typically get oral PUVA treatments 2 to 3 times a week and may begin to see improvement after 6 to 10 treatments. Studies have shown similar efficacy between oral PUVA and bath PUVA and superiority of bath PUVA over NB–UV-B for the treatment of psoriasis.[107,108]

## Treatment Protocol

A typical oral PUVA treatment protocol is listed in **Table 5**. Patients undergoing oral PUVA treatment are usually given 8-MOP 90 minutes before UV-A exposure. 5-MOP, which produces less gastrointestinal side effects and is less phototoxic than 8-MOP, is also used in Europe; however, 5-MOP is not available in the United States. Generally, food should be avoided for 1 hour before and 1 hour after dosing of 8-MOP, as food can slow or decrease absorption. However, in patients with nausea, it may be necessary to have patients take psoralen after a light meal; but a consistent

amount should be given for each treatment so dosing can be standardized and incrementally increased over time. Treatments are usually given 2 to 3 times a week, with at least 48 hours between consecutive treatments to allow for proper assessment of side effects, such as erythema, hyperpigmentation, or blistering. The starting doses of UV-A are typically determined by Fitzpatrick skin type. Generally, if there is no erythema, the UV-A dose should be increased at the next session. If there is erythema that clears before the next session, then the treatment dose should be maintained; if there is erythema that persists for 48 hours or more, then the next treatment session should be canceled.

There is currently no consensus on the protocol for maintenance therapy for PUVA. Although maintenance may be beneficial to prevent relapse, the increased risk of carcinogenesis must be considered. Similar to NB–UV-B, PUVA requires a significant time commitment, yet maintenance therapy is typically much less than NB–UV-B. PUVA maintenance can be as infrequent as once per month versus NB–UV-B, which is usually at least once per week. An alternative recommendation is PUVA maintenance for 3 to 6 months after clearance, usually once weekly without increases in dose. Given the increased risk of nonmelanoma skin cancers after more than 200 treatments, it is recommended that PUVA treatments do not exceed 200 in fair-skinned individuals. Treatment protocols for topical, bath, and soak PUVA are listed in **Box 1**.[109,110]

There are typically 3 different dosing levels of UV-A1: low dose (10–20 J/cm$^2$ per treatment), medium dose (50–70 J/cm$^2$), and high dose (70–130 J/cm$^2$). For most disease processes, the medium dose is the most widely used, as it has been shown to be superior to low dose and is as efficacious as high-dose UVA1. **Table 6** lists representative UV-A1 treatment protocols.[111]

## Side Effects

The most common adverse effects with PUVA therapy are erythema, pruritus, hyperpigmentation, dry skin, nausea, and/or vomiting. Melanonychia, onycholysis, hypertrichosis, lentigines, and blistering may also occur.[54] Photoaging is a side effect of chronic PUVA therapy. As psoralens are photosensitizers, care should be taken when patients are taking other medications that are photosensitizers, such as nonsteroidal antiinflammatory drugs; diuretics; neuroleptics; antibiotics, such as fluoroquinolones or tetracyclines; and antifungals.[112] Hepatic toxicity is uncommonly reported in those who have been treated with PUVA.

**Table 5**
**Oral PUVA treatment protocol**[a]

| Dosing of Oral 8-MOP | | |
| --- | --- | --- |
| Patient Weight | | |
| Pounds | Kilograms | Dose (mg) |
| <66 | <30 | 10 |
| 66–143 | 30–65 | 20 |
| 144–200 | 66–91 | 30 |
| >200 | >91 | 40 |

| Dose of UV-A for Oral PUVA | | | |
| --- | --- | --- | --- |
| Skin Type | Initial Dose (J/cm$^2$) | Increase (J/cm$^2$) | Maximum Dose (J/cm$^2$) |
| I | 0.5–1.5 | 0.5–1.0 | 8–12 |
| II | 1.0–2.5 | 0.5–1.0 | 8–14 |
| III | 1.5–3.5 | 0.5–1.5 | 12–18 |
| IV | 2.0–4.5 | 0.5–2.0 | 12–22 |
| V | 2.5–5.5 | 1.0–2.5 | 20–26 |
| VI | 3.0–6.5 | 1.0–3.0 | 20–30 |

Missed Treatment Protocol
  8–9 d: Increase per standard protocol
  10–14 d: Keep same dose
  15–20 d: Decrease dose by 1–2 J/cm$^2$
  21–24 d: Decrease dose by 2–3 J/cm$^2$
  25–28 d: Decrease dose by 3–4 J/cm$^2$
  >28 d: Start over

[a] This protocol is a representative protocol for psoriasis. Although no consensus exists, PUVA phototherapy protocols for other indications are generally similar to those used in psoriasis.

*Adapted from* Menter A, Korman NJ, Elmets CA, et al. Guidelines of care for the management of psoriasis and psoriatic arthritis: section 5. Guidelines of care for the treatment of psoriasis with phototherapy and photochemotherapy. J Am Acad Dermatol 2010;62(1):126; with permission.

**Box 1**
**Topical, soak, and bath PUVA treatment protocol**

*Topical PUVA*

1. Apply 0.005% 8-MOP solution in aqueous gel to diseased areas using gloves. Ensure repeat applications are given to same areas

2. Irradiate with UV-A within 15 to 20 minutes

3. Initial UV-A dose: either 40% of minimal phototoxic dose, or 0.5 to 1.0 $J/cm^2$

4. Subsequent UV-A doses: 0.5 to 2 $J/cm^2$ depending on the site

5. Frequency: twice weekly

*Soak PUVA*

1. Soak hands and/or feet in 0.03% 8-MOP (made by dissolving one 10-mg tablet or 1 mL of 1% solution of 8-MOP in 3 L of warm water) for 20 to 30 minutes

2. Irradiate with UV-A within 15 to 20 minutes

3. Initial UV-A dose: 1 to 2 $J/cm^2$

4. Subsequent UV-A doses: increase by 0.5 to 1.0 $J/cm^2$ at each successive treatment

5. Frequency: twice weekly

*Bath PUVA*

1. Soak in tub of 0.000075% 8-MOP (made by dissolving six 10-mg 8-MOP tablets in 80 L of warm water) for 20 to 30 minutes

2. Irradiate with UV-A within 15 to 20 minutes

3. Initial UV-A dose: 0.2 to 0.5 $J/cm^2$

4. Subsequent UV-A doses: increase by 20% to 40% of initial dose at each successive treatment

5. Frequency: twice weekly

*Adapted from* Halpern SM, Anstey AV, Dawe RS, et al. Guidelines for topical PUVA: a report of a workshop of the British photodermatology group. Br J Dermatol 2000;142(1):22–31; and Tsui CL, Levitt J. Practical pearls in phototherapy. Int J Dermatol 2013;52(11):1395–7.

It has been suggested through case reports that PUVA increases the risk of cataracts. In a prospective 25-year follow-up study by Malanos and Stern,[113] PUVA was not found to increase the risk of cataracts in patients who used eye protection during treatment. When outdoors, patients should wear eye protection during treatment and for the remainder of the day following treatment.

It has been well established that patients exposed to PUVA have a dose-related increased risk of SCC and, to a lesser extent, BCC.[84,114–121] A study by Stern and colleagues[120] followed 1373 patients since 1975 who were treated with PUVA therapy for psoriasis. Over 25 years, they have found SCC to be strongly associated with high-dose PUVA (>200 treatments), with the risk greatest in those with Fitzpatrick skin types I and II.[121] According to a meta-analysis by Stern and Lunder,[119] the overall incidence among patients exposed to high-dose PUVA (>200 treatments or 2000 $J/cm^2$) was 14-fold higher than in those patients exposed to low-dose PUVA (<100 treatments or 1000 $J/cm^2$). However, the increased risk of nonmelanoma skin cancer in those who have received long-term PUVA therapy has not been clearly established in nonwhite populations.[122] Based on data collected in the United States, the genital area in men with psoriasis exposed to high-dose PUVA is particularly susceptible to developing invasive SCC.[123] It is, therefore, particularly important to use genital shields in patients during phototherapy treatment. There is an additional risk of developing skin cancers in those patients treated with radiation and PUVA, so particular caution should be taken in patients with a previous history of radiation exposure.[116,120] Although studies are limited by sample size and period of follow-up, bath PUVA therapy has not been shown to increase the risk of skin cancer.[124,125]

There is conflicting evidence regarding whether PUVA increases the risk of melanoma in patients. In the same cohort of patients followed by Stern and colleagues[126] since 1975, a 5.5-fold increased risk of malignant melanoma was observed after 15 years of follow-up in patients who received 250 treatments or more. Further follow-up of this cohort has maintained an increased risk of melanoma in this population over time, after adjusting for age, sex, and temporal increase in incidence of melanoma in the aging population.[127] Risk was most pronounced in those with Fitzpatrick skin types I and II. These results stand in contrast to several other cohort studies that have not found this increased risk of melanoma with PUVA therapy,[114,128–131] including a large-scale Swedish study of 4799 patients given PUVA therapy since 1974, whose researchers did not report an increased risk of malignant melanoma with a mean follow-up of 16 years.[131]

Few serious side effects have been reported with UV-A1. The most common side effects include erythema, pruritus, hyperpigmentation, blister formation, photoaging, polymorphic light eruptions, and herpes simplex virus reactivation.[18,132,133] The risk of developing skin cancer with UV-A1 is not yet known. Cases of Merkel

**Table 6**
**UV-A1 treatment protocols**

| Indication | Dose (J/cm$^2$) | Frequency | Duration |
|---|---|---|---|
| Atopic dermatitis | 60 | 3–5 times per wk | 3–6 wk |
| Dyshidrotic dermatitis | 60 | 3–5 times per wk | 3–6 wk |
| CTCL | 60 | 3–5 times per wk | 3–6 wk |
| Localized scleroderma | 60 | 3–5 times per wk | 40 sessions |
| Lichen sclerosus | 50 | 5 times per wk | 40 sessions |
| Systemic lupus erythematosus | 10 | 5 times per wk | 3 wk |
| Subacute prurigo | 50 | 5 times per wk | 4 wk |
| Urticaria pigmentosa | 60 | 5 times per wk | 3 wk |
| Pityriasis rosea | 30 | 3 times per wk | 3 wk |

*Adapted from* Gambichler T, Terras S, Kreuter A. Treatment regimens, protocols, dosage, and indications for UVA1 phototherapy: facts and controversies. Clin Dermatol 2013;31(4):438–54; with permission.

cell carcinoma and melanoma during UV-A1 phototherapy have been reported[134,135]; but until larger studies are conducted, the risk of skin cancer with UV-A1 phototherapy remains unknown.

## SUMMARY

UV phototherapy has evolved into a powerful tool for the treatment of both common and rare dermatoses. Given its efficacy and good side-effect profile, it should be strongly considered as a treatment modality by the practitioner in the appropriate clinical setting.

## REFERENCES

1. Fitzpatrick TB, Pathak MA. Historical aspects of methoxsalen and other furocoumarins. J Invest Dermatol 1959;32(2 Pt 2):229–31.
2. Pathak MA, Fitzpatrick TB. The evolution of photochemotherapy with psoralens and UVA (PUVA): 2000 BC to 1992 AD. J Photochem Photobiol B 1992;14(1–2):3–22.
3. Fahmy IR, Abu-Shady H. Ammi majus Linn.; pharmacognostical study and isolation of a crystalline constituent, ammoidin. Q J Pharm Pharmacol 1947;20(3):281–91 [discussion: 426].
4. Fahmy IR, Abu-Shady H. The isolation and properties of ammoidin, ammidin and majudin, and their effect in the treatment of leukodermia. Q J Pharm Pharmacol 1948;21(4):499–503.
5. Fahmy IR, Abushady H, Schonberg A, et al. A crystalline principle from Ammi majus L. Nature 1947;160(4066):468.
6. Roelandts R. The history of phototherapy: something new under the sun? J Am Acad Dermatol 2002;46(6):926–30.
7. Parrish JA, Fitzpatrick TB, Tanenbaum L, et al. Photochemotherapy of psoriasis with oral methoxsalen and longwave ultraviolet light. N Engl J Med 1974; 291(23):1207–11.
8. Goeckerman WH. Treatment of psoriasis. Northwest Med 1925;24:229–31.
9. Ingram JT. The approach to psoriasis. Br Med J 1953;12(2):591–4.
10. Wiskemann A. UVB-Phototherapie der Psoriasis mit einer fur die PUVA-Therapie entwickelten Stehbox. [UVB-phototherapy of psoriasis using a standing box developed for PUVA-therapy]. Z Hautkr 1978; 53(18):633–6 [in German].
11. Gilchrest BA, Rowe JW, Brown RS, et al. Ultraviolet phototherapy of uremic pruritus. Long-term results and possible mechanism of action. Ann Intern Med 1979;91(1):17–21.
12. Alsins J, Claesson S, Fischer T, et al. Development of high intensity narrow-band lamps and studies of the irradiation effect on human skin. Irradiation with high intensity lamps. Acta Derm Venereol 1975; 55(4):261–71.
13. Fischer T, Alsins J, Berne B. Ultraviolet-action spectrum and evaluation of ultraviolet lamps for psoriasis healing. Int J Dermatol 1984;23(10):633–7.
14. Parrish JA, Jaenicke KF. Action spectrum for phototherapy of psoriasis. J Invest Dermatol 1981; 76(5):359–62.
15. van Weelden H, De La Faille HB, Young E, et al. A new development in UVB phototherapy of psoriasis. Br J Dermatol 1988;119(1):11–9.
16. Green C, Ferguson J, Lakshmipathi T, et al. 311 nm UVB phototherapy–an effective treatment for psoriasis. Br J Dermatol 1988;119(6):691–6.
17. Krutmann J, Czech W, Diepgen T, et al. High-dose UVA1 therapy in the treatment of patients with atopic dermatitis. J Am Acad Dermatol 1992;26(2 Pt 1):225–30.

18. Kroft EB, Berkhof NJ, van de Kerkhof PC, et al. Ultraviolet A phototherapy for sclerotic skin diseases: a systematic review. J Am Acad Dermatol 2008;59(6):1017–30.

19. Schlaak JF, Buslau M, Jochum W, et al. T cells involved in psoriasis vulgaris belong to the Th1 subset. J Invest Dermatol 1994;102(2):145–9.

20. Uyemura K, Yamamura M, Fivenson DF, et al. The cytokine network in lesional and lesion-free psoriatic skin is characterized by a T-helper type 1 cell-mediated response. J Invest Dermatol 1993; 101(5):701–5.

21. Enk CD, Sredni D, Blauvelt A, et al. Induction of IL-10 gene expression in human keratinocytes by UVB exposure in vivo and in vitro. J Immunol 1995;154(9):4851–6.

22. Skov L, Hansen H, Allen M, et al. Contrasting effects of ultraviolet A1 and ultraviolet B exposure on the induction of tumour necrosis factor-alpha in human skin. Br J Dermatol 1998;138(2):216–20.

23. Johnson-Huang LM, Suarez-Farinas M, Sullivan-Whalen M, et al. Effective narrow-band UVB radiation therapy suppresses the IL-23/IL-17 axis in normalized psoriasis plaques. J Invest Dermatol 2010;130(11):2654–63.

24. Piskin G, Tursen U, Sylva-Steenland RM, et al. Clinical improvement in chronic plaque-type psoriasis lesions after narrow-band UVB therapy is accompanied by a decrease in the expression of IFN-gamma inducers – IL-12, IL-18 and IL-23. Exp Dermatol 2004;13(12):764–72.

25. Racz E, Prens EP, Kurek D, et al. Effective treatment of psoriasis with narrow-band UVB phototherapy is linked to suppression of the IFN and Th17 pathways. J Invest Dermatol 2011;131(7): 1547–58.

26. Walters IB, Ozawa M, Cardinale I, et al. Narrowband (312-nm) UV-B suppresses interferon gamma and interleukin (IL) 12 and increases IL-4 transcripts: differential regulation of cytokines at the single-cell level. Arch Dermatol 2003;139(2):155–61.

27. Duthie MS, Kimber I, Norval M. The effects of ultraviolet radiation on the human immune system. Br J Dermatol 1999;140(6):995–1009.

28. Kammeyer A, Teunissen MB, Pavel S, et al. Photoisomerization spectrum of urocanic acid in human skin and in vitro: effects of simulated solar and artificial ultraviolet radiation. Br J Dermatol 1995; 132(6):884–91.

29. Zanolli M. Phototherapy treatment of psoriasis today. J Am Acad Dermatol 2003;49(Suppl 2): S78–86.

30. Krueger JG, Wolfe JT, Nabeya RT, et al. Successful ultraviolet B treatment of psoriasis is accompanied by a reversal of keratinocyte pathology and by selective depletion of intraepidermal T cells. J Exp Med 1995;182(6):2057–68.

31. Ozawa M, Ferenczi K, Kikuchi T, et al. 312-nanometer ultraviolet B light (narrow-band UVB) induces apoptosis of T cells within psoriatic lesions. J Exp Med 1999;189(4):711–8.

32. Weatherhead SC, Farr PM, Jamieson D, et al. Keratinocyte apoptosis in epidermal remodeling and clearance of psoriasis induced by UV radiation. J Invest Dermatol 2011;131(9):1916–26.

33. Kolgen W, Both H, van Weelden H, et al. Epidermal Langerhans cell depletion after artificial ultraviolet B irradiation of human skin in vivo: apoptosis versus migration. J Invest Dermatol 2002;118(5): 812–7.

34. McLoone P, Woods GM, Norval M. Decrease in Langerhans cells and increase in lymph node dendritic cells following chronic exposure of mice to suberythemal doses of solar simulated radiation. Photochem Photobiol 2005;81(5):1168–73.

35. Wong T, Hsu L, Liao W. Phototherapy in psoriasis: a review of mechanisms of action. J Cutan Med Surg 2013;17(1):6–12.

36. van Praag MC, Mulder AA, Claas FH, et al. Long-term ultraviolet B-induced impairment of Langerhans cell function: an immunoelectron microscopic study. Clin Exp Immunol 1994;95(1):73–7.

37. DeSilva B, McKenzie RC, Hunter JA, et al. Local effects of TL01 phototherapy in psoriasis. Photodermatol Photoimmunol Photomed 2008;24(5): 268–9.

38. Seite S, Zucchi H, Moyal D, et al. Alterations in human epidermal Langerhans cells by ultraviolet radiation: quantitative and morphological study. Br J Dermatol 2003;148(2):291–9.

39. Mork NJ, Austad J. Short-wave ultraviolet light (UVB) treatment of allergic contact dermatitis of the hands. Acta Derm Venereol 1983;63(1):87–9.

40. Sjovall P, Christensen OB. Local and systemic effect of ultraviolet irradiation (UVB and UVA) on human allergic contact dermatitis. Acta Derm Venereol 1986;66(4):290–4.

41. Yoshikawa T, Rae V, Bruins-Slot W, et al. Susceptibility to effects of UVB radiation on induction of contact hypersensitivity as a risk factor for skin cancer in humans. J Invest Dermatol 1990;95(5): 530–6.

42. Miyauchi H, Horio T. Ultraviolet B-induced local immunosuppression of contact hypersensitivity is modulated by ultraviolet irradiation and hapten application. J Invest Dermatol 1995; 104(3):364–9.

43. Skov L, Hansen H, Dittmar HC, et al. Susceptibility to effects of UVB irradiation on induction of contact sensitivity, relevance of number and function of Langerhans cells and epidermal macrophages. Photochem Photobiol 1998;67(6):714–9.

44. Soyland E, Heier I, Rodriguez-Gallego C, et al. Sun exposure induces rapid immunological

changes in skin and peripheral blood in patients with psoriasis. Br J Dermatol 2011;164(2):344–55.

45. Novak Z, Bonis B, Baltas E, et al. Xenon chloride ultraviolet B laser is more effective in treating psoriasis and in inducing T cell apoptosis than narrow-band ultraviolet B. J Photochem Photobiol B 2002;67(1):32–8.

46. Adrian RM, Parrish JA, Momtaz TK, et al. Outpatient phototherapy for psoriasis. Arch Dermatol 1981;117(10):623–6.

47. Larko O, Swanbeck G. Home solarium treatment of psoriasis. Br J Dermatol 1979;101(1):13–6.

48. Walters IB, Burack LH, Coven TR, et al. Suberythemogenic narrow-band UVB is markedly more effective than conventional UVB in treatment of psoriasis vulgaris. J Am Acad Dermatol 1999; 40(6 Pt 1):893–900.

49. Almutawa F, Alnomair N, Wang Y, et al. Systematic review of UV-based therapy for psoriasis. Am J Clin Dermatol 2013;14(2):87–109.

50. Picot E, Meunier L, Picot-Debeze MC, et al. Treatment of psoriasis with a 311-nm UVB lamp. Br J Dermatol 1992;127(5):509–12.

51. Storbeck K, Holzle E, Schurer N, et al. Narrowband UVB (311 nm) versus conventional broadband UVB with and without dithranol in phototherapy for psoriasis. J Am Acad Dermatol 1993;28(2 Pt 1): 227–31.

52. Dawe RS, Cameron H, Yule S, et al. A randomized controlled trial of narrowband ultraviolet B vs bath-psoralen plus ultraviolet A photochemotherapy for psoriasis. Br J Dermatol 2003;148(6): 1194–204.

53. Schindl A, Klosner G, Honigsmann H, et al. Flow cytometric quantification of UV-induced cell death in a human squamous cell carcinoma-derived cell line: dose and kinetic studies. J Photochem Photobiol B 1998;44(2):97–106.

54. Menter A, Korman NJ, Elmets CA, et al. Guidelines of care for the management of psoriasis and psoriatic arthritis: section 5. Guidelines of care for the treatment of psoriasis with phototherapy and photochemotherapy. J Am Acad Dermatol 2010; 62(1):114–35.

55. Berneburg M, Rocken M, Benedix F. Phototherapy with narrowband vs broadband UVB. Acta Derm Venereol 2005;85(2):98–108.

56. Guckian M, Jones CD, Vestey JP, et al. Immunomodulation at the initiation of phototherapy and photochemotherapy. Photodermatol Photoimmunol Photomed 1995;11(4):163–9.

57. Hofer A, Hassan AS, Legat FJ, et al. Optimal weekly frequency of 308-nm excimer laser treatment in vitiligo patients. Br J Dermatol 2005; 152(5):981–5.

58. Hofer A, Hassan AS, Legat FJ, et al. The efficacy of excimer laser (308 nm) for vitiligo at different body sites. J Eur Acad Dermatol Venereol 2006;20(5): 558–64.

59. Cameron H, Dawe RS, Yule S, et al. A randomized, observer-blinded trial of twice vs. three times weekly narrowband ultraviolet B phototherapy for chronic plaque psoriasis. Br J Dermatol 2002; 147(5):973–8.

60. Dawe RS, Wainwright NJ, Cameron H, et al. Narrowband (TL-01) ultraviolet B phototherapy for chronic plaque psoriasis: three times or five times weekly treatment? Br J Dermatol 1998;138(5):833–9.

61. Wainwright NJ, Dawe RS, Ferguson J. Narrowband ultraviolet B (TL-01) phototherapy for psoriasis: which incremental regimen? Br J Dermatol 1998; 139(3):410–4.

62. Youssef RM, Mahgoub D, Mashaly HM, et al. Different narrowband UVB dosage regimens in dark skinned psoriatics: a preliminary study. Photodermatol Photoimmunol Photomed 2008;24(5): 256–9.

63. Kleinpenning MM, Smits T, Boezeman J, et al. Narrowband ultraviolet B therapy in psoriasis: randomized double-blind comparison of high-dose and low-dose irradiation regimens. Br J Dermatol 2009;161(6):1351–6.

64. Schneider LA, Hinrichs R, Scharffetter-Kochanek K. Phototherapy and photochemotherapy. Clin Dermatol 2008;26(5):464–76.

65. Boztepe G, Akinci H, Sahin S, et al. In search of an optimum dose escalation for narrowband UVB phototherapy: is it time to quit 20% increments? J Am Acad Dermatol 2006;55(2):269–71.

66. Stern RS, Armstrong RB, Anderson TF, et al. Effect of continued ultraviolet B phototherapy on the duration of remission of psoriasis: a randomized study. J Am Acad Dermatol 1986;15(3): 546–52.

67. Boztepe G, Karaduman A, Sahin S, et al. The effect of maintenance narrow-band ultraviolet B therapy on the duration of remission for psoriasis: a prospective randomized clinical trial. Int J Dermatol 2006;45(3):245–50.

68. Walker D, Jacobe H. Phototherapy in the age of biologics. Semin Cutan Med Surg 2011;30(4):190–8.

69. Mudigonda T, Dabade TS, Feldman SR. A review of targeted ultraviolet B phototherapy for psoriasis. J Am Acad Dermatol 2012;66(4):664–72.

70. Housman TS, Pearce DJ, Feldman SR. A maintenance protocol for psoriasis plaques cleared by the 308 nm excimer laser. J Dermatolog Treat 2004;15(2):94–7.

71. Lapolla W, Yentzer BA, Bagel J, et al. A review of phototherapy protocols for psoriasis treatment. J Am Acad Dermatol 2011;64(5):936–49.

72. Gordon PM, Diffey BL, Matthews JN, et al. A randomized comparison of narrow-band TL-01 phototherapy and PUVA photochemotherapy for

psoriasis. J Am Acad Dermatol 1999;41(5 Pt 1): 728–32.

73. Henseler T, Wolff K, Honigsmann H, et al. Oral 8-methoxypsoralen photochemotherapy of psoriasis. The European PUVA study: a cooperative study among 18 European centres. Lancet 1981; 1(8225):853–7.

74. Markham T, Rogers S, Collins P, et al. (TL-01) phototherapy vs oral 8-methoxypsoralen psoralen-UV-A for the treatment of chronic plaque psoriasis. Arch Dermatol 2003;139(3):325–8.

75. Melski JW, Tanenbaum L, Parrish JA, et al. Oral methoxsalen photochemotherapy for the treatment of psoriasis: a cooperative clinical trial. J Invest Dermatol 1977;68(6):328–35.

76. Yones SS, Palmer RA, Garibaldinos TT, et al. Randomized double-blind trial of the treatment of chronic plaque psoriasis: efficacy of psoralen-UV-A therapy vs narrowband UV-B therapy. Arch Dermatol 2006;142(7):836–42.

77. Bonis B, Kemeny L, Dobozy A, et al. 308 nm UVB excimer laser for psoriasis. Lancet 1997; 350(9090):1522.

78. Feldman SR, Mellen BG, Housman TS, et al. Efficacy of the 308-nm excimer laser for treatment of psoriasis: results of a multicenter study. J Am Acad Dermatol 2002;46(6):900–6.

79. Trehan M, Taylor CR. Medium-dose 308-nm excimer laser for the treatment of psoriasis. J Am Acad Dermatol 2002;47(5):701–8.

80. Lavker RM, Gerberick GF, Veres D, et al. Cumulative effects from repeated exposures to suberythemal doses of UVB and UVA in human skin. J Am Acad Dermatol 1995;32(1):53–62.

81. Prystowsky JH, Keen MS, Rabinowitz AD, et al. Present status of eyelid phototherapy. Clinical efficacy and transmittance of ultraviolet and visible radiation through human eyelids. J Am Acad Dermatol 1992;26(4):607–13.

82. George SA, Ferguson J. Lesional blistering following narrow-band (TL-01) UVB phototherapy for psoriasis: a report of four cases. Br J Dermatol 1992;127(4):445–6.

83. Lee E, Koo J, Berger T. UVB phototherapy and skin cancer risk: a review of the literature. Int J Dermatol 2005;44(5):355–60.

84. Stern RS, Laird N. The carcinogenic risk of treatments for severe psoriasis. Photochemotherapy Follow-up Study. Cancer 1994;73(11):2759–64.

85. Hearn RM, Kerr AC, Rahim KF, et al. Incidence of skin cancers in 3867 patients treated with narrowband ultraviolet B phototherapy. Br J Dermatol 2008;159(4):931–5.

86. Man I, Crombie IK, Dawe RS, et al. The photocarcinogenic risk of narrowband UVB (TL-01) phototherapy: early follow-up data. Br J Dermatol 2005; 152(4):755–7.

87. Tauscher AE, Fleischer AB Jr, Phelps KC, et al. Psoriasis and pregnancy. J Cutan Med Surg 2002;6(6):561–70.

88. Vun YY, Jones B, Al-Mudhaffer M, et al. Generalized pustular psoriasis of pregnancy treated with narrowband UVB and topical steroids. J Am Acad Dermatol 2006;54(Suppl 2):S28–30.

89. Coven TR, Walters IB, Cardinale I, et al. PUVA-induced lymphocyte apoptosis: mechanism of action in psoriasis. Photodermatol Photoimmunol Photomed 1999;15(1):22–7.

90. Esaki K, Mizuno N. Effect of psoralen + ultraviolet-A on the chemotactic activity of polymorphonuclear neutrophils towards anaphylatoxin C5a des Arg. Photochem Photobiol 1992;55(5):783–8.

91. Ravic-Nikolic A, Radosavljevic G, Jovanovic I, et al. Systemic photochemotherapy decreases the expression of IFN-gamma, IL-12p40 and IL-23p19 in psoriatic plaques. Eur J Dermatol 2011;21(1): 53–7.

92. Singh TP, Schon MP, Wallbrecht K, et al. 8-methoxypsoralen plus ultraviolet A therapy acts via inhibition of the IL-23/Th17 axis and induction of Foxp3+ regulatory T cells involving CTLA4 signaling in a psoriasis-like skin disorder. J Immunol 2010; 184(12):7257–67.

93. Coimbra S, Oliveira H, Reis F, et al. Interleukin (IL)-22, IL-17, IL-23, IL-8, vascular endothelial growth factor and tumour necrosis factor-alpha levels in patients with psoriasis before, during and after psoralen-ultraviolet A and narrowband ultraviolet B therapy. Br J Dermatol 2010;163(6):1282–90.

94. Rotsztejn H, Zalewska A, Trznadel-Budzko E, et al. Influence of systemic photochemotherapy on regulatory T cells and selected cytokine production in psoriatic patients: a pilot study. Med Sci Monit 2005;11(12):CR594–8.

95. Godar DE. UVA1 radiation triggers two different final apoptotic pathways. J Invest Dermatol 1999; 112(1):3–12.

96. Szegedi A, Simics E, Aleksza M, et al. Ultraviolet-A1 phototherapy modulates Th1/Th2 and Tc1/Tc2 balance in patients with systemic lupus erythematosus. Rheumatology (Oxford) 2005;44(7):925–31.

97. Krutmann J, Grewe M. Involvement of cytokines, DNA damage, and reactive oxygen intermediates in ultraviolet radiation-induced modulation of intercellular adhesion molecule-1 expression. J Invest Dermatol 1995;105(Suppl 1):67S–70S.

98. Gruss C, Reed JA, Altmeyer P, et al. Induction of interstitial collagenase (MMP-1) by UVA-1 phototherapy in morphea fibroblasts. Lancet 1997; 350(9087):1295–6.

99. Ju M, Chen K, Chang B, et al. UVA1 irradiation inhibits fibroblast proliferation and alleviates pathological changes of scleroderma in a mouse model. J Biomed Res 2012;26(2):135–42.

100. Kreuter A, Hyun J, Skrygan M, et al. Ultraviolet A1-induced downregulation of human beta-defensins and interleukin-6 and interleukin-8 correlates with clinical improvement in localized scleroderma. Br J Dermatol 2006;155(3):600–7.

101. Spuls PI, Witkamp L, Bossuyt PM, et al. A systematic review of five systemic treatments for severe psoriasis. Br J Dermatol 1997;137(6): 943–9.

102. Garbis H, Elefant E, Bertolotti E, et al. Pregnancy outcome after periconceptional and first-trimester exposure to methoxsalen photochemotherapy. Arch Dermatol 1995;131(4):492–3.

103. Gunnarskog JG, Kallen AJ, Lindelof BG, et al. Psoralen photochemotherapy (PUVA) and pregnancy. Arch Dermatol 1993;129(3):320–3.

104. Stern RS, Lange R. Outcomes of pregnancies among women and partners of men with a history of exposure to methoxsalen photochemotherapy (PUVA) for the treatment of psoriasis. Arch Dermatol 1991;127(3):347–50.

105. Marqueling AL, Cordoro KM. Systemic treatments for severe pediatric psoriasis: a practical approach. Dermatol Clin 2013;31(2):267–88.

106. Krutmann J, Schopf E. High-dose-UVA1 phototherapy: a novel and highly effective approach for the treatment of acute exacerbation of atopic dermatitis. Acta Derm Venereol Suppl (Stockh) 1992; 176:120–2.

107. Berneburg M, Herzinger T, Rampf J, et al. Efficacy of bath psoralen plus ultraviolet A (PUVA) vs. system PUVA in psoriasis: a prospective, open, randomized, multicentre study. Br J Dermatol 2013; 169(3):704–8.

108. Salem SA, Barakat MA, Morcos CM. Bath psoralen + ultraviolet A photochemotherapy vs. narrow band-ultraviolet B in psoriasis: a comparison of clinical outcome and effect on circulating T-helper and T-suppressor/cytotoxic cells. Photodermatol Photoimmunol Photomed 2010;26(5): 235–42.

109. Halpern SM, Anstey AV, Dawe RS, et al. Guidelines for topical PUVA: a report of a workshop of the British photodermatology group. Br J Dermatol 2000;142(1):22–31.

110. Tsui CL, Levitt J. Practical pearls in phototherapy. Int J Dermatol 2013;52(11):1395–7.

111. Gambichler T, Terras S, Kreuter A. Treatment regimens, protocols, dosage, and indications for UVA1 phototherapy: facts and controversies. Clin Dermatol 2013;31(4):438–54.

112. Stern RS, Kleinerman RA, Parrish JA, et al. Phototoxic reactions to photoactive drugs in patients treated with PUVA. Arch Dermatol 1980;116(11): 1269–71.

113. Malanos D, Stern RS. Psoralen plus ultraviolet A does not increase the risk of cataracts: a 25-year prospective study. J Am Acad Dermatol 2007; 57(2):231–7.

114. Chuang TY, Heinrich LA, Schultz MD, et al. PUVA and skin cancer. A historical cohort study on 492 patients. J Am Acad Dermatol 1992;26(2 Pt 1): 173–7.

115. Lindelof B, Sigurgeirsson B, Tegner E, et al. PUVA and cancer: a large-scale epidemiological study. Lancet 1991;338(8759):91–3.

116. Stern RS, Laird N, Melski J, et al. Cutaneous squamous-cell carcinoma in patients treated with PUVA. N Engl J Med 1984;310(18):1156–61.

117. Stern RS, Lange R. Non-melanoma skin cancer occurring in patients treated with PUVA five to ten years after first treatment. J Invest Dermatol 1988; 91(2):120–4.

118. Stern RS, Liebman EJ, Vakeva L. Oral psoralen and ultraviolet-A light (PUVA) treatment of psoriasis and persistent risk of nonmelanoma skin cancer. PUVA Follow-up Study. J Natl Cancer Inst 1998;90(17): 1278–84.

119. Stern RS, Lunder EJ. Risk of squamous cell carcinoma and methoxsalen (psoralen) and UV-A radiation (PUVA). A meta-analysis. Arch Dermatol 1998; 134(12):1582–5.

120. Stern RS, Thibodeau LA, Kleinerman RA, et al. Risk of cutaneous carcinoma in patients treated with oral methoxsalen photochemotherapy for psoriasis. N Engl J Med 1979;300(15):809–13.

121. Nijsten TE, Stern RS. The increased risk of skin cancer is persistent after discontinuation of psoralen + ultraviolet A: a cohort study. J Invest Dermatol 2003;121(2):252–8.

122. Murase JE, Lee EE, Koo J. Effect of ethnicity on the risk of developing nonmelanoma skin cancer following long-term PUVA therapy. Int J Dermatol 2005;44(12):1016–21.

123. Stern RS. Genital tumors among men with psoriasis exposed to psoralens and ultraviolet A radiation (PUVA) and ultraviolet B radiation. The Photochemotherapy Follow-up Study. N Engl J Med 1990; 322(16):1093–7.

124. Hannuksela A, Pukkala E, Hannuksela M, et al. Cancer incidence among Finnish patients with psoriasis treated with trioxsalen bath PUVA. J Am Acad Dermatol 1996;35(5 Pt 1):685–9.

125. Hannuksela-Svahn A, Sigurgeirsson B, Pukkala E, et al. Trioxsalen bath PUVA did not increase the risk of squamous cell skin carcinoma and cutaneous malignant melanoma in a joint analysis of 944 Swedish and Finnish patients with psoriasis. Br J Dermatol 1999;141(3):497–501.

126. Stern RS, Nichols KT, Vakeva LH. Malignant melanoma in patients treated for psoriasis with methoxsalen (psoralen) and ultraviolet A radiation (PUVA). The PUVA Follow-Up Study. N Engl J Med 1997; 336(15):1041–5.

127. Stern RS, PUVA Follow up Study. The risk of melanoma in association with long-term exposure to PUVA. J Am Acad Dermatol 2001;44(5):755–61.

128. Forman AB, Roenigk HH Jr, Caro WA, et al. Long-term follow-up of skin cancer in the PUVA-48 cooperative study. Arch Dermatol 1989;125(4):515–9.

129. Lindelof B. Risk of melanoma with psoralen/ultraviolet A therapy for psoriasis. Do the known risks now outweigh the benefits? Drug Saf 1999;20(4):289–97.

130. Morison WL, Baughman RD, Day RM, et al. Consensus workshop on the toxic effects of long-term PUVA therapy. Arch Dermatol 1998;134(5):595–8.

131. Lindelof B, Sigurgeirsson B, Tegner E, et al. PUVA and cancer risk: the Swedish follow-up study. Br J Dermatol 1999;141(1):108–12.

132. Gambichler T, Othlinghaus N, Tomi NS, et al. Medium-dose ultraviolet (UV) A1 vs. narrowband UVB phototherapy in atopic eczema: a randomized crossover study. Br J Dermatol 2009;160(3):652–8.

133. Kroft EB, van de Kerkhof PC, Gerritsen MJ, et al. Period of remission after treatment with UVA-1 in sclerodermic skin diseases. J Eur Acad Dermatol Venereol 2008;22(7):839–44.

134. Calzavara-Pinton P, Monari P, Manganoni AM, et al. Merkel cell carcinoma arising in immunosuppressed patients treated with high-dose ultraviolet A1 (320-400 nm) phototherapy: a report of two cases. Photodermatol Photoimmunol Photomed 2010;26(5):263–5.

135. Wallenfang K, Stadler R. Assoziation zwischen UVA1 bzw. Bade-PUVA-Bestrahlung und Melanomentwicklung?. [Association between UVA1 and PUVA bath therapy and development of malignant melanoma] Hautarzt 2001;52(8):705–7 [in German].

# Photodynamic Therapy

Ali M. Rkein, MD, David M. Ozog, MD*

KEYWORDS

- Photodynamic therapy • Aminolevulinic acid • Methyl aminolevulinate • Nonmelanoma skin cancer
- Light-based therapies

KEY POINTS

- Over the past 100 years, photodynamic therapy (PDT) has evolved into a safe and effective treatment option for actinic keratosis, superficial nonmelanoma skin cancer (NMSC), and more recently, photoaging, acne, and verrucae.
- PDT is the interaction among 3 ingredients: light, a photosensitizer, and oxygen. This interaction generates reactive oxygen species (ROS), especially singlet oxygen radicals, which cause cell death by necrosis or apoptosis.
- The 2 commonly used photosensitizers, aminolevulinic acid (ALA) and methyl aminolevulinate (MAL), are metabolized by cells into the photoactive porphyrin, protoporphyrin IX (PpIX). Thus, an incubation period is required.
- Red or blue light are commonly used light sources to activate the photosensitizer.

## INTRODUCTION

PDT relies on the interaction between a photosensitizer, the appropriate wavelength, and oxygen. The reaction generates ROS in cells that take up the photosensitizer, causing cell death by necrosis or apoptosis, but spares the surrounding tissue. Initially, PDT relied on systemic administration of the photosensitizer, but the advent of a topical application revolutionized the field. Over the past 100 years, PDT has evolved into a safe and effective dermatologic treatment option for actinic keratosis/cheilitis, superficial NMSC, and more recently, photoaging, acne, sebaceous hyperplasia, and verrucae.[1,2] Furthermore, PDT has also expanded outside dermatology, and it is now used as adjuvant therapy to treat pulmonary, respiratory tract, neural, and urinary tract tumors, as well as vitreoretinal disease.

## HISTORICAL PERSPECTIVE

Ancient civilizations have known for thousands of years that they could combine different plants with sunlight to treat various skin diseases. It was not until about 100 years ago that Hermann von Tappeiner[3] coined the term photodynamic action to describe an oxygen-dependent reaction after photosensitization. He noted that in the absence of oxygen, dye and light alone did not cause cell death. He continued to develop the concept of PDT, and eventually described the first cases in humans, using eosin as the photosensitizer to treat various skin conditions, including condyloma lata and NMSC.

Over the years, many photosensitizers have been used, and the most studied agent is hematoporphyrin. However, hematoporphyrin had to be administered intravenously and was cleared from tissue slowly, resulting in prolonged phototoxicity. It was not until 1990 that Kennedy and colleagues[4] reported the use of 5-ALA and visible light for topical PDT treatment of the skin. ALA was revolutionary, because it easily penetrated damaged or abnormal stratum corneum and rapidly cleared. Using a single application to treat basal cell carcinoma (BCC), Kennedy and colleagues[4] were able to achieve a 90% complete response rate.

Funding Sources: None.
Conflict of Interest: None.
Department of Dermatology, Henry Ford Hospital, 3031 West Grand Boulevard, Suite 800, Detroit, MI, USA
* Corresponding author.
E-mail address: DOZOG1@hfhs.org

Dermatol Clin 32 (2014) 415–425
http://dx.doi.org/10.1016/j.det.2014.03.009

derm.theclinics.com

## MECHANISM OF ACTION

PDT is the interaction among 3 ingredients: light, a photosensitizer, and oxygen (**Fig. 1**). After exposure of the photosensitizer to light containing its action spectrum, ROS, especially singlet oxygen radicals, are generated. The ROS affect all intracellular components, including proteins and DNA, resulting in necrosis or apoptosis.[2] Thus, only cells with intracellular photosensitizer are selectively damaged, and the surrounding tissue is spared, resulting in an outstanding cosmetic result.

## SENSITIZER

The multiple early photosensitizers, including eosin red and the hematoporphyrin derivatives, were not widely used in dermatology because they had an unfavorable side effect profile.[3] The advent of 5-ALA revolutionized PDT. The photosensitizer 5-ALA has a low molecular weight, which allows it to easily penetrate the stratum corneum and be cleared from the skin within 24 to 48 hours of application.[2] ALA is the first compound synthesized in the porphyrin-heme pathway (see **Fig. 1**) and is converted endogenously into the photosensitizer PpIX. Once PpIX is exposed to its action spectra (including 400–410 nm and 635 nm), ROS are generated, which destroy the

target cell. Although the heme synthesis pathway is controlled by ALA synthase, exogenous ALA bypasses this rate-limiting enzyme and overwhelms the cell's ability to convert PpIX into heme. ALA is thought to preferentially target tumors of epithelial origin because of their defective epidermal barrier and slower conversion of PpIX into heme. In the United States, ALA is available as a 20% solution and is marketed under the trade name Levulan.

An alternative to ALA is the methyl ester form, MAL.[2] The presence of methyl ester group makes the molecule more lipophilic and enhances penetration; however, it must be converted back to ALA by intracellular enzymes. Although this may limit the availability of ALA, MAL has been shown to have better tumor selectivity and to reach maximal intracellular concentrations of PpIX quickly, allowing a shorter incubation period. In the United States, MAL was available for a brief period as a 16.8% cream under the trade name Metvixia. However, it is currently unavailable in the US market because of economic reasons, but remains widely used in Europe.

## LIGHT SOURCE

Several light sources, including coherent and incoherent light, have been used in PDT. PpIX has a strong absorption peak at 405 nm, along with

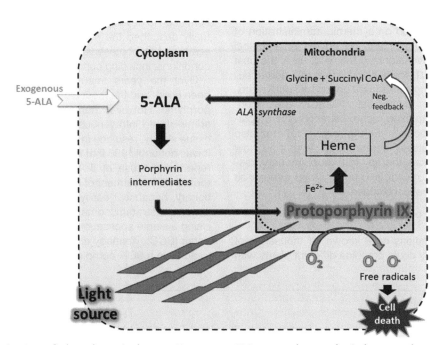

**Fig. 1.** Mechanism of photodynamic therapy. Exogenous ALA enters the porphyrin-heme pathway and is converted endogenously into the photosensitizer PpIX. Once PpIX is activated by the proper wavelength of light, it produces singlet oxygen free radicals, which destroy the target cell.

several smaller Q bands; the last peak is at 635 nm. Blue light, which includes the wavelength 405 nm, efficiently excites PpIX and is commonly used. However, because of its relatively short wavelength, it does not penetrate deeply. For thicker lesions, red light, which includes the wavelength 635 nm, is frequently used. This wavelength targets the last Q band; because red light does not excite PpIX as efficiently as blue light, a higher fluence (dose) is needed.[2] Multiple other light sources that take advantage of the action spectrum of PpIX have been used, including intense pulsed light (IPL), pulsed dye laser (585 nm), and natural sunlight.

It is important to consider the fluence (Joules per square centimeter) and irradiance (milliwatts per square centimeter) that are used in PDT. The effective photosensitizing dose for a light source of approximately 405 nm is 10 J/cm$^2$, and a 10-fold increase, or 100 J/cm$^2$ for a light source of 635 nm. Because PDT consumes oxygen, it is important to use an appropriate rate of fluence (ie, irradiance), because a high irradiance may consume the oxygen molecules too quickly, leading to a decrease in efficiency.[2] For this reason, a typical PDT treatment with blue light takes about

15 minutes and a treatment with red light takes about 30 minutes. Red light requires a longer irradiation period because it does not excite PpIX as efficiently as blue light.

## THERAPEUTIC APPLICATIONS AND EXPECTED OUTCOMES

Since the advent of PDT, the list of indications has continued to grow. The following section focuses on the treatment and expected outcomes of photorejuvenation, acne, verrucae, actinic keratosis, and NMSC. The readers are referred to **Tables 1** and **2** as well as **Box 1**, which outline therapeutic applications and expected outcomes of PDT and a general PDT protocol as well as typical settings used in PDT, respectively.

### Photorejuvenation

Multiple clinical studies have consistently demonstrated excellent cosmetic results with the use of PDT. Babilas and colleagues,[5] in a prospective, randomized controlled, split-face study, treated with MAL 25 patients with sun-damaged skin followed by irradiation with either a light-emitting diode (635 nm, 37 J/cm$^2$) or an IPL

**Table 1**
**Indications and expected outcomes**

| Indication | Summary of Recommendations |
|---|---|
| Photorejuvenation | Excellent cosmetic results for all facets of photodamage<br>Multiple other proven and accepted modalities, which are less expensive and require less time |
| Acne vulgaris | Highly effective in the treatment of inflammatory papules, but not comedones<br>Excellent option for moderate to severe acne when isotretinoin is not an option<br>Drawbacks include time commitment, discomfort during treatment, posttreatment erythema, and crusting |
| Verrucae | Very effective<br>Reported clearance rates of hand and foot warts ranging from 56%–100%<br>Reported clearance rates of condyloma accuminata ranging from 66%–79% |
| Actinic keratosis | Highly effective<br>When treating head and neck, efficacy similar to, or exceeds other FDA-approved modalities<br>Better cosmetic outcome when compared with cryotherapy |
| Bowen disease | Efficacy likely superior to cryotherapy and 5-FU<br>Good cosmetic outcome |
| Superficial basal cell carcinoma | Highly effective and similar to simple excisions<br>Useful in treating multiple lesions<br>Main disadvantage is time commitment |
| Nodular basal cell carcinoma | Not recommended at this time |

*Abbreviations:* FDA, US Food and Drug Administration; 5-FU, 5-fluorouracil.

**Table 2**
**PDT-specific treatment protocols for different indications**

| Indication | Topical Photosensitizer | Incubation Period | Light Source | Dose | Comments |
|---|---|---|---|---|---|
| Photorejuvenation | ALA | 30 min–3 h | Blue light IPL | 10 J/cm$^2$ 37 J/cm$^2$ | 2–3 treatments, repeated monthly |
| | MAL | 30 min–1 h | Red light | 37 J/cm$^2$ | |
| Acne vulgaris | ALA | 3 h | Blue light Red light | 10 J/cm$^2$ 37 J/cm$^2$ | 2–3 treatments, repeated monthly |
| | MAL | 3 h | Red light | 37 J/cm$^2$ | |
| Verrucae | ALA | 4 h | Red light | ≥100 J/cm$^2$ | 4–5 treatments, repeated biweekly |
| Actinic keratosis | ALA | 4 h | Blue light Red light | 10 J/cm$^2$ 75–150 J/cm$^2$ | Requires 1–2 sessions of PDT for optimal results |
| | MAL | 3 h | Red light | 37–75 J/cm$^2$ | |
| Bowen disease | ALA | 4 h | Red light | ≥100 J/cm$^2$ | Requires 2–3 sessions of PDT for optimal results |
| | MAL | 3 h | Red light | 75–100 J/cm$^2$ | |
| Superficial basal cell carcinoma | ALA | 3–6 h | Red light | ≥60 J/cm$^2$ | Requires 2–3 sessions of PDT for optimal results |
| | MAL | 3 h | Red light | 37–75 J/cm$^2$ | |

device (610–950 nm, 80 J/cm$^2$). At 3 months, the investigators found significant improvement in wrinkling and pigmentation, irrespective of the light source used. Gold and colleagues[6] evaluated short-contact (30–60 minutes) ALA-PDT using IPL as a light source, versus IPL alone in 16 patients in a side-by-side design. Patients were exposed to PDT for a total of 3 monthly treatments and followed up at months 1 and 3. The IPL treatment parameters were 34 J/cm$^2$; cutoff filters used were 550 nm for Fitzpatrick skin types I to III and 570 nm for Fitzpatrick skin type IV. The investigators found greater improvement in the ALA-PDT-IPL group, compared to patients who received IPL alone for all facets of photodamage.

The practical challenge with using PDT for photorejuvenation is the availability of multiple other proven and accepted modalities such as chemical peels, laser, and IPL. The additional time and supply costs of PDT limit it from becoming a widely used treatment option for photorejuvenation.

### Acne Vulgaris

*Propionibacterium acnes* produce an endogenous porphyrin, coproporphyrin III, which makes it ideal for treatment with PDT. In addition, both ALA and MAL are strongly absorbed by the pilosebaceous unit. Two studies used biopsies to examine the effect of PDT on sebaceous glands. One used a high-dose light source (550–700 nm at 150 J/cm$^2$), and the other used a low-dose light source (600–700 nm at 13 J/cm$^2$). Both regimens caused sebocyte suppression, but suppression by the high-dose light source lasted longer.[7,8] Furthermore, Wiegell and Wulf[9,10] compared the efficacy of ALA-PDT to MAL-PDT for the treatment of acne in a randomized, split-face, investigator-blinded study. Patients underwent one treatment and were followed up for 12 weeks. Both photosensitizers were applied for 3 hours under occlusion, followed by irradiation with red light (635 nm, 37 J/cm$^2$). The investigators found an average reduction of 59% in inflammatory lesions, in both the ALA and MAL treatment groups, but no

**Box 1**
**PDT general treatment protocol**

- Patient washes the area to be treated with soap and water
- Acetone or Alcohol soaked 4 × 4 gauze is used to remove any remaining debris and oil
- The photosensitizer is evenly applied to the entire area to be treated. A second coat of the photosensitizer can be applied, after the first coat has dried.
- Allow the photosensitizer to incubate for 2–3 hours (see below for more comprehensive recommendations).
- Activate the photosensitizer with the appropriate light source.
- The patient must stay out of the any direct sunlight for 48 hours
- The treatment is repeated as needed in 2–3 weeks

reduction in the number of noninflammatory lesions; there was no statistical difference between the 2 drugs. Finally, in a review of PDT studies for treatment of acne, Sakamoto and colleagues[11] concluded that incubation periods of at least 3 hours were associated with long-term remission, high-dose ALA-PDT and MAL-PDT (with an incubation period of at least 3 hours, high fluence, and red light) have similar efficacy, and red light is more likely to destroy sebaceous glands than blue or pulsed light.

In clinical practice, treatment of acne with PDT is an important modality (**Fig. 2**). The efficacy of PDT for inflammatory lesions is superior to that of antibiotics in most cases, but inferior to that of isotretinoin. Thus, it is a useful treatment option for patients with moderate to severe inflammatory acne who are poor candidates for isotretinoin. Noninflammatory lesions do not seem to be affected, which can be treated with adjunctive retinoids or physical extraction. Limitations include time commitment, discomfort during treatment, posttreatment erythema, cost, and crusting.

## Verrucae

Several studies have demonstrated the high efficacy of PDT in the treatment of verrucae. Clearance rates of hand and foot verrucae have been reported in the range of 56% to 100%. In one study, patients were randomized to 6 repetitive ALA-PDT or placebo-PDT treatments, performed every 1 to 2 weeks. The warts were pared down before treatment, and ALA was applied under occlusion for 4 hours before irradiation with red light (590–700 nm, 70 J/cm$^2$). At 1 and 2 months posttreatment, the median relative reduction in area with clinically apparent verrucae was 98% and 100% in the ALA-PDT group versus 52% and 71% in the placebo group, respectively. It was concluded that ALA-PDT is superior to placebo-PDT in the treatment of verrucae.[12] In another

study, Schroeter and colleagues[13] treated periungual and subungual verrucae with ALA-PDT. ALA was applied under occlusion for an average of 4.6 hours (3–6 hours) and then irradiated with red light (580–700 nm, 70 J/cm$^2$, with a range of 30–180 J/cm$^2$). The investigators found that after an average of 4.5 treatments, total clearance was achieved in 90% of the patients.

Several studies have also examined the efficacy of PDT in the treatment of genital warts. Stefanaki and colleagues[14] treated males with condyloma accuminata with ALA under occlusion for 6 to 11 hours and then irradiated with broadband visible light (400–800 nm, 70 J/cm$^2$ or 100 J/cm$^2$). Repeat treatment was done 1 week later for lesions that did not achieve at least a 50% improvement. At 1 year, the overall cure rate was 79.2%. In another study, Fehr and colleagues[15] examined the efficacy of PDT in the treatment of vulvar and vaginal condylomata. ALA was applied under occlusion for an average of 2.5 hours (2–4 hours), and lesions were then irradiated with pulsed dye laser (635 nm, 116 J/cm$^2$, with a range of 100–132 J/cm$^2$). Almost 8 weeks after the treatment, a complete clearance rate of 66% was reported.

## Actinic Keratosis

The initial US Food and Drug Administration (FDA) phase 2 and 3 studies of ALA-PDT (Levulan Kerastick) in the treatment of nonhyperkeratotic actinic keratosis on the face and scalp had a clearance rate of 85% to 90% after 1 to 2 treatment sessions. The ALA was applied for 14 to 18 hours, followed by irradiation with a blue light source (10 J/cm$^2$) for 1000 seconds. Since then, different protocols have been developed to improve the efficacy for other indications and to reduce the discomfort and time associated with the administration of PDT.[2] In a European multicenter, randomized, prospective study with 119 subjects and 1500 lesions, MAL-PDT was compared with cryosurgery in the

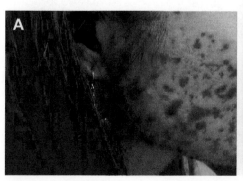
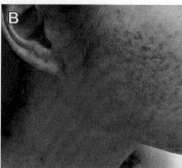

**Fig. 2.** Acne (*A*) before and (*B*) after treatment with several sessions of photodynamic therapy using 20% aminolevulinic acid and blue light.

treatment of actinic keratosis. Patients were randomized to either a single treatment with MAL-PDT (3 hours) incubation with illumination with broad-spectrum red light (75 J/cm$^2$) or a double freeze-thaw cycle of liquid nitrogen. No significant difference between the 2 treatment modalities was found, but MAL-PDT provided a superior cosmetic result.[16] Touma and colleagues[17] examined the effect of pretreatment with urea (to enhance ALA penetration) and concluded that urea did not influence the therapeutic outcome. Finally, a recent Cochrane review found that ALA-PDT, or MAL-PDT, with blue or red light, resulted in similar efficacy in the treatment of actinic keratosis; however, for ALA-PDT, longer incubation (4 hours) resulted in better results compared to shorter incubation time (<2 hours).[18] The review also found that 4-hour incubation with ALA-PDT was significantly more efficacious than cryotherapy but that 1-hour incubation with ALA-PDT (blue light or pulsed dye laser) was not significantly different from 0.5% 5-fluorouracil (5-FU) incubation. Last, the review found that MAL-PDT had similar efficacy regardless of the light source used (red light, broadband visible light with water-filtered infrared A, and daylight).

In summary, treatment of actinic keratosis on the face and scalp with PDT (**Fig. 3**) has an expected outcome equal to or better than other FDA-approved treatment modalities. In addition, many patients who have previously undergone treatment with cryotherapy, topical 5-FU, or imiquimod ultimately prefer PDT. This preference may be because of decreased pain compared to cryotherapy, shorter total treatment and recovery time compared to topical agents, and/or improved cosmetic outcome. This fact was demonstrated by Tierney and colleagues,[19] who completed a survey to assess patient perceptions and preferences in the management of actinic keratosis and found that PDT had faster recovery and improved

cosmetic outcome when compared with surgical excision and cryotherapy. Furthermore, patients preferred PDT to 5-FU or imiquimod.

For actinic keratosis on the trunk and extremities, there is a marked decrease in clinical efficacy with PDT. Measures such as increased incubation time, curetting of lesions or using fractional ablative lasers before the administration of ALA, occlusion, and/or pretreatment with topical agents are used to improve outcomes in these areas.

## NMSC
### Bowen Disease

Multiple studies have demonstrated that PDT is effective in treating Bowen disease. Morton and colleagues[20] conducted several clinical trials to optimize ALA-PDT for the treatment of Bowen disease. The investigators concluded that red light (630 nm) was superior to green light (540 nm) in both complete clearance and recurrence rates. They also conducted a placebo-controlled, randomized, multicenter study that compared the efficacy of MAL-PDT to cryotherapy and 5-FU in the treatment of Bowen disease. MAL was incubated for 3 hours, followed by irradiation with a broadband red light (75 J/cm$^2$, 570–670 nm). Treatment was repeated 1 week later. At 3 months, repeat treatment was performed on lesions with a partial response. At 1 year, the estimated sustained lesion complete response rate of MAL-PDT was superior to those of cryotherapy (80% vs 67%) and 5-FU (80% vs 69%). Furthermore, Salim and colleagues[21] compared ALA-PDT with topical 5-FU in the treatment of Bowen disease. ALA was incubated for 4 hours followed by irradiation with narrow-band red light (630 nm, 100 J/cm$^2$). Both ALA-PDT and 5-FU were repeated 6 weeks later as necessary. After 1 year, the investigators found that 82% of the lesions treated with PDT showed complete response, versus 42% with 5-FU.

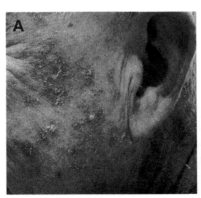 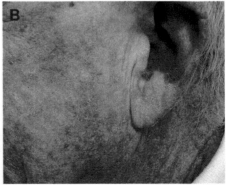

**Fig. 3.** Actinic keratosis on left cheek (*A*) before and (*B*) after treatment with photodynamic therapy using 20% aminolevulinic acid and blue light.

In clinical practice, these are acceptable clearance rates for Bowen disease, and PDT may be superior to 5-FU at 1 year posttreatment (**Fig. 4**). Recurrent lesions can be either treated again with PDT or surgically treated by excision, electrodessication and curettage, or Mohs surgery depending on size and location. In addition, in the United States, PDT may have significantly lower out-of-pocket costs for patients without prescription coverage or with a high prescription deductible.

## BCC

Multiple studies have examined the efficacy of ALA and MAL-PDT in the treatment of BCC. The average weighted complete clearance rates from 12 studies with follow-up periods between 3 and 36 months was 87% for superficial BCC and 53% for nodular BCC.[2] Morton and colleagues[22] found that an incubation of 6 hours with ALA was better than a 4-hour incubation and red light (630 nm) was more efficacious than green light (540 nm). Szeimies and colleagues[23] compared MAL-PDT to simple excision in the treatment of superficial BCC. The investigators treated 196 patients with 2 sessions of MAL-PDT, repeated 1 week apart, and again at 3 months, as necessary. MAL was applied under occlusion for 3 hours followed by irradiation with narrow-band red light (630 nm, 37 J/cm²). They concluded that MAL-PDT and simple excision offer similarly high efficacy but MAL-PDT provided a much better cosmetic outcome.

In clinical practice, PDT is commonly used to treat small, uncomplicated superficial BCCs. The main advantage of PDT over electrodessication and curettage is markedly improved appearance of PDT-treated areas, including less hypopigmentation and clinical scarring. Recalcitrant lesions may be given a repeat PDT treatment, or treated with other modalities. The main disadvantage is the time commitment (3-hour incubation period), pain, and the need for 2 treatment sessions versus 1 for electrodessication and curettage. These disadvantages are often outweighed when patients have multiple superficial BCCs, Gorlin syndrome, or propensity for hypertrophic scarring. To improve efficacy in these instances, one of the authors (D.M.O.) has used pulsed dye laser as an alternate light source. The typical settings on a 595-nm device are 7.5 J/cm², 10 × 3 mm spot size, and 10-ms pulse duration. Each lesion is pulse stacked 7 to 10 times for a total fluence of 52.5 to 75 J/cm² with a 3- to 4-mm margin around lesion. Hundreds of lesions have been treated in the authors' clinics, with low recurrence rates (David Ozog, unpublished data, 2013). The authors' group[24] has previously demonstrated the utility of pulsed dye laser-PDT in various dermatologic disorders.

## MANAGEMENT OF ADVERSE EVENTS
### Pain

The mechanism of action of pain in PDT is yet to be clarified, but it is thought to be secondary to the interaction between the inflammation caused by cell necrosis and myelinated A delta or unmyelinated C fibers. Pain is often described by patients as a burning sensation and peaks during the first few minutes of treatment. Several studies, using the *visual analog scale* (VAS) for pain, have demonstrated that about 20% of patients experience a pain rated at 6 or more, which is considered significant and may lead to reduced compliance.[25]

Multiple factors play an important role in the amount of pain experienced. These factors include

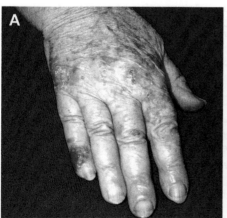
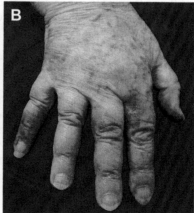

**Fig. 4.** (*A*) Right hand with multiple Bowen disease. (*B*) After 2 sessions of photodynamic therapy using 20% aminolevulinic acid and blue light combined with pulsed dye laser. The residual lesion on fifth digit was surgically excised using Mohs surgery.

the type of photosensitizer used, location of lesions, type of lesion, amount and rate of energy delivered, type of light source, and number of sessions. Several studies have shown that MAL-PDT is less painful than ALA-PDT. This may be explained by the fact that MAL is more selectively absorbed by abnormal cells when compared with ALA.[25] In addition, it is also believed that the ALA is transported into nerve endings, whereas MAL is not. Treatment of lesions located in areas with many nerve endings, such as the head and hands, along with larger surface areas (>130 mm$^2$) has been found to be more painful. Furthermore, the type of lesion treated may lead to more pain; an actinic keratosis is more painful than Bowen disease or BCCs. As expected, the greater the rate and the overall energy delivered, ie, irradiance and fluence, the greater the amount of pain. Studies comparing pain with different PDT light sources have generated inconsistent results; thus no firm conclusion can be made.[25] Finally, the second session is usually the most painful, with the first session serving as a predictor of the amount of pain that the patient will experience.

Several strategies have been studied that have been found to be helpful in reducing the level of pain, but not completely eliminating it, including using cold air, administering topical/injectable anesthetics, reducing irradiance, and interrupting the PDT session (**Table 3**).

### Cold air

Cooling of the skin is the most common method of managing pain during the treatment of PDT. This method may work by reducing metabolism, leading to a reduction of tissue damage. In addition, cold air stimulates the A delta fiber, which inhibits pain transmission. In fact, Stangeland and Kroon found a statistically significant difference in overall pain scores at 3 and 9 minutes, when air-cooled devices were used during the treatment of actinic keratosis.[26] However, Tyrell and colleagues[27]

found that when compared with controls, patients using cooling devices had significantly less PpIX photobleaching and reduced clinical clearance rates at 3 months. The investigators concluded that although air cooling devices are an effective method of pain control during PDT treatment, they should be sparingly used. However, in clinical practice, cold air cooling has a clear role in decreasing patient discomfort and completing treatment sessions. To compensate for possible decreased efficacy of PDT treatment with cold air cooling, the incubation time of the sensitizer or the duration of treatment may be increased.

### Injectable anesthetics

Using either nerve blocks or local infiltration with anesthesia, without the addition of a vasoconstrictor, has been found to be helpful in managing pain in PDT treatment. Using anesthesia without a vasoconstrictor allows an adequate flow of oxygen to the treated area. Paoli and colleagues[28] performed unilateral facial nerve blocks in the treatment of 16 patients with symmetrically distributed facial actinic keratosis (AKs) mainly on the forehead. Pain during PDT treatment was assessed by VAS. The investigators found that pain was significantly reduced on the side treated with the facial block; the mean VAS score on the blocked side of the face was 1.3 compared with 7.5 on the nonanesthetized side. Serra-Guillen and colleagues,[29] compared the efficacy of supratrochlear and supraorbital nerve block with cold air analgesia in reducing pain experienced during PDT. They found that nerve block is superior to cold air. However, because of both additional time and cost, use of injectable anesthetics is typically reserved for cases in which other noninvasive methods for anesthesia have failed.

### Interruption of treatment

Interrupting PDT for an interval of 3 minutes and spraying the patient with cold water to help cool

### Table 3
### Strategies to manage pain in PDT

| Method | Efficacy | Limitations |
|---|---|---|
| Cool air | Effective in reducing pain, but does not eliminate it | May reduce clinical efficacy |
| Injectable anesthetics (without vasoconstrictor) | Significantly reduces pain | Additional time and cost |
| Interruption of treatment (3-min break with cold spray) | Effective in reducing pain<br><br>Cold spray does not decrease efficacy | Using cold packs may decrease efficacy<br>Prolong session |
| Topical anesthetics | Not effective | — |

the treated area significantly reduces pain and does not decrease the efficacy of the treatment. This fact was demonstrated by Wigell and colleagues[30] who treated 24 patients with actinic keratosis; treatments were separated by a 3-minute pause in illumination, at which time the treated sites were cooled with either cold water spray or cold water pack (CoolPack). Using the VAS, the investigators found that pain intensity was reduced by 1.2 points using the water spray and 1.3 points by the Cool-Pack but was decreased even more after a pause in treatment (by 3.7 points in patients who received the water spray and 3.0 points in those who received the CoolPack). They concluded that the combination of cooling and a 3-minute pause resulted in a greater reduction in pain, when compared with cooling alone. Although this study did not show a decrease in efficacy with the use of cold packs, this potential effect, which has been shown with the use of cold air (described earlier) should be considered. Therefore, initial attempts to decrease discomfort should be performed with interruption but without the use of cold packs.

## Topical anesthetics

Topical anesthetics have shown disappointing results. topical eutectic mixture of local anesthetics, lidocaine, tetracaine, and capsaicin have all been used; however, none of them demonstrated any benefit.[25]

## Phototoxicity

Phototoxicity manifesting as erythema and edema are common side effects of PDT therapy. A review by Lehmann[31] of 2031 patients treated with PDT over a 5-year period found that 89% of patients experienced erythema and edema. The erythema peaks at about 1 to 2 hours after irradiation and usually resolves within 1 to 2 weeks. In rare cases, the erythema may persist for longer than 3 months. Histamine has been found to be released after ALA-PDT and peaks at 30 minutes after irradiation. However, a study by Brooke and colleagues[32] found that although cetirizine doubled the median minimal urticating dose, it did not influence the 24-hour minimal phototoxic dose or erythema dose response. Ibboston[33] found that 34% of patients undergoing PDT developed urticaria, but others[34] have found much lower rates, ranging from 0.9% to 3.8%. Thus, although some investigators have recommended use of prophylactic antihistamines, they are not widely used.

## Infection

The risk of infection is quite small, possibly because of inherent PDT antimicrobial activity.

The risk has been estimated to be less than 1%.[2] However, the development of sterile pustules is commonly seen in patients with acne vulgaris treated with PDT. Although rare, Wolfe and colleagues[35] reported 4 cases of cellulitis in the treatment of more than 700 patients with PDT. All 4 patients presented with increased pain and burning 1 to 4 days after PDT treatment, and cultures of treated sites were positive for Staphylococcus aureus. Thus, in a patient who presents with increased pain and burning after PDT treatment, culture of the treated site and prophylactic antibiotics against S aureus are recommended. The recurrence of herpes simplex has been rarely reported, and prophylactic antiviral treatment is not recommended at this time.

## Immunosuppression

In a murine model, topical PDT has been shown to reduce the number of epidermal Langerhans cells starting at 1 day after application, which continues to decrease and reaches a minimum level about 5 days later. In the same animal model, PDT has been found to reduce the delayed hypersensitivity response to 2,4-dinitrofluorobenzene at treated sites (ie, local immunosuppression); when higher fluence was used, systemic immunosuppression was observed.[36] However, it should be noted that patients undergoing transplant are often successfully treated with PDT for NMSC and that in human subjects, no report of clinically relevant immunosuppression has been reported.

## Scarring

PDT therapy is usually the treatment of choice when cosmesis is of concern in the treatment of superficial NMSC.[2] However, atrophic and hypertrophic scars have been reported, and the risk is estimated to be less than 1%. Depending on the severity of the phototoxic reaction, milia and epidermoid cysts have been observed, but these resolve over time.[2] Because these side effects may occur as a result of phototoxicity, it is important to be conservative in incubation time, irradiance and fluence used, and length of irradiation. As with other treatment modalities, such as laser and chemical peels, scarring can occur if patients excoriate their lesions during the healing process. Patients should be counseled accordingly, and this information should be included in a patient information handout.

## Pigmentation

Because PDT is known to cause inflammation in the treated area, changes in pigmentation are an expected outcome. Both hyperpigmentation and hypopigmentation have been reported with both MAL and ALA, but a higher incidence has been reported with ALA.[2] This risk may be greater in patients with skin types IV to VI. As in other cases with postinflammatory pigmentation, this usually resolves with time. Patients should be educated about photoprotection, including the use of broad-spectrum sunscreens with sun protection factor greater than 30 once the acute phototoxic response has subsided. Patients should be informed that this discoloration, which can resemble a windburn or bronzing, will gradually fade with time.

### Risk of Carcinogenesis

Finland and colleagues[37] examined the effects of PDT and Psoralen plus ultraviolet light therapy (PUVA) on human skin using an in vivo model. The investigators concluded that PUVA results in accumulation and phosphorylation of p53, which can lead to DNA damage that may lead to tumorigenesis, whereas ALA-PDT does not. However, there have been several case reports of skin cancers developing after PDT treatments, including a melanoma on an elderly patient's scalp after multiple PDT treatments, and keratoacanthoma developing after multiple treatments with ALA blue light PDT for facial actinic keratosis. However, it is difficult to prove causation in each case and development of skin cancer may be coincidental. PDT is still new to medicine, with widespread use starting in the early 1990s. Thus, long-term follow-up of patients receiving multiple PDT treatments is recommended.

## SUMMARY

The field of PDT continues to advance. Sufficient data exist at this time that demonstrate the utility of PDT in the treatment of actinic keratosis, superficial NMSC, photoaging, acne, and verrucae. PDT offers efficacy similar to standard treatments, with high patient tolerance and excellent cosmesis. However, PDT, unlike surgical excision, does not provide histologic control in the treatment of NMSC, and thus it is prudent to select appropriate lesions for treatment with this modality. PDT is generally well tolerated. While pain remains the most common adverse event reported, various effective strategies have been developed to manage pain.

## REFERENCES

1. Rivard J, Ozog D. Henry Ford Hospital dermatology experience with Levulan Kerastick and blue light photodynamic therapy. J Drugs Dermatol 2006; 5(6):556–61.

2. Babilas P, Schreml S, Landthaler M, et al. Photodynamic therapy in dermatology: state-of-the-art. Photodermatol Photoimmunol Photomed 2010;26(3): 118–32.

3. Szeimies RM, Drager J, Abels C, et al. History of photodynamic therapy in dermatology. Photodynamic therapy and fluorescence diagnosis in dermatology. Amsterdam: Elsevier; 2001. p. 3–16.

4. Kennedy JC, Pottier RH, Pross DC. Photodynamic therapy with endogenous protoporphyrin IX: basic principles and present clinical experience. J Photochem Photobiol B 1990;6(1–2):143–8.

5. Babilas P, Travnik R, Werner A, et al. Split-face-study using two different light sources for topical PDT of actinic keratoses: non-inferiority of the LED system. J Dtsch Dermatol Ges 2008;6:25–32.

6. Gold MH, Bradshaw VL, Boring MM, et al. Split-face comparison of photodynamic therapy with 5-aminolevulinic acid and intense pulsed light versus intense pulsed light alone for photodamage. Dermatol Surg 2006;32:795–801 [discussion: 801–3].

7. Hongcharu W, Taylor CR, Chang Y, et al. Topical ALA-photodynamic therapy for the treatment of acne vulgaris. J Invest Dermatol 2000;115:183–92.

8. Itoh Y, Ninomiya Y, Tajima S, et al. Photodynamic therapy of acne vulgaris with topical delta-aminolaevulinic acid and incoherent light in Japanese patients. Br J Dermatol 2001;144:575–9.

9. Wiegell SR, Wulf HC. Photodynamic therapy of acne vulgaris using methyl aminolaevulinate: a blinded, randomized, con-trolled trial. Br J Dermatol 2006; 154:969–76.

10. Wiegell SR, Wulf HC. Photodynamic therapy of acne vulgaris using 5-aminolevulinic acid versus methyl aminolevulinate. J Am Acad Dermatol 2006;54: 647–51.

11. Sakamoto FH, Torezan L, Anderson RR. Photodynamic therapy for acne vulgaris: a critical review from basics to clinical practice Part 2 Understanding parameters for acne treatment with photodynamic therapy. J Am Acad Dermatol 2010;63:195–211.

12. Stender IM, Na R, Fogh H, et al. Photodynamic therapy with 5-aminolaevulinic acid or placebo for recalcitrant foot and hand warts: randomised double-blind trial. Lancet 2000;355:963–6.

13. Schroeter CA, Kaas L, Waterval JJ, et al. Successful treatment of periungual warts using photodynamic therapy: a pilot study. J Eur Acad Dermatol Venereo 2007;21:1170–4.

14. Stefanaki IM, Georgiou S, Themelis GC, et al. In vivo fluorescence kinetics and photodynamic therapy in condylomata acuminata. Br J Dermatol 2003;149: 972–6.

15. Fehr MK, Hornung P, Schwarz VA, et al. Photodynamic therapy of vulvar and vaginal condylomata and intraepithelial neoplasia using topical 5-aminolaevulinic acid. Lasers Surg Med 2002;30:273–9.

16. Morton C, Campbell S, Gupta G, et al. Intraindividual, right-left comparison of topical methyl aminolaevulinate-photodynamic therapy and cryotherapy in subjects with actinic keratoses: a multicentre, randomized controlled study. Br J Dermatol 2006;155:1029–36.

17. Touma D, Yaar M, Whitehead S, et al. A trial of short incubation, broad-area photodynamic therapy for facial actinic keratoses and diffuse photodamage. Arch Dermatol 2004;140:33–40.

18. Gupta AK, Paquet M, Villanueva E, et al. Interventions for actinic keratoses. Cochrane Database Syst Rev 2012;(12):CD004415.

19. Tierney EP, Eide MJ, Jacobsen G, et al. Photodynamic therapy for actinic keratoses: survey of patient perceptions of treatment satisfaction and outcomes. J Cosmet Laser Ther 2008;10(2):81–6.

20. Morton C, Horn M, Leman J, et al. Comparison of topical methyl aminolevulinate photodynamic therapy with cryotherapy or fluorouracil for treatment of squamous cell carcinoma in situ: results of a multicenter randomized trial. Arch Dermatol 2006;142:729–35.

21. Salim A, Leman JA, McColl JH, et al. Randomized comparison of photodynamic therapy with topical 5-fluorouracil in Bowen's disease. Br J Dermatol 2003;148:539–43.

22. Morton CA, MacKie RM, Whitehurst C, et al. Photodynamic therapy for basal cell carcinoma: effect of tumor thickness and duration of photosensitizer application on response. Arch Dermatol 1998;134:248–9.

23. Szeimies RM, Ibbotson S, Murrell DF, et al. A clinical study comparing methyl aminolevulinate photodynamic therapy and surgery in small superficial basal cell carcinoma (8–20 mm), with a 12-month follow-up. J Eur Acad Dermatol Venereol 2008;22:1302–11.

24. Liu A, Moy RL, Ross EV, et al. Pulsed dye laser and pulsed dye laser-mediated photodynamic therapy in the treatment of dermatologic disorders. Dermatol Surg 2012;38(3):351–66.

25. Chaves Y, Torezan L, Niwa AB, et al. Pain in photodynamic therapy: mechanism of action and management strategies. An Bras Dermatol 2012;87(4):521–6 [quiz: 527–9].

26. Stangeland KZ, Kroon S. Cold air analgesia as pain reduction during photodynamic therapy of actinic keratosis. J Eur Acad Dermatol Venereol 2012;26(7):849–54.

27. Tyrrell J, Campbell SM, Curnow A. The effect of air cooling pain relief on protoporphyrin IX photobleaching and clinical efficacy during dermatological photodynamic therapy. J Photochem Photobiol B 2011;103(1):1–7.

28. Paoli J, Halldin C, Ericson MB, et al. Nerve blocks provide effective pain relief during topical photodynamic therapy for extensive facial actinic keratoses. Clin Exp Dermatol 2008;33(5):559–64.

29. Serra-Guillen C, Hueso L, Nagore E, et al. Comparative study between cold air analgesia and supraorbital and supratrochlear nerve block for the management of pain during photodynamic therapy for actinic keratoses of the frontotemporal zone. Br J Dermatol 2009;161(2):353–6.

30. Wiegell SR, Haedersdal M, Wulf HC. Cold water and pauses in illumination reduces pain during photodynamic therapy: a randomized clinical study. Acta Derm Venereol 2009;89:145–9.

31. Lehmann P. Side effects of topical photodynamic therapy. Hautarzt 2007;58:597–603.

32. Brooke RCC, Sinha A, Sidhu MK, et al. Histamine is released following aminolevulinic acid-photodynamic therapy of human skin and mediates an aminolevulinic acid dose-related immediate inflammatory response. J Invest Dermatol 2006;126:2296–301.

33. Ibbotson SH. Adverse effects of topical photodynamic therapy. Photodermatol Photoimmunol Photomed 2011;27(3):116–30.

34. Kaae J, Philipsen PA, Haedersdal M, et al. Immediate whealing urticaria in red light exposed areas during photodynamic therapy. Acta Derm Venereol 2008;88(5):480–3.

35. Wolfe CM, Hatfield K, Cognetta AB. Cellulitis as a postprocedural complication of topical 5-aminolevulinic acid photodynamic therapy in the treatment of actinic keratosis. J Drugs Dermatol 2007;6:544–8.

36. Hayami J, Okamoto H, Sugihara A, et al. Immunosuppressive effects of photodynamic therapy by topical aminolevulinic acid. J Dermatol 2007;34:320–7.

37. Finlan LE, Kernohan NM, Thomson G, et al. Differential effects of 5-aminolaevulinic acid photodynamic therapy and psoralen plus ultraviolet A therapy on p53 phosphorylation in normal human skin in vivo. Br J Dermatol 2005;153:1001–10.

# Sunscreens
# A Review of Health Benefits, Regulations, and Controversies

Silvia E. Mancebo, BS[a], Judy Y. Hu, MD[b],
Steven Q. Wang, MD[a],*

## KEYWORDS

- Photoprotection • Skin cancer prevention • Sunscreen controversies • Sunscreen regulations

## KEY POINTS

- Regular sunscreen use prevents the development of actinic keratosis (AK), squamous cell carcinoma (SCC), melanoma, and photoaging associated with sun exposure.
- Food and Drug Administration (FDA) final ruling on labeling and effectiveness testing adopted the critical wavelength (CW) test to assess ultraviolet (UV)-A filtering capacity; only products with CW greater than or equal to 370 nm can claim broad-spectrum status.
- Safety profiles of sunscreens have been called into question, but current studies show that sunscreens are safe and effective.
- Appropriate application and improved compliance remain the major challenges that limit the effectiveness of sunscreen use.

## INTRODUCTION

Skin cancer is the most common cancer in the United States. Over the past decades, both the incidence and the mortality of skin cancer have been rising. Current estimates of nonmelanoma skin cancer suggest that more than 2 million Americans are affected annually and 1 in 5 Americans will be affected in their lifetime.[1,2] UV light plays a major role in the development of skin cancer.[3] Exposure to sunlight has been attributed to nearly 90% of nonmelanoma and 65% of melanoma skin cancers.[4,5] Therefore, protecting from UV light is a major strategy in the prevention of skin cancer.

UV light is classified into different wavelengths: UV-C (270–290 nm), UV-B (290–320 nm), UV-A2 (320–340 nm), and UV-A1 (340–400 nm).[6] UV-C is filtered by the ozone layer and does not reach the surface of the earth. Compared to UV-B radiation, UV-A penetrates deeper into the skin and reaches the dermis. The intensity of UV radiation that reaches the skin depends on several environmental factors including latitude, altitude, season, cloudiness, and time of day.[7] As UV radiation travels through the skin, DNA, lipids, and proteins absorb UV energy causing direct and indirect damage to nearby structures.[8,9] High-energy UV-B rays cause direct damage to DNA by creating covalent bonds between pyrimidine bases.[10,11] These bonds have a high mutagenic potential and need to be corrected by DNA repair mechanisms. Indirect damage is caused by both UV-A and UV-B light, resulting in the formation of reactive oxygen species, oxidative DNA damage, and activation of inflammatory cytokines.[12–14] Ultimately, these molecular insults result in sunburns, pigment darkening, suppression of cellular immunity, premature aging, and photocarcinogenesis.[15–17]

Conflict of Interest: No conflicts of interest.
[a] Dermatology Service, Memorial Sloan Kettering Cancer Center, 160 East 53rd Street, New York, NY 10022, USA; [b] Global Health Research LLC, Chatham, NJ, USA
* Corresponding author. Dermatology Service, Memorial Sloan Kettering Cancer Center, 136 Mountain View Boulevard, Basking Ridge, NJ 07920.
E-mail address: wangs@mskcc.org

Dermatol Clin 32 (2014) 427–438
http://dx.doi.org/10.1016/j.det.2014.03.011
0733-8635/14/$ – see front matter © 2014 Elsevier Inc. All rights reserved.

derm.theclinics.com

Over the past decades, there has been an increased effort by the health care community to promote healthy sun-related attitudes and behaviors. Comprehensive sun protection includes minimizing sun exposure by using photoprotective gear such as long-sleeved shirts, wide-brimmed hats, and sunglasses and by applying sunscreen regularly (**Box 1**). Among these measures, sunscreens are one of the most popular protective methods used by the public.[18] This review discusses the health benefits afforded by sunscreen use, reviews the impact of the 2011 FDA ruling on sunscreen labeling and effectiveness testing, and addresses the controversies and limitations associated with sunscreen use.

## MECHANISM OF ACTION

Sunscreens provide temporary protection against UV radiation. The active ingredients are classified into organic and inorganic UV filters based on chemical composition and mechanism of action. Organic filters are aromatic compounds that work by absorbing UV light, and inorganic filters are minerals that can absorb, reflect, and scatter UV light (**Fig. 1**). There are advantages and disadvantages associated with both kinds of filters, and it is not infrequent to see both types of filters present in commercially available formulations.

Organic UV filters exert their protective effects by absorbing high-energy photons from UV radiation. The energy absorbed is transmitted to electrons, which jump to an excited state, and on return to ground state, release their energy in the form of heat or light in longer wavelength.[19–21] p-Aminobenzoic acid was the first UV filter

available in the United States but had many undesirable properties. It was known for its potential to cause photoallergic, contact dermatitis and stain clothes.[22] Newer generations of organic filters have improved safety and sensory profiles and extended coverage to the UV-A range.

At present, there are 15 organic UV filters approved for use in the United States (**Table 1**). At this time, avobenzone is the only organic filter approved by the FDA that has long-range UV-A (340–400 nm) protection. Its absorption profile ranges from 310 nm to 400 nm, with an absorption peak around 360 nm.[23] Avobenzone is known for being intrinsically unstable and degrades after 1 hour of UV exposure.[24] To maintain its efficacy, it must be combined with a photostabilizer, which facilitates the transition from an excited state back to ground state.[25] Without the presence of a photostabilizer, the avobenzone molecule in its excited state can isomerize and fragment into compounds that are less effective at filtering UV light.[26]

Zinc oxide ($ZnO$) and titanium dioxide ($TiO_2$) are the only inorganic UV filters approved for use in the United States (see **Table 1**). Early generations of these products lacked popularity because of inherent flaws in their sensory profiles. These early-generation products contained larger particles with higher refractive indices resulting in a thick, white coat that had poor particle dispersion and comedogenic potential.[27] Over the past few decades, manufacturers have modified formulations to include microsized and nanosized $ZnO$ and $TiO_2$, which scatter less visible light and create more transparent films that provide improved cosmetic appearance.[28] The reduction in particle size has also led to changes in the absorption profile. Nanosized $TiO_2$ has an enhanced ability to absorb UV light in the UV-B range (ie, 290–320 nm).[29] However, this increase in UV-B absorption may result in decreased protection from UV-A radiation and potential loss of broad-spectrum coverage.[30] Compared to organic filters, these filters are less susceptible to degradation from UV exposure and have a lower potential of causing allergic reactions.[27]

## HEALTH BENEFITS OF USING SUNSCREEN

Sunscreen use has been shown to impart many health benefits. Studies have demonstrated that using sunscreen on a daily basis can prevent the development of AK, SCC, and melanoma.[31–33] Furthermore, there is evidence suggesting that sunscreens can diminish the appearance of premature aging and prevent exacerbations of photodermatoses.[34,35] Much of the information

---

**Box 1**

**Patient recommendations for comprehensive photoprotection**

- Seek shade and minimize sun exposure, especially between 10 AM and 2 PM

- Wear photoprotective clothing, including a wide-brimmed hat, long-sleeve shirt, pants, and sunglasses

- Use a broad-spectrum sunscreen with an SPF of 15 or more daily

- For extended outdoor activity, use a water-resistant, broad-spectrum sunscreen with an SPF of 30 or more

- Apply 1 oz of sunscreen to the entire body 15 minutes before going outside

- When outdoor, reapply sunscreen at least every 2 hours, or immediately after swimming or excessive sweating

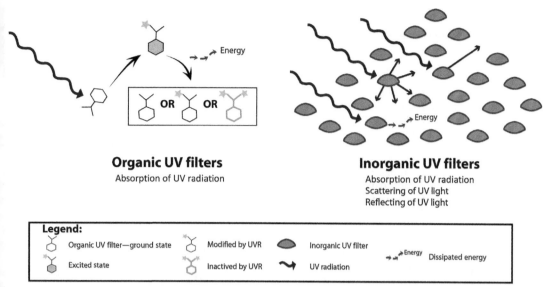

**Organic UV filters**
Absorption of UV radiation

**Inorganic UV filters**
Absorption of UV radiation
Scattering of UV light
Reflecting of UV light

Legend:

Organic UV filter—ground state       Modified by UVR       Inorganic UV filter       Energy  Dissipated energy

Excited state       Inactived by UVR       UV radiation

**Fig. 1.** Sunscreens' mechanism of action. Organic UV filters absorb energy from UV radiation causing electrons in the filter to jump to an excited state. On return to ground state, energy is released in the form of heat or light in longer wavelength. Transition back to ground state has the potential of causing chemical modifications, resulting in filters that are less effective at filtering UV light. Inorganic UV filters can absorb, reflect, and scatter UV light. Compared to organic filters, these products are more stable to degradation from UV exposure.

that we have today on the protective effects of sunscreens has been derived from the Nambour Skin Cancer Prevention Trial in Australia. This series of studies, initiated in 1992, was conducted using a sunscreen with sun protection factor (SPF) 16 containing 2% 4-*tert*-butyl-4′-methoxy-4-dibenzolymethane (avobenzone) and 8% 2-ethylhexyl-*p*-methoxycinnamate (octinoxate) as active ingredients.[36] This formulation is not photostable and will not pass the new FDA standards to be labeled broad spectrum.[37] Nonetheless, the fact that this sunscreen reduced the incidence of skin cancer suggests that modern-day sunscreens with a higher SPF value and broad-spectrum protection may likely provide even greater health benefits.

### Prevention of AK and SCC

AKs are well-known risk factors for the development of nonmelanoma skin cancer, and nearly 65% of SCCs arise from previously diagnosed actinic lesions.[38] Several studies have explored the effect of sunscreen use on the development of AKs. Thompson and colleagues[39] used a randomized controlled trial to study the incidence, prevalence, and remission rates of AKs. These investigators supplied participants with broad-spectrum SPF 17 sunscreen containing 2% avobenzone and 8% octinoxate or a base cream containing no active ingredients. Over the span of 7 months, the study showed that daily sunscreen use reduced the emergence of new

lesions, decreased the total number of AKs, and induced greater remission rates, all in a dose-dependent manner.[39] Darlington and colleagues[31] also evaluated the prevalence of AKs. These investigators assessed the rate of change in the incidence of AKs among participants from the Nambour Skin Cancer Prevention Trial in Australia. They found that daily use of broad-spectrum, SPF 16 sunscreen resulted in a 24% reduction in the average rate of AK development. In addition, their study revealed a greater reduction in the rate of AK acquisition among participants who had fewer baseline AKs, suggesting that sunscreen use might be more effective at preventing, rather than inducing remission of AKs.[31,40]

SCC commonly occurs on sun-exposed areas of the body in fair-skinned individuals. Both AK and SCC are associated with high-dose cumulative UV exposure.[41] There is strong evidence supporting the use of sunscreen as a safe and effective method to prevent SCC. In a randomized controlled trial of 1621 adults who lived in Nambour, Australia, participants were assigned either to an intervention group that was provided with SPF 16 sunscreen containing 2% avobenzone and 8% octinoxate for daily use or to a control group that was allowed to use sunscreen at their discretion.[36] After a 4.5-year intervention, the study showed a statistically significant 38% reduction in the incidence of SCC tumors among participants assigned to the sunscreen group. Both cohorts were followed up for another

**Table 1**
**Ultraviolet light filters approved by FDA for use In United States**

| | | | Active Ingredient | Maximum λ (nm) Absorption | UV Spectrum Coverage |
|---|---|---|---|---|---|
| Organic UV filters | UV-B filters | **Aminobenzoates** | | | |
| | | | para-Aminobenzoic acid | 283 | UV-B |
| | | | Padimate O (octyl dimethyl PABA) | 311 | UV-B |
| | | **Cinnamates** | | | |
| | | | Cinoxate (2-ethoxyethyl p-methoxycinnamate) | 289 | UV-B |
| | | | Octinoxate (octyl methoxycinnamate) | 311 | UV-B |
| | | **Salicylates** | | | |
| | | | Trolamine salicylate (triethanolamine salicylate) | 260–355 | UV-B |
| | | | Homosalate (homomenthyl salicylate) | 306 | UV-B |
| | | | Octisalate (octyl salicylate) | 307 | UV-B |
| | | **Others** | | | |
| | | | Octocrylene (2-ethylhexyl 2-cyano-3, 3- diphenylacrylate) | 303 | UV-B, UV-A2 |
| | | | Ensulizole (phenylbenzimidazole sulfonic acid) | 310 | UV-B |
| | UV-A filters | **Benzophenones** | | | |
| | | | Oxybenzone (benzophenone-3) | 288, 325 | UV-B, UV-A2 |
| | | | Dioxybenzone (benzophenone-8) | 352 | UV-B, UV-A2 |
| | | | Sulisobenzone (benzophenone-4) | 366 | UV-B, UV-A2 |
| | | **Dibenzoylmethanes** | | | |
| | | | Avobenzone (butyl methoxydibenzoylmethane, Parsol 1789) | 360 | UV-A1 |
| | | **Anthralates** | | | |
| | | | Meradimate (menthyl anthranilate) | 340 | UV-A2 |
| | | **Camphors** | | | |
| | | | Ecamsule (terephthalylidene dicamphor sulfonic acid, Mexoryl SX) | 345 | UV-B, UV-A |
| Inorganic UV filters | | | Zinc oxide | Depends on particle size | UV-B, UV-A |
| | | | Titanium dioxide | Depends on particle size | UV-B, UV-A |

*Abbreviation:* PABA, para-Aminobenzoic acid.

*Data from* U.S. Food and Drug Administration. Sunscreen drug products for over-the-counter human use [stayed indefinitely]. 21 CFR 352. Available at: http://www.gpo.gov/fdsys/pkg/CFR-2002-title21-vol5/pdf/CFR-2002-title21-vol5-sec352-10.pdf. Revised April 1, 2013. Effective June 4, 2004. Accessed September 1, 2013.

8 years after the completion of the first 4.5 years; the same investigators reported similar protective effects of daily sunscreen use in the same cohort of participants.[32] Although most of this effect may be attributed to the use of sunscreen during the original trial, many of the participants in the intervention group continued to use sunscreen more frequently during the follow-up period.[42]

### Reduction of Basal Cell Carcinoma

Basal cell carcinoma (BCC) accounts for up to 80% of all skin cancers, and sun exposure has been identified as a risk factor for the development of these tumors.[1] The relationship between UV light and BCC development is complex. Most BCC tumors arise on chronically sun-damaged skin involving the face, head, and neck areas, but about one-third of tumors develop in areas with minimal sun exposure, such as the trunk and lower limbs, suggesting that other factors are involved in tumorigenesis.[43] To date, the previously mentioned Nambour Skin Cancer Prevention Trial in Australia has been the only randomized controlled study to look at the effect of sunscreen use on BCC development.[36] The results of this study did not reveal a significant difference in BCC prevalence between the groups studied. However, the follow-up study conducted by van der Pols and colleagues[32] 8 years later showed a

25% reduction in BCC incidence among participants previously assigned to the sunscreen group. This trend was also not statistically significant. Several explanations have been proposed to explain these results. First, BCC has a latency period of more than 20 years from the time of UV damage to the clinical onset of disease.[43] The study by van der Pols and colleagues,[32] demonstrated a trend toward decreased BCC incidence, indicating that longer periods of follow-up may be needed to observe the protective effect of sunscreen use in BCC development. In addition, the design of both studies allowed participants in the control group to use sunscreen at their discretion. In fact, about 25% of the participants in the control group used sunscreen as regularly as participants in the intervention group, implying that the results of the study may have been diluted by the behavior of the control group.[42] In conclusion, sunscreens may be beneficial in preventing BCC development; however, further studies are needed to clearly delineate this effect.

## Prevention of Melanoma

Melanoma results from a multifactorial process involving both genetic and environmental predispositions. UV radiation has been identified as the only modifiable risk factor for the development of melanoma.[33] High-dose intermittent sun exposure associated with sunburns carries a lifetime relative risk for melanoma of up to 1.6 across all age groups.[44] Despite the established etiologic role of UV exposure on the development of melanoma, evidence to support the use of sunscreen as a preventative method has been historically ambiguous and controversial.[42,45] A meta-analysis was conducted by Dennis and colleagues[46] evaluating all cohort and case-control studies published between 1966 and 2003. This study revealed neither a protective nor a harmful association between sunscreen use and melanoma. In 2010, Green and colleagues[33] published the first randomized control study to evaluate the protective effects of sunscreen use on the development of melanoma. This study looked at melanoma as a secondary endpoint, 10 years after the conclusion of the Nambour Skin Cancer Prevention Trial. The investigators found a 50% reduction in new primary melanomas and a 73% reduction in invasive melanoma rates among participants previously assigned to the sunscreen group. This landmark study demonstrated that regular sunscreen use reduces the risk of developing melanoma. It is important to highlight that the investigators followed up the cohort for more than 15 years in this study.

## Prevention of Skin Aging

Photoaging is a complex and progressive process exacerbated by UV exposure. Among the treatments available, sunscreens are considered the most effective at preventing photoaging. Data to support this concept comes from a randomized controlled trial conducted by Hughes and colleagues[34] among participants in the Nambour Skin Cancer Prevention Trial, who were younger than 55 years. These investigators obtained skin surface replicas of the dorsal part of the left hand of the participants and graded the microtopography. Each unit increase in microtopography grade correlates with visible signs of skin aging, such as deterioration of skin texture and increase in visible small blood vessels and comedones on the face, as well as with the risk of developing AKs and nonmelanoma skin cancer.[47–49] Hughes and colleagues[34] found that daily sunscreen use reduces the likelihood of having higher microtopography grades and also decreases the risk of developing AKs and skin cancer.

## Management of Photodermatoses

Polymorphous light eruption (PMLE) is a common photodermatosis characterized by highly pruritic and polymorphous skin lesions resulting from exposure to sunlight.[50] The disease reduces quality of life because of physical appearance of lesions and pruritus. The mainstay in management of PMLE includes sun avoidance, regardless of the severity of disease.[50] Patients are encouraged to adopt a comprehensive sun protection regimen if they must be outside, including daily use of broad-spectrum sunscreen with SPF greater than 30 that is applied generously and frequently.[51] Schleyer and colleagues[52] analyzed the efficacy of sunscreens with high UV-A and UV-B protection in the development of PMLE lesions after standardized photoprovocation. A total of 12 patients were treated with UV-A, UV-B, or both UV-A and UV-B light at sites where either broad-spectrum sunscreen containing several UV-A and UV-B filters or vehicle cream without active ingredients were applied. In 10 of these patients, PMLE lesions were provoked in the placebo sites, while sites pretreated with sunscreen were fully protected from PMLE. Ultimately, the results of this study show that high-SPF, broad-spectrum sunscreen can successfully prevent the development of PMLE.[52,53]

## FDA REGULATION ON SUNSCREEN LABELING AND EFFECTIVENESS TESTING

The harmful effects of UV-A radiation have been long recognized. UV-A radiation has been implied in molecular and cellular damage that results in photoaging, immunosuppression, and skin cancer development.[54] Exposure to UV-A radiation has been associated with oxidative damage that causes increased melanin synthesis, cell membrane lipid peroxidation, activation of matrix metalloproteinases, and release of inflammatory cytokines and growth factors.[7,13,14] Ultimately, the resulting effect is lasting damage to cells, vessels, and tissues that may permanently alter skin integrity.[55]

Historically, in the United States, sunscreens containing one or more UV-A filters were permitted to claim the broad-spectrum status, although the level of UV-A protection varied significantly among these products.[56] In 2011, the FDA published the final ruling on labeling and effectiveness testing for sunscreens (**Table 2**). A pass/fail system using the in vitro CW test was adopted as the only method for assessing UV-A filtering capacity. The CW test measures UV absorption along the UV spectrum (ie, 290–400 nm) and defines the CW as the wavelength at which 90% of UV absorption occurs (**Fig. 2**).[57] According to the new FDA standards, sunscreen products must have a CW greater than or equal to 370 nm to carry the

**Table 2**
**Highlights of 2011 FDA final ruling on labeling and effectiveness testing**

| | |
|---|---|
| Active Ingredients | 17 active ingredients approved for use in sunscreens in the United States (see **Table 2**)<br>8 active ingredients being evaluated under TEA process<br>Combination of avobenzone and ensulizole not currently allowed |
| Labeling Requirements | |
| Broad Spectrum and SPF Greater than 15 | *Uses and Benefit Claim:* "Helps prevent sunburn" and "if used as directed with other sun protection measures (see Directions), decreases the risk of skin cancer and early skin aging caused by the sun"<br>*Sun Protection Measures:* "Spending time in the sun increases your risk of skin cancer and early skin aging. To decrease this risk, regularly use a sunscreen with broad spectrum SPF value of 15 or higher and other sun protection measures including, limit time in the sun, especially from 10 AM – 2 PM and wear long-sleeved shirts, pants, hats, and sunglasses" |
| Not Broad Spectrum or SPF Less than 15 | *Uses:* "Helps prevent sunburn"<br>*Skin Cancer/Skin Aging Alert:* "Spending time in the sun increases your risk of skin cancer and early skin aging. This product has been shown only to help prevent sunburn, *not* skin cancer or early skin aging" |
| Water Resistant | *Directions:* "Reapply after 40 (or 80) min of swimming or sweating, immediately after towel drying or at least every 2 h" |
| Not Water Resistant | *Directions:* "Reapply at least every 2 h and use a water-resistant sunscreen if swimming or sweating" |
| All Sunscreen Products | *Directions:* "Apply liberally/generously 15 min before sun exposure" |
| Label Claims Not Allowed | "Sunblock," "sweatproof," "waterproof," "instant protection," "all day," or extended wear claims, unless FDA approved |
| Effectiveness Testing | |
| SPF Testing | In vivo MED test on 10–13 patients with more than 10 valid results |
| Broad-Spectrum Testing | In vitro, pass/fail CW test; product must have CW $\geq$370 nm |
| Pending Issues | • Maximum label to be capped at "SPF 50+"<br>• Dosage forms may not be eligible for review: wipes, towelettes, powders, body washes, shampoos<br>• Sprays: remaining concerns about effectiveness and safety<br>• 8 UV filters under review of TEA process may provide broader options for manufacturers |

*Abbreviations:* MED, minimum erythema dose; TEA, time and extent application.
*Data from* U.S. Food and Drug Administration. Labeling and effectiveness testing: sunscreen drug products for over-the-counter human use — small entity compliance guide. 2012. Available at: http://www.fda.gov/drugs/guidancecomplianceregulatoryinformation/guidances/ucm330694.htm. Accessed September 1, 2013.

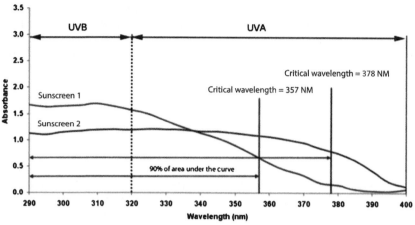

**Fig. 2.** Critical wavelength method. CW represents the wavelength at which 90% of the absorbance curve resides. Sunscreen 1 has an SPF of 30 and a CW of 357 nm. Sunscreen 2 has an SPF of 15 and a CW of 378 nm. According to the 2011 final rule, only Sunscreen 2 can claim broad-spectrum status. (*From* Wang SQ, Tanner PR, Lim HW, et al. The evolution of sunscreen products in the United States: a 12-year cross sectional study. Photochem Photobiol Sci 2013;12:197–202; with permission from the European Society for Photobiology, the European Photochemistry Association, and The Royal Society of Chemistry.)

broad-spectrum label. In addition, the final ruling has established criteria to assure the reliability of the CW test. These criteria include testing a specific amount of sunscreen, preirradiating sunscreen samples to account for photodegradation, determining the mean UV transmittance at each wavelength, and using the sum of this data to calculate the CW.[57] As can be seen in **Fig. 2**, the CW is a measurement of the breadth of UV coverage. It does not measure the amplitude of UV protection and therefore should be used in combination with the SPF, which measures the amplitude of UV-B protection.[58]

The FDA has also adopted new benefit and warning statements. For the first time, sunscreens providing broad-spectrum coverage with an SPF greater than 15 can claim to decrease the risk of skin cancer and early aging caused by the sun.[57] The benefit statement is based on evidence implicating UV radiation in the development of precancerous and cancerous lesions, as well as on cumulative data supporting the beneficial role of sunscreens in the prevention of skin cancer and skin aging.[58] While this claim validates the protective effects of broad-spectrum sunscreens, the FDA cautiously emphasizes that clinical benefits can only be obtained when sunscreens are "used with other sun protection measures" and if "reapplied at least every 2 hours."[58] Furthermore, a warning statement is reserved for sunscreens that do not provide broad-spectrum coverage or have an SPF less than 15, highlighting that "spending time in the sun increases the risk of skin cancer and early skin aging" and also that "this product has been shown only to prevent

sunburns, not skin cancer or early skin aging."[58] This statement intends to alert the public about the harms of sun exposure, as well as to increase awareness about the risk of using sunscreens that do not provide adequate UV-A and UV-B protection.

There are several pending issues not addressed by the final ruling in 2011. Currently, there is no limit to the maximum allowed SPF label. Sunscreen manufacturers have marketed products with SPF exceeding 100, claiming that higher SPF values provide superior protection.[58] The benefit of using higher SPF products is to compensate for inadequate application of sunscreen by consumers, resulting in much lowered protection.[59] While these claims are valid, there is a tendency for products with a high SPF value to instill a false sense of security. Consumers may overrely on these products as their only source of sun protection, staying outdoors longer and therefore increasing their UV exposure dose.[58] As a result, the FDA has proposed to cap the maximum label at SPF 50+, stating there is insufficient evidence to support the clinical benefits of products with SPF above this level.[60] This decision is not final, and the FDA is open to evaluate evidence supporting the use of high-SPF sunscreens.

Another issue that has not been fully addressed by the final ruling concerns the evaluation of nonconventional sunscreen formulations. The FDA published the "Advance Notice of Proposed Rulemaking (ANPR): Sunscreen Drug Products for Over-The-Counter Human Use; Request for Data and Information Regarding Dosage Forms," which approves oils, lotions, creams, gels, butters, pastes, and ointments for continued marketing.[61] However, sunscreens in the form of wipes, towelettes, powders, body washes, and shampoos may not be eligible for review in the future. If the ANPR becomes final, these products would no longer be marketed in the United States. Sunscreens in the form of sprays may be eligible for review in the future. However, there is concern that sprays can result in unintentional inhalation and do not provide the same protection as conventional formulations (ie, creams) because of the diffuse manner in which they are dispensed.[58]

Last, the FDA still needs to evaluate several UV filters waiting to be approved. Currently, there are 17 UV filters approved for use as active ingredients in the United States, including ecamsule, which is only approved for use in one specific formulation. Among the filters available, very few filters provide broad-spectrum coverage and even fewer have the ability to filter longer-wavelength UV-A rays. There are 8 UV filters being considered for review under the time and extent application process (Table 3). These filters have been in the European, Australian, or Asian market for at least 5 years, and if approved, would provide manufacturers with more options to create higher-quality formulations.[58]

## CONTROVERSIES ASSOCIATED WITH SUNSCREENS
### Safety of Oxybenzone

Oxybenzone is an organic filter that absorbs both UV-B and short-range UV-A rays. To date, this compound has received much attention because of concerns regarding its hormonal disrupting potential. Oxybenzone is systemically absorbed and excreted in the urine and feces. Several in vitro and in vivo animal studies have demonstrated the estrogenic and antiandrogenic activity of oxybenzone.[62–65] However, the dose exposures in these animal studies were extremely high. Wang and colleagues[66] showed that it would take more than 277 years of daily application of sunscreen to attain the same levels of oxybenzone exposure. Also, a study by Janjua and colleagues[67] evaluating the effect of topical application of oxybenzone suggests that this compound does not accumulate in the plasma. These investigators supplied 15 men and 17 postmenopausal women participants with 10% (wt/wt) oxybenzone sunscreen for 1 week. The results of the study reveal maximum oxybenzone systemic absorption 3 hours after application. Oxybenzone plasma concentrations 24 hours and 96 hours after the first application were not significantly different, indicating that there was no accumulation of oxybenzone in the plasma during the treatment week. In addition, this study evaluated sex hormone levels at the beginning and end of the study. There was a small, but statistically significant, difference in testosterone, inhibin B, and serum estradiol levels. However, these differences were neither biologically significant nor related to exposure to oxybenzone.[67] Last, the binding affinity of oxybenzone for estrogen receptors is orders of magnitude weaker than that of estrogen and estradiol.[65]

### Safety of Nanoparticles

In recent years, the safety of nanosized titanium dioxide ($TiO_2$) and zinc oxide (ZnO) has also been called to question. Inorganic filters have generally

**Table 3**
**Active ingredients pending FDA approval under the time and extent application (TEA) process**

| Active Ingredients | Maximum λ (nm) Absorption | UV Spectrum Coverage | Date of TEA Application |
| --- | --- | --- | --- |
| Enzacamene (methylbenzylidene camphor) | 300 | UV-B | July 11, 2003 |
| Amiloxate (isoamyl methoxycinnamates) | 310 | UV-B | July 11, 2003 |
| Octyl triazone (ethylhexyl triazone) | 314 | UV-B | July 11, 2003 |
| Tinosorb M/Bisoctrizole (Methylene-*bis*-benzotriazolyl tetramethylbutylphenol) | 305, 360 | UV-B, UV-A | December 5, 2005 |
| Tinosorb S/Bemotrizinol (*bis*-ethylhexyloxyphenol) | 310, 343 | UV-B, UV-A | December 5, 2005 |
| Iscotrizinol (diethylhexyl butamido triazone) | 312 | UV-B | July 26, 2006 |
| Ecamsule (terephthalylidene diacamphor sulfinic acid) | 345 | UV-B, UV-A | September 12, 2008 |
| Mexoryl XL (drometrizole trisiloxane) | 303, 344 | UV-B, UV-A | June 2, 2010 |

*Data from* U.S. Food and Drug Administration. Status of OTC rulemakings – rulemaking history of OTC time and extent applications. Available at: http://www.fda.gov/Drugs/DevelopmentApprovalProcess/DevelopmentResources/Over-the-CounterOTCDrugs/StatusofOTCRulemakings/ucm072455.htm. Updated April 11, 2012. Accessed September 1, 2013.

been considered safe, with minimal absorption past the stratum corneum.[68] However, as the size of the particles decreased, there was rising concern that metal oxides can penetrate the skin and cause local and systemic toxicities, specifically related to damage from UV-induced free radicals. Several in vivo and in vitro studies have shown no percutaneous penetration of nanoparticles in normal adult human skin.[69] In addition, studies evaluating the direct effect of nanoparticles on cellular and molecular structures reveal that nanoparticles are safe and do not cause damage to mammalian cells.[70] To address the potential for free radical formation, manufacturers have encapsulated these nanosized particles with magnesium and other materials to reduce the emission of free radicals. Last, human skin has an intrinsic and elaborate antioxidant defense system to neutralize free radicals.

### Sunscreen-Induced Vitamin D Deficiency

Vitamin D is a fat-soluble vitamin that is primarily formed from cutaneous exposure to the UV-B portion of sunlight. Vitamin D is thought to exert a beneficial effect on human physiology, and over the past years, concerns regarding the inhibitory effect of sunscreen in vitamin D synthesis have been raised.[22,71] Theoretically, the use of sunscreens at 2 mg/cm$^2$ can reduce the formation of vitamin D because sunscreens effectively block UV-B from reaching the epidermis.[72–74] However, clinical data indicate that inadequate application of sunscreens results in increased exposure to sunlight, leading to enhanced production of vitamin D among sunscreen users.[69] It is recommended that individuals should be dissuaded from attaining vitamin D through excessive UV exposure. Instead, dietary supplementation of vitamin D provides a reliable route to attain adequate serum levels.[75] The Institute of Medicine recommends a daily dietary allowance of 600 IU of vitamin D for children and adults up to 70 years of age. Adults older than 71 years can increase their daily recommended allowance to 800 IU of vitamin D per day.[76]

## LIMITATIONS OF SUNSCREEN USE

Modern-day sunscreens provide superior UV protection. However, UV absorption profiles are only one aspect in creating an effective product. Other attributes, such as fragrance, color, appearance, sensory profile, packaging, and cost are often ignored in academic discussions, but play vital roles in the efficacy of the final products. Sunscreens that fail to meet consumer demands in these areas may lead to poor user compliance

resulting in poor UV protection.[77] It should not be a surprise that the best sunscreen product is the one that is readily used by consumers.

There are many challenges faced by manufacturers in creating a sunscreen formulation with a refined sensory profile. Most of the organic filters available in the market are oil-soluble molecules that result in a greasy sensation. In addition, water-resistant sunscreens contain polymers, such as bis-polyethylene glycol-18 methyl ether dimethyl silane, trimethylsiloxysilicate, and butylated polyvinylpyrrolidone that can create a sticky sensation. To address some of these issues, manufacturers have included a variety of slipping agents and polymeric surfactants that improve the overall tactile and sensory profile.[77]

Aside from formulation challenges, inappropriate use of sunscreen by consumers is a major limiting factor that negatively affects sunscreen effectiveness. Consumers tend to use sunscreens as their sole protection when outdoors, and they also tend to stay out in the sun longer, engaging in practices such as sunbathing and tanning.[78–80] In addition, the application dosage is much lower. Instead of applying 2 mg/cm$^2$, the actual amount of sunscreen used by most consumers is closer to 0.5 mg/cm$^2$, which results in a marked decrease in the effective SPF.[59,81] Last, consumers should reapply sunscreen at least every 2 hours to maintain the level of effectiveness, a practice that is uncommon among the average user.[82]

## SUMMARY

Over the past decades, the role of sunscreens has progressed from merely preventing sunburns to reducing the risk of skin cancer and skin aging. Although significant technical advancements have been made to improve the overall UV protection, improvement in texture and sensory profile can increase user compliance. As the general public becomes increasingly aware of the detrimental effects of sun exposure, clinicians and dermatologists need to continue their effort to educate the public about the proper measures to protect from UV damage. Sunscreens are only one type of photoprotection, and other measures, such as avoiding the sun, seeking shade, and wearing protective gear should be equally used.

## REFERENCES

1. Rogers HW, Weinstock MA, Harris AR, et al. Incidence estimate of nonmelanoma skin cancer in the United States, 2006. Arch Dermatol 2010; 146(3):283–7.

2. Robinson JK. Sun exposure, sun protection, and vitamin D. JAMA 2005;294(12):1541–3.

3. International Agency for Research on Cancer. Solar and ultraviolet radiation. Lyon (France): International Agency for Research on Cancer; 1992.

4. Sayre RM, Dowdy JC, Lott DL, et al. Commentary on 'UVB-SPF': the SPF labels of sunscreen products convey more than just UVB protection. Photodermatol Photoimmunol Photomed 2008;24(4):218–20.

5. Armstrong BK, Kricker A. How much melanoma is caused by sun exposure? Melanoma Res 1993;3(6):395–401.

6. Coblentz WW. The Copenhagen Meeting of the Second International Congress on Light. Science 1932;76(1975):412–5.

7. Kullavanijaya P, Lim HW. Photoprotection. J Am Acad Dermatol 2005;52(6):937–58 [quiz: 959–62].

8. Calzavara-Pinton P, Sala R, Arisi MC, et al. Photobiology, photodermatology and sunscreens: a comprehensive overview. Part 1: damage from acute and chronic solar exposure. G Ital Dermatol Venereol 2013;148(1):89–106.

9. Marrot L, Meunier JR. Skin DNA photodamage and its biological consequences. J Am Acad Dermatol 2008;58(5 Suppl 2):S139–48.

10. Budden T, Bowden NA. The role of altered nucleotide excision repair and UVB-induced DNA damage in melanomagenesis. Int J Mol Sci 2013;14(1):1132–51.

11. Ravanat JL, Douki T, Cadet J. Direct and indirect effects of UV radiation on DNA and its components. J Photochem Photobiol B 2001;63(1–3):88–102.

12. Djavaheri-Mergny M, Mergny JL, Bertrand F, et al. Ultraviolet-A induces activation of AP-1 in cultured human keratinocytes. FEBS Lett 1996;384(1):92–6.

13. Darr D, Fridovich I. Free radicals in cutaneous biology. J Invest Dermatol 1994;102(5):671–5.

14. Runger TM, Kappes UP. Mechanisms of mutation formation with long-wave ultraviolet light (UVA). Photodermatol Photoimmunol Photomed 2008;24(1):2–10.

15. Moyal D, Fourtanier A. Acute and chronic effects of UV on skin. In: Rigel DS, Weiss RA, Lim HW, et al, editors. Photoaging. New York: Marcel Dekker, Inc; 2004. p. 15–32.

16. Gil EM, Kim TH. UV-induced immune suppression and sunscreen. Photodermatol Photoimmunol Photomed 2000;16(3):101–10.

17. Sklar LR, Almutawa F, Lim HW, et al. Effects of ultraviolet radiation, visible light, and infrared radiation on erythema and pigmentation: a review. Photochem Photobiol Sci 2013;12(1):54–64.

18. National Cancer Institute. Sun protection. Cancer trends progress report 2011/2012 Update. 2012. Available at: http://progressreport.cancer.gov/doc_detail.asp?pid=1&did=2009&chid=91&coid=911&mid=#trends. Accessed July 31, 2013.

19. Gantz GM, Sumner WG. Stable ultraviolet light absorbers. Textile Res J 1957;27:244–51.

20. Knox JM, Guin J, Cockerell EG. Benzophenones. Ultraviolet light absorbing agents1. J Invest Dermatol 1957;29(6):435–44.

21. Kanof NH. Protection of the skin against the harmful effects of sunlight. Arch Dermatol Res 1956;74:46.

22. Celleno L, Calzavara-Pinton P, Sala R, et al. Photobiology, photodermatology and sunscreens: a comprehensive overview. Part 2: topical and systemic photoprotection. G Ital Dermatol Venereol 2013;148(1):107–33.

23. Kockler J, Robertson S, Oelgemöller M, et al. Butyl methoxy dibenzoylmethane. Profiles of drug substances, excipients, and related methodology 2013;38(2013):87–111.

24. Deflandre A, Lang G. Photostability assessment of sunscreens. Benzylidene camphor and dibenzoylmethane derivatives. Int J Cosmet Sci 1988;10(2):53–62.

25. Beasley D, Meyer T. Characterization of the UVA protection provided by avobenzone, zinc oxide, and titanium dioxide in broad-spectrum sunscreen products. Am J Clin Dermatol 2010;11(6):413–21.

26. Bonda C. The photostability of organic sunscreen actives: a review. In: Shaath N, editor. Sunscreens: regulations and commercial development. 3rd edition. Boca Raton (FL): Taylor & Francis; 2005. p. 321–49.

27. Wang SQ, Balagula Y, Osterwalder U. Photoprotection: a review of the current and future technologies. Dermatol Ther 2010;23(1):31–47.

28. Mitchnick MA, Fairhurst D, Pinnell SR. Microfine zinc oxide (Z-cote) as a photostable UVA/UVB sunblock agent. J Am Acad Dermatol 1999;40(1):85–90.

29. Chen L, Tooley I, Wang S. Nanotechnology in photoprotection. In: Nasir A, Friedman A, Wang S, editors. Nanotechnology in dermatology. New York: Springer; 2013. p. 9–18.

30. Wang SQ, Tooley IR. Photoprotection in the era of nanotechnology. Semin Cutan Med Surg 2011;30(4):210–3.

31. Darlington S, Williams G, Neale R, et al. A randomized controlled trial to assess sunscreen application and beta carotene supplementation in the prevention of solar keratoses. Arch Dermatol 2003;139(4):451–5.

32. van der Pols JC, Williams GM, Pandeya N, et al. Prolonged prevention of squamous cell carcinoma of the skin by regular sunscreen use. Cancer Epidemiol Biomarkers Prev 2006;15(12):2546–8.

33. Green AC, Williams GM, Logan V, et al. Reduced melanoma after regular sunscreen use: randomized trial follow-up. J Clin Oncol 2011;29(3):257–63.

34. Hughes MC, Williams GM, Baker P, et al. Sunscreen and prevention of skin aging: a randomized trial. Ann Intern Med 2013;158(11):781–90.

35. Bissonnette R, Nigen S, Bolduc C. Influence of the quantity of sunscreen applied on the ability to protect against ultraviolet-induced polymorphous light eruption. Photodermatol Photoimmunol Photomed 2012;28(5):240–3.

36. Green A, Williams G, Neale R, et al. Daily sunscreen application and betacarotene supplementation in prevention of basal-cell and squamous-cell carcinomas of the skin: a randomised controlled trial. Lancet 1999;354(9180):723–9.

37. Chesnut C, Kim J. Is there truly no benefit with sunscreen use and Basal cell carcinoma? A critical review of the literature and the application of new sunscreen labeling rules to real-world sunscreen practices. J Skin Cancer 2012;2012:480985.

38. Criscione VD, Weinstock MA, Naylor MF, et al. Actinic keratoses: natural history and risk of malignant transformation in the Veterans Affairs Topical Tretinoin Chemoprevention Trial. Cancer 2009; 115(11):2523–30.

39. Thompson SC, Jolley D, Marks R. Reduction of solar keratoses by regular sunscreen use. N Engl J Med 1993;329(16):1147–51.

40. Green AC, McBride P. Squamous cell carcinoma of the skin (non-metastatic). Clin Evid (Online) 2010; 2010:1–8.

41. de Gruijl FR. Photobiology of photocarcinogenesis. Photochem Photobiol 1996;63(4):372–5.

42. Green AC, Williams GM. Point: sunscreen use is a safe and effective approach to skin cancer prevention. Cancer Epidemiol Biomarkers Prev 2007; 16(10):1921–2.

43. Situm M, Buljan M, Bulat V, et al. The role of UV radiation in the development of basal cell carcinoma. Coll Antropol 2008;32(Suppl 2):167–70.

44. Dennis LK, Vanbeek MJ, Beane Freeman LE, et al. Sunburns and risk of cutaneous melanoma: does age matter? A comprehensive meta-analysis. Ann Epidemiol 2008;18(8):614–27.

45. Berwick M. Counterpoint: sunscreen use is a safe and effective approach to skin cancer prevention. Cancer Epidemiol Biomarkers Prev 2007;16(10): 1923–4.

46. Dennis LK, Beane Freeman LE, VanBeek MJ. Sunscreen use and the risk for melanoma: a quantitative review. Ann Intern Med 2003;139(12):966–78.

47. Green AC, Hughes MC, McBride P, et al. Factors associated with premature skin aging (photoaging) before the age of 55: a population-based study. Dermatology 2011;222(1):74–80.

48. Holman CD, Armstrong BK, Evans PR, et al. Relationship of solar keratosis and history of skin cancer to objective measures of actinic skin damage. Br J Dermatol 1984;110(2):129–38.

49. Kricker A, Armstrong BK, English DR, et al. Pigmentary and cutaneous risk factors for non-melanocytic skin cancer–a case-control study. Int J Cancer 1991;48(5):650–62.

50. Fesq H, Ring J, Abeck D. Management of polymorphous light eruption: clinical course, pathogenesis, diagnosis and intervention. Am J Clin Dermatol 2003;4(6):399–406.

51. Lenane P, Murphy GM. Sunscreens and the photodermatoses. J Dermatolog Treat 2001;12(1):53–7.

52. Schleyer V, Weber O, Yazdi A, et al. Prevention of polymorphic light eruption with a sunscreen of very high protection level against UVB and UVA radiation under standardized photodiagnostic conditions. Acta Derm Venereol 2008;88(6): 555–60.

53. Medeiros VL, Lim HW. Sunscreens in the management of photodermatoses. Skin Therapy Lett 2010; 15(6):1–3.

54. Seite S, Reinhold K, Jaenicke T, et al. Broad-spectrum moisturizer effectively prevents molecular reactions to UVA radiation. Cutis 2012;90(6):321–6.

55. Moyal D. Need for a well-balanced sunscreen to protect human skin from both Ultraviolet A and Ultraviolet B damage. Indian J Dermatol Venereol Leprol 2012;78(Suppl 1):S24–30.

56. Wang SQ, Tanner PR, Lim HW, et al. The evolution of sunscreen products in the United States–a 12-year cross sectional study. Photochem Photobiol Sci 2013;12(1):197–202.

57. U.S. Food and Drug Administration. Final monograph: labeling and effectiveness testing; sunscreen drug products for over-the-counter human use. 2011. Available at: http://www.gpo.gov/fdsys/pkg/FR-2011-06-17/pdf/2011-14766.pdf. Accessed September 1, 2013.

58. Wang SQ, Lim HW. Current status of the sunscreen regulation in the United States: 2011 Food and Drug Administration's final rule on labeling and effectiveness testing. J Am Acad Dermatol 2011; 65(4):863–9.

59. Diffey BL. Chapter 27 sunscreens: use and misuse. In: Paolo UG, editor. Comprehensive series in photosciences, vol. 3. Amsterdam: Elsevier; 2001. p. 521–34.

60. Mease PJ. Spondyloarthritis: is methotrexate effective in psoriatic arthritis? Nat Rev Rheumatol 2012; 8(5):251–2.

61. U.S. Food and Drug Administration. Sunscreen drug products for over-the- counter human use; request for data and information regarding dosage forms. 2011. Available at: http://www.gpo.gov/fdsys/pkg/FR-2011-06-17/pdf/2011-14768.pdf. Accessed September 1, 2013.

62. Nakagawa Y, Suzuki T. Metabolism of 2-hydroxy-4-methoxybenzophenone in isolated rat hepatocytes and xenoestrogenic effects of its metabolites on

MCF-7 human breast cancer cells. Chem Biol Interact 2002;139(2):115–28.

63. Ma R, Cotton B, Lichtensteiger W, et al. UV filters with antagonistic action at androgen receptors in the MDA-kb2 cell transcriptional-activation assay. Toxicol Sci 2003;74(1):43–50.

64. Heneweer M, Muusse M, van den Berg M, et al. Additive estrogenic effects of mixtures of frequently used UV filters on pS2-gene transcription in MCF-7 cells. Toxicol Appl Pharmacol 2005;208(2):170–7.

65. Schlumpf M, Cotton B, Conscience M, et al. In vitro and in vivo estrogenicity of UV screens. Environ Health Perspect 2001;109(3):239–44.

66. Wang SQ, Burnett ME, Lim HW. Safety of oxybenzone: putting numbers into perspective. Arch Dermatol 2011;147(7):865–6.

67. Janjua NR, Mogensen B, Andersson AM, et al. Systemic absorption of the sunscreens benzophenone-3, octyl-methoxycinnamate, and 3-(4-methyl-benzylidene) camphor after whole-body topical application and reproductive hormone levels in humans. J Invest Dermatol 2004; 123(1):57–61.

68. Nash JF. Human safety and efficacy of ultraviolet filters and sunscreen products. Dermatol Clin 2006; 24(1):35–51.

69. Burnett ME, Wang SQ. Current sunscreen controversies: a critical review. Photodermatol Photoimmunol Photomed 2011;27(2):58–67.

70. Nohynek GJ, Lademann J, Ribaud C, et al. Grey goo on the skin? Nanotechnology, cosmetic and sunscreen safety. Crit Rev Toxicol 2007;37(3): 251–77.

71. Matsuoka LY, Ide L, Wortsman J, et al. Sunscreens suppress cutaneous vitamin D3 synthesis. J Clin Endocrinol Metab 1987;64(6):1165–8.

72. McLaughlin M, Raggatt PR, Fairney A, et al. Seasonal variations in serum 25-hydroxycholecalciferol in healthy people. Lancet 1974;1(7857):536–8.

73. Webb AR, Kift R, Durkin MT, et al. The role of sunlight exposure in determining the vitamin D status of the U.K. white adult population. Br J Dermatol 2010;163(5):1050–5.

74. Webb AR, Pilbeam C, Hanafin N, et al. An evaluation of the relative contributions of exposure to sunlight and of diet to the circulating concentrations of 25-hydroxyvitamin D in an elderly nursing home population in Boston. Am J Clin Nutr 1990;51(6): 1075–81.

75. Halpern AC. Vitamin D: a clinical perspective. Pigment Cell Melanoma Res 2013;26(1):5–8.

76. Rosen CJ, Abrams SA, Aloia JF, et al. IOM committee members respond to Endocrine Society vitamin D guideline. J Clin Endocrinol Metab 2012;97(4): 1146–52.

77. Wang SQ, Hu JY. Challenges in making effective sunscreen. In: Halpern AC, Marghoob AA, editors. The melanoma letter, vol. 30. New York: Skin Cancer Foundation; 2012. p. 4–6.

78. Autier P, Dore JF, Negrier S, et al. Sunscreen use and duration of sun exposure: a double-blind, randomized trial. J Natl Cancer Inst 1999;91(15): 1304–9.

79. Autier P, Dore JF, Reis AC, et al. Sunscreen use and intentional exposure to ultraviolet A and B radiation: a double blind randomized trial using personal dosimeters. Br J Cancer 2000;83(9): 1243–8.

80. Autier P. Sunscreen abuse for intentional sun exposure. Br J Dermatol 2009;161(Suppl 3):40–5.

81. Autier P, Boniol M, Severi G, et al. Quantity of sunscreen used by European students. Br J Dermatol 2001;144(2):288–91.

82. Thieden E, Philipsen PA, Sandby-Moller J, et al. Sunscreen use related to UV exposure, age, sex, and occupation based on personal dosimeter readings and sun-exposure behavior diaries. Arch Dermatol 2005;141(8):967–73.

# Photoprotection
## Clothing and Glass

Fahad Almutawa, MD[a],*, Hanan Buabbas, PhD[b]

### KEYWORDS

- Ultraviolet • Photoprotection • Glass • Window films • Sunglasses • Clothing

### KEY POINTS

- Physical methods of photoprotection include glass, window films, sunglasses, and clothing.
- All types of glass block UV-B.
- UV-A transmission depends on the type of the glass.
- Window films added to glass greatly decrease the UV-A transmission of the glass.
- Fabric characteristics can greatly affect the level of photoprotection offered by clothing.

## INTRODUCTION

All people are exposed to ultraviolet (UV) radiation (UVR) from the sun. UVR is divided into UV-C (100–290 nm), UV-B (290–320 nm), and UV-A (320–400 nm). All of UV-C and most UV-B (approximately 90%) are absorbed by the ozone layer, which results in mainly UV-A and a small percentage of UV-B reaching the surface of the earth.[1] UVR has known effects on the skin and eyes. With regards to the skin, the acute effects include erythema, edema, pigment darkening, delayed tanning, epidermal hyperplasia, and vitamin D biosynthesis. The chronic effects include immunosuppression, photoaging, and photocarcinogenesis.[2] On the eyes, UVR exposure has been strongly associated with the development of pterygium, photokeratitis, climatic droplet keratopathy, and cortical cataracts.[3] Photoprotection in the form of seeking shade between 10 AM and 2 PM, wearing a wide-brimmed hat, and applying sunscreen is widely promoted to the public. However, little attention is given to educate the public on physical methods of photoprotection, which include clothing, glass, and sunglasses.

## PHOTOPROTECTION BY GLASS

Glass is a combination of sand or silica and other components, which are melted together at a very high temperature. At room temperature, it becomes a solid, whereas at higher temperatures, it softens to become a liquid.[4] Flat glass is the basic material used to make industrial and automotive glass. It is produced by the float process. During the float process, sand, limestone, soda ash, dolomite, iron oxide, and salt cake are mixed together with broken glass (cullet). These ingredients are melted at 1600 °C to produce a flat glass.[5] The flat glass is then treated in different ways to produce the different types of glasses that are discussed in the next section (Table 1).

### Main Types of Glass

Annealed glass is the basic flat glass, which is the first result of the float process. It is the starting material in the glass industry to produce more advanced glass. It breaks into large pieces.[5]

Toughened or tempered glass is produced by heating the flat glass, followed by rapid cooling of the glass surface by air, which results in glass that withstands more compression than flat glass. It breaks into small regular pieces.[5]

Coated glass is made by applying a surface coating to the glass that results in additional advantages, such as decrease in the transmission

Disclosures: No conflict of interest.
[a] Department of Medicine, Kuwait University, PO Box 24923, Al-Jabriya, Safat 13110, Kuwait; [b] Medical Photophysics Laboratory, Asaad al Hamad Dermatology Center, PO Box 17296, Khaldeyah 72453, Kuwait City, Kuwait
* Corresponding author.
E-mail address: fahad.almutawa@hsc.edu.kw

## Table 1
## Common types of glass

| Types of Glass | Comments |
|---|---|
| Annealed glass | Basic flat glass<br>Breaks into large pieces |
| Toughened (tempered) glass | Withstands more compression than annealed glass<br>Breaks into small regular pieces |
| Coated glass | Made by applying a surface coating to the glass<br>Decreases the transmission of light and heat, resistance to scratch, or resistance to corrosion |
| Laminated glass | Made up of $\geq$2 layers of glass with interlayers of plastic<br>Decreases transmission of UVR, transmission of sound, and improves security<br>Broken pieces are held together by the interlayer |
| Patterned glass | Flat glass with a surface that shows a regular pattern |

of light or heat, resistance to scratch, or resistance to corrosion.[5]

Laminated glass comprises 2 or more layers of glass with 1 or more interlayers of polymeric material (plastic) such as polyvinyl butyral. It is used in car windshields and facades of buildings. Technology can be incorporated in laminated glass to provide UV filtering, decreasing of sound transmission, adding colors, or resistance to fire. When it breaks, the broken pieces are held together by the interlayer, which provides safety.[5]

Patterned glass is a type of flat glass with a surface that shows a regular pattern.[5]

### UV Transmission Through Residential Glass

Almost all glass blocks UV-B radiation, regardless of type or properties of the glass.[6] However, the transmission of UV-A radiation varies according to the type, thickness, and color of the glass. Duarte and colleagues[6] looked at the transmission of UV-A through various types of residential glass (annealed, patterned, tempered [toughened], and laminated). In most studies on glass, UV-A transmission is measured up to 380 nm, because at wavelength greater than 380 nm, glass would have to be opaque or heavily tinted to provide photoprotection. The transmission was measured by a photometer (UV-A-400C, NBC, OH) at zero distance from the UV-A source. These investigators showed that annealed and tempered glass transmit 74% and 72% of

UV-A, respectively; patterned glass transmits less UV-A (45%), whereas laminated glass blocks all UV-A. The color of the glass also plays a major role in the transmission of UV-A. Of 5 different colors of patterned glass (green, yellow, wine, blue, and colorless), green was found to be the most protective, followed by yellow. Colorless and wine have similar properties, whereas blue glass offered the least photoprotection.[6] The thickness of the glass has a small effect on the UV-A transmission. Increasing the thickness of the glass 5 times (from 0.2 cm to 1.0 cm) resulted in a modest decrease in the transmission of UV-A, from 76% to 51%.[6]

### UV Exposure in Automobiles

People spend approximately 1 to 2 hours per day in their automobiles, based on an epidemiologic study that evaluated 169 individuals from different parts of the United States.[7] When Kimlin and colleagues[8] evaluated UV exposure in cars both with open and closed windows, they found that the exposure is high enough to be considered in calculating the total lifetime UV exposure.

There is some clinical evidence to suggest that UV exposure in automobiles might have a biological significance. Hampton and colleagues[9] found that a 30 to 60 minutes exposure to solar radiation in midday summer in the United Kingdom through automobile tempered glass can reach a dose of 5 J/cm$^2$, which is sufficient to induce eruptions in patients with severe photosensitivity disorders. Two studies from Australia, which separately evaluated actinic keratosis and lentigo maligna, found these 2 conditions to be more common on the right side (the driver's side in Australia).[10,11] Skin cancers such as basal cell carcinomas, squamous cell carcinomas, melanomas, and Merkel cell carcinomas were found to be slightly more common on the left side from 2 retrospective studies performed in the United States.[12,13]

### Automobile Glass

Of the flat glass industry market, 15% to 20% goes to the production of automobile glazing.[5] Automobile glazing is made up of laminated or tempered (toughened) glass. Either type can be tinted to improve the comfort and decrease visible light and infrared transmission. Most automobile glasses are tinted. The most commonly used tint is green, although gray and blue have also been used.[9] Windshields are made up of laminated glass for safety reasons to prevent ejection of the passengers in the event of frontal impacts whereas side and back windows are usually made up of tempered (toughened) glass.[14]

## UV transmission through automobile glass

Similar to residential glass, both laminated and tempered glass used for automobiles block UV-B. The transmission of UV-A depends on the type and color of the glass.

Laminated glass, which is used in windshields, blocks most UV-A radiation. Bernstein and colleagues[15] measured the UV irradiance (by ELSEC UV monitor [Littlemore Scientific Engineering, Dorset, UK]) of solar radiation in a sunny September day in New Jersey both directly and through a laminated glass (windshield of a 2006 Volvo) and found that laminated glass blocked 98% of the UVR. Moehrle and colleagues[16] examined green-tinted, blue-tinted, and infrared reflective glass of the laminated types used in windshields of 3 Mercedes-Benz models for their UV transmission characteristics and found that all of them blocked UV-A up to 380 nm. Comparing 3 different colors of laminated glass used in windshields, gray was the most protective, with transmission of only 0.06% of UV-A, followed by green, which transmits 9% of UV-A, and clear laminated glass, which transmits 9.7% of UV-A radiation.[9] Laminated glass used in windshields allows minimal transmission of UV-A radiation (up to 380 nm), and gray has been shown to be the most effective.

Tempered glass is used in most side and back windows. Similar to other types of glass, it blocks UV-B but transmits variable amounts of UV-A radiation. Bernstein and colleagues[15] found that the side window (tempered glass) of a 2006 Volvo transmitted 79% of the UV-A radiation. Hampton and colleagues[9] evaluated 4 different colors of tempered glass used in side windows. These investigators found the transmission of UV-A as follows: clear (63%), light green (36%), dark green (23%), and gray (11%). Another study[16] evaluated 3 different types of tempered glass: double-glazed green, double-glazed blue, and double-glazed infrared reflective glass. The study showed that the average amount of UV-A transmission was 17.5% in double-glazed green glass, 22.4% in double-glazed blue glass, and 0.8% in double-glazed infrared reflective glass. From these studies, the amount of UV-A transmission through tempered glass depends on the color of the glass. In addition, the thickness of the glass offers additional protective benefit, with double-glazed glass transmitting less UV-A than a single pane of the same color. Using infrared reflective technology in the tempered glass adds great advantage in regards to UV-A protection and decrease of infrared transmission.

These studies show how the characteristics of glass affect the transmission of UVR, but how can this be applied to day-to-day life? Mean UVR exposure to a car passenger is 3% to 4% of the ambient UVR, with the highest UV exposure to the left arm (in those countries with left-sided driver's seats) and lateral head of the driver.[16] Whether the UV-A exposure through the tempered glass is sufficient to induce rash in photosensitive patients is dependent on the distance of the body part from the window and time spent in the car. In the worst-case scenario, when the arm is elevated and thus in direct contact with sunlight, exposure of 30 minutes through a tempered, clear, side window resulted in measurements of 5 J/cm$^2$ of UV-A. This dose is sufficient to induce clinical lesions in highly photosensitive patients with conditions such as polymorphous light eruption or chronic actinic dermatitis.[9]

## Window films

The use of window films started in the 1960s. They were used for the reflection of solar radiation but allowing vision. During the energy crisis of the 1970s, interest also developed in reducing heat loss to the outside.[17]

Film is composed of polyester substrate with adhesive layer on 1 side and scratch-resistant coat on the other side. All the components of the film must have a high optical quality to allow for vision through the film.[17]

A standard film has the following components: (1) protective release layer, which is a thin polyester layer, which must be removed before application; (2) adhesive layer to bind the film to the glass; (3) multiple layers of polyester with laminating adhesive in between; (4) hard acrylic coating to protect the film from scratching; and (5) dyes, metals, alloys, or UV filters which are added to offer specific advantages to the film.[17]

The UV blocking ability of films can be achieved by different ways. The metals, alloys, and dyes, which are incorporated into films to reflect the solar radiation, can offer some UV protection by reflection or absorption of UVR. However, the primary method of UV protection is by either adding UV inhibitors to the adhesive layer or having a separate layer of UV inhibitors.[14] Having a separate layer of UV inhibitors may offer better performance and longevity, but there is no evidence to support this statement.[18] Most manufacturers claim UV protection of up to 99%; however, this claim is based on the measurement of UVR up to 380 nm. A study evaluated 40 different films from 8 different brands and found that UVR blocking of the film when applied to glass ranged from 86% to 99%. Most of the tested products blocked more than 90% of UVR up to 400 nm, but only 2 products blocked 99% of UVR.[18]

Applying film to glass results in decrease in the transmission of UVR. Two studies evaluated window films on tempered glass and found more than 99% reduction in the transmission of UVR.[6,15] Duarte and colleagues[6] applied a sunlight control film (G5, Insulfilm, Brazil) to a tempered glass, which resulted in total blockage of the transmission of UV-A as measured by a UV-A photometer (NBC, OH). Bernstein and colleagues[15] measured the UV transmission through the windshield, side window, and side window plus Formula One UV absorbing film (Formula One®, Solutia, St. Louis, MO, USA). The measurement was made on a sunny day in New Jersey by a UV monitor (ELSEC UV, Dorset, UK). These investigators found that the windshield blocked 98% of UVR, whereas the side window blocked only 21% of the UVR, which increased to 99.6% after the addition of window film.

## PHOTOPROTECTION WITH SUNGLASSES
### UV Exposure and the Eye

UV-B is absorbed mainly by the cornea, whereas UV-A is absorbed by the cornea, aqueous, and the lens.[3] The time of maximum UV exposure to the eyes is from 8 to 10 AM and 2 to 4 PM, when the rays of the sun are parallel to the eyes, in contrast to the time of maximum UV exposure to the skin, which is from 10 AM to 2 PM.[19]

Exposure to UV-A and UV-B can affect the eyes. There is strong evidence to support the association of UVR exposure and the following eye conditions: pterygium, photokeratitis, climatic droplet keratopathy, and cortical cataract.[3] Several studies[20,21] showed an association between UV-B and UV-A exposure and the formation of pterygium in a dose-dependent fashion. Acute exposure to UV-B can result in photokeratitis, which is a painful, superficial burn of the cornea similar to skin sunburn, whereas chronic exposure to UV-A and UV-B is associated with the formation

of climatic droplet keratopathy.[3] UV-B has also been strongly associated with the development of cortical cataracts; doubling the UV-B exposure resulted in 60% increase in the risk of developing cortical cataracts.[22] A recent meta-analysis[23] has suggested an association between sunlight exposure and the development of age-related macular degeneration. However, this association is most likely caused by blue light rather than UV-A or UV-B.[24] On the other hand, there is limited evidence to support the association of UVR and the development of pinguecula, nuclear and posterior subcapsular cataract, and ocular melanoma.[3]

### Sunglasses Guidelines

Three national standards for sunglasses exist: (1) the American standard ANSI Z80.3, last updated in 2010; (2) the European standard EN 1836:2005; and (3) the Australia/New Zealand standard AS/NZS 1067:2003. The European and the Australian are similar with regards to UVR requirements, but they differ in the definition of UV-A and the maximum allowed UV-B transmission (**Table 2**).[25,26] The American standard is summarized in **Table 3**. In the American standard, the allowed UV transmission depends on whether it is for normal use (such as inside cars, or from car to home or office) or for prolonged use.[26]

Compliance with the Australian and European standards by eyeglass manufacturers is mandatory. Australian guidelines also require compliance testing by a third party. A study conducted in 2003 to 2004, during the time when compliance with European standard was not mandatory, testing 646 pairs of eyeglasses that carried the CE mark (which stands for compliance with the European standard) found that 17% of the tested sunglasses failed to meet the European standard (EN 1836). The investigators concluded that self-regulation was not working.[27]

Table 2
Summary of the European standard (EN 1836:2005) and the Australian standard (AS/NZS 1067:2003)

| Lens Category | Luminous Transmittance (LT) (%) AS/NZS 1067 and EN 1836 | UV-B (% LT) EN (280–315 nm) | UV-B (% LT) AS (280–315 nm) | UV-A EN (315–380 nm) | UV-A AS (315–400 nm) |
|---|---|---|---|---|---|
| 0 (very light tint) | 80–100 | 10 | 5 | LT | LT |
| 1 (light tint) | 43–80 | 10 | 5 | LT | LT |
| 2 (medium tint) | 18–43 | 10 | 5 | LT | LT |
| 3 (dark tint) | 8–18 | 10 | 5 | 50% LT | 50% LT |
| 4 (very dark tint) | 3–8 | 10 | 5 | 50% LT | 50% LT |

*Data from* European Committee for Standardization. Sunglass standard revision. EN 1836:2005; and Standards Australia, Standards New Zealand. Sunglasses and fashion spectacles. AS/NZS 1067:2003.

**Table 3**
**Summary of the US standard (ANSI Z80.3)**

| Lens Color | Purpose | Luminous Transmittance (LT) (%) | UV-B (280–315 nm) (% LT) Normal Use | UV-B (280–315 nm) (% LT) Prolonged Use | UV-A (315–380 nm) Normal Use | UV-A (315–380 nm) Prolonged Use (% LT) |
|---|---|---|---|---|---|---|
| Light | Cosmetic | >40 | 12.5 | 1 | LT | 50 |
| Medium to dark | General purpose | 8–40 | 12.5 | 1 | LT | 50 |
| Very dark | Special purpose | 3–8 | 1 | 1 | 50% LT | 50 |
| Strongly colored | Special purpose | >8 | 1 | 1 | 50% LT | 50 |

*Data from* American National Standards Institute. Nonprescription sunglasses and fashion eyewear–requirements. ANSI Z80.3:2010.

Size, style, and position of the sunglasses are other factors that should be considered. Small lenses increase the probability of UVR reaching the eyes from the side of the lens. Based on this factor, the Australian standard has a minimum requirement of the lens size, which is 28 mm for adult and 24 mm for children. The eye can also be exposed to UVR through the reflection of solar radiation coming from the back on the posterior surface of the lens, as shown by Sakamoto and colleagues.[28] This study showed the importance of using a wraparound style or side shields to decrease the amount of UVR reflection. In regards to the position of the eyeglasses, moving the sunglasses a small distance (6 mm) away from the forehead results in more than 20% increase in the amount of UVR reaching the eyes.[29]

However, sunglasses may indirectly increase UV exposure to the eyes. Sunglasses, especially those with darker shades, cause the pupil to dilate, making the eye structures more susceptible to UV if the lens has poor UV protection ability or the style or position of the lens allows UVR to be reflected from the sides. Similar to sunscreen, sunglasses may provide a false sense of security, resulting in increase in outdoor exposure.[29]

The public should be aware to choose sunglasses that are in compliance with 1 of the 3 national standards, choose a wraparound style or sunglasses with side shields, and position the sunglasses as close as possible to the forehead.

## PHOTOPROTECTION BY CLOTHING

Clothing offers a simple and effective method of photoprotection. Its advantages over sunscreen are standardized coverage and constant level of protection throughout the day. However, there are several factors that affect the level of photoprotection offered by clothing, which are discussed later. UV protection factor (UPF) has been developed as an analogue to sun protection factor of sunscreen to measure the level of UV protection by textiles. It was used for the first time in Australia in 1996.[30] UPF is defined as the average of effective UV irradiance of unprotected skin over the average of effective UV irradiance of protected skin by the fabrics.[31] UPF can be determined by in vitro and in vivo methods. The in vitro method is most commonly used to determine UPF. It is an accurate and reproducible method, especially for textiles with UPF higher than 50. UPF is measured under the worst-case scenario, in which a collimated light source is applied at a right angle to the fabric. Thus, in real life, the UPF of the fabric is usually greater than the measured UPF.[31]

### Methods for Assessing the UPF of Textiles

#### In vitro method

The in vitro method is most commonly used to determine the UPF of textiles. Two methods are available to evaluate UPF using in vitro measurements: either by radiometry or by spectrophotometry. Radiometry requires a UV light source that mimics solar radiation, such as a xenon arc lamp to illuminate a fabric sample, band pass filters to choose between UV-A only and UV-A + UV-B spectrum, fabric samples, and a detector that behaves like human skin. UV transmission through fabric is then measured using a radiometer (**Fig. 1**). This technique is used when a researcher wants to determine the relative variability of different fabrics. The best method to measure UPF is spectrophotometry, which measures the intensity of UVR as transmitted by fabric as a function of wavelength. A lamp provides the UVR source (xenon arc or deuterium lamp). The beam of light strikes the monochromator (diffraction grating), which acts like a prism and separates the light into individual wavelengths; while the monochromator rotates, only a specific wavelength of light reaches the exit slit. Then, the light

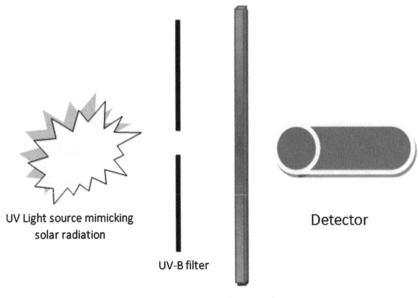

UV Light source mimicking
solar radiation

UV-B filter

Detector

Textiles sample

**Fig. 1.** Radiometric measurements for UPF.

interacts with fabric, and the detector measures the transmission of radiation through the fabric.

To calculate the UPF, the spectral irradiance of the UV source and the spectral irradiance transmitted through the fabric are weighted against the erythema action spectrum in the following formula[31]:

$$UPF = \frac{\sum_{\lambda=280}^{\lambda=400} E_\lambda \times S_\lambda \times \Delta\lambda}{\sum_{\lambda=280}^{\lambda=400} E_\lambda \times S_\lambda \times T_\lambda \times \Delta\lambda} \tag{1}$$

where

$E_\lambda$ = CIE erythemal spectral effectiveness (unitless), where CIE is the International Commission on Illumination

$S_\lambda$ = solar spectral irradiance ($W.m^{-2}.nm^{-1}$ at wavelength $\lambda$ nm)

$T_\lambda$ = average spectral transmission of the specimen

$\Delta\lambda$ = measured wavelength interval (nm)

From this formula, the UPF calculation depends on the erythema action spectrum; because UV-B is 1000 times more erythemogenic than UV-A, the UPF reflects mainly the protection against UV-B.[32]

### In vivo method

The in vivo method is less commonly used than the in vitro method, because it is more costly and impractical. It is generally used to confirm the in vitro UPF measurement.[31] It is calculated by determining the minimal erythema dose (MED) of unprotected skin and dividing it on the MED of

the protected skin by the fabric. For determination of the MED, different doses of UVR, using solar simulator usually in a geometric series, are applied to uninvolved skin of individuals, and the visible reaction of the skin is recorded at 24 hours.

The in vivo measurement can be performed as either on skin or off skin.[31,33] On skin is performed when the fabric is placed directly on the skin, whereas off skin is performed by placing the fabric 2 mm away from the skin.[31,33]

Gambichler and colleagues[34] compared the in vitro method with the in vivo method both in laboratory and in real-life scenarios with moving individuals. These investigators found that the UPF measured by the in vitro method was significantly higher than the UPF measured by the in vivo method in the laboratory. However, the UPF measured in real-life scenarios with moving individuals was lower than that measured by in vitro. Therefore, the in vitro measurement using spectrophotometry, which is most commonly used, provides valid UPF values for real-life situations.

The inverse of UPF is called erythema weighted transmittance (EWT), or penetration. Fabrics have good protection if the EWT approaches zero.[35] EWT is expressed mathematically as Equation 2:

$$EWT = \frac{1}{UPF} \tag{2}$$

EWT values are measured between 0 and 1 or 0% and 100%.

There are several international standards for rating UPF for fabrics,[35] such as:

1. Australian/New Zealand Standard AS/NZS 4399:1996. *Sun Protective Clothing. Evaluation and Classification* (**Table 4**)
2. European standard EN 13758-1:2002 *Sun Protective Clothing, Method of Test for Apparel Fabrics*
3. European standard 13,758-2:2003 *Solar UV Properties–Classification and Marking of Apparel*
4. American Association of Textile Chemists and Colorists (AATCC) test method 183-2004 *Transmittance or Blocking of Erythemally Weighted UVR Through Fabrics*
5. US standard D6603-00 *Guide for Labeling of UV-Protective Textiles*
6. US standard D6544-00 *Standard Practice for Preparation of Textiles Prior to Ultraviolet (UV) Transmission Testing*

All of the standards apply UPF Equation 1 for measuring UPF. The differences between these standards are the position of the fabrics to the instrument, scanning interval, erythema action spectrum, marking (labels), and classification system of UPF.

## Influence of Fabric Parameters on UPF

Several fabric characteristics can affect the UPF, such as porosity, weight, thickness, type of fabric, laundering, hydration, stretch, fabric processing, UV absorbers, color, and fabric to skin distance.[36]

### Porosity, Weight, and Thickness

Porosity of the fabric (also known as fabric openness, cover factor, and tightness of weave) is the most important factor that affects transmission of UVR through fabric. It depends on the fabric construction and weight. Knitted fabrics have larger spaces between the yarns (threads) than weaved fabrics. As a result, UV transmission is higher in knitted than weaved fabrics. The closer the knit or weave of a fabric, the smaller the space between the yarns and the greater the UV protection.[37,38] Heavy fabrics, in general, have less space between the yarns, which result in higher UV protection.[39] Thicker fabrics also have less space between the yarns and have been shown to have higher UV protection.[39,40]

### Type of Fabric

It is difficult to compare the UPF between different materials. The reason is that different materials go through different production steps, such as dyeing and finishing. Thus, comparing fabrics means comparing the combinations of material, dye, and finish.[31] Crews and colleagues[40] subdivided fabrics based on UV absorbing properties to 3 groups and found that cotton and rayon (cellulosic fibers) have the least UV absorbing capacity (UPF<15), whereas polyester has the highest. Wool, silk, and nylon lie between these 2 groups.

### Color of Fabrics

Srinivasan and Gatewood[41] showed that there is no relationship between hue and UPF. They and other groups[42,43] have shown that black fabric does not have the highest UPF. This factor is the result of the transmission and absorption characteristic of the specific colors. However, in general, colored fabric has better UV protection than white fabric, and darker colors have better UV protection than lighter colors, because of increased UV absorption.[32,44]

### Laundry

UPF increases after first washing, because of shrinkage of the fabric, especially cotton, which results in a decrease in the space between the yarns (porosity).[44]

### Moisture Content

Moisture from perspiration or water can significantly affect UPF. This situation depends on 2 factors: (1) the absorption of water by the textile fibers results in swelling of the fibers, which leads to a decrease in the spaces between the yarns; (2) the presence of water in the spaces between the yarns can decrease the UV scattering, which results in an increase in UV transmission.[37] Gambichler and colleagues[45] tested the effect of wetness on different types of fabrics, namely cotton, linen, viscose (rayon), and polyester, and found no significant difference in UPF for fabrics

**Table 4**
**UPF classification system according to Australian/New Zealand Standard (AS/NZS 4399:1996)**

| UPF | Protection Category | Effective UVR Transmission (%) | UPF Rating |
|---|---|---|---|
| 15–24 | Good protection | 6.7 to 4.2 | 15, 20 |
| 25–39 | Very good | 4.1 to 2.6 | 25, 30, 35 |
| 40–50, 50+ | Excellent | Less than 2.5 | 40, 45, 50, 50+ |

*Data from* Standards Australia/Standards New Zealand. Sun protective clothing. AS/NZS 4399:1996.

moistened with tap water versus salt water. Wetting significantly decreases the UPF of cotton fabrics. However, UPF of linen, viscose, and polyester showed no significant change with wetting. Wetting of fabrics can change their UPF; thus, moisture content should be tested and added to garment labels.

### Stretch

Distance between yarns increases when the fabric is stretched, thus increasing the transmission of UVR, as occurs with elastane and Lycra. When elastane is stretched by 10%, UPF decreases by 50%.[46]

### Fabric to Skin Distance

Skin is more photoprotected when the distance between fabric and skin is high. A loose shirt has higher UPF than a tight shirt, because the more distance between clothing and the skin, the more diffusion of UVR.

### Fabric Processing

Fabric processing can change the UV protection of the fabrics. Sizing and bleaching of fabric result in a decrease in the UV protection of the fabric.[39] On the other hand, application of optical whitening agents that have fluorescent-like properties results in re-emission of absorbed UVR in the visible range, which increases UV protection.[39] Knit fabrics with a rough surface sometimes undergo a chemical processing with an enzyme called cellulase to smooth the surface of the fabric. This process results in increase in UV protection of the fabric, most likely because of a decrease in the spaces between the yarns (porosity).[39]

### UV Absorbers

Adding broadband UVR absorbers, such as Tinosorb FD, during laundry enhances UVR blocking properties of fabrics. Tinosorb FD, a photoprotective agent present in some laundry additives, absorbs broadband UVR and can increase the UPF up to 400% after 5 washings.[32] The increase in UPF can be maintained even after 20 washes (**Table 5**).[47]

Recently, increased attention has been given to the protection of fabrics against the visible light range, a subject rarely addressed in past decades.[48] Visible light sensitivity is an important phenomenon in patients with photosensitive disorders aggravated by visible light and patients treated with photodynamic therapy.

Visible light protection factor (VPF) can be measured in 2 ways. The first involves using a

**Table 5**
**Influence of Fabric characteristics on UPF**

| Factor | Comment |
|---|---|
| Type of fabric | Cotton and rayon (cellulosic fibers) have the least UPF. Wool, silk and nylon have moderate UPF. Polyester has highest UPF |
| Color | Colored fabrics have higher UPF |
| Thickness | Thick fabrics have higher UPF |
| Laundry | UPF increases after washing |
| Weight | Heavy fabrics have higher UPF |
| Stretch | Stretched fabrics have lower UPF |
| Wetness | Dry fabrics have higher UPF |
| Fabric to skin distance | Loose fit has higher UPF |
| Porosity | Tight weave has higher UPF |
| UV absorbing agent | Increase UPF |

spectrophotometer, which produces visible light from xenon lamp and measures direct and diffuse transmitted radiation using this equation:

$$VPF(\lambda) = \frac{1}{T(\lambda)} \qquad (3)$$

where

$T(\lambda)$ is the transmission coefficient at a particular wavelength.

Another way to determine VPF is by calculating the ratio of intensity at selective wavelengths in the visible range (400–700 nm) with and without fabrics, which can be achieved by using a combination of xenon light source to produce visible light and a monochromator.

### SUMMARY

UVR has well-known adverse effects on the skin and eyes. This article focuses on physical means of photoprotection, including glass, window films, sunglasses, and clothing. In general, all types of glass block UV-B. However, the degree of UV-A transmission depends on the type, thickness, and color of the glass. Adding window films to glass greatly decreases the transmission of UV-A. When choosing sunglasses, it is important to choose sunglasses that comply with 1 of the 3 national standards, to choose a wraparound style or side shields, and to wear them as close as possible to the eyes. In addition, it is important to choose clothing that covers as much skin as possible. Factors that can affect the transmission of UVR through cloth include tightness of weave, thickness, weight, type of fabrics, laundering, hydration, stretch, fabric processing, UV absorbers, color, and fabric to skin distance.

## REFERENCES

1. World Health Organization. Global solar UV index: a practical guide. Geneva (Switzerland): World Health Organization; 2002.
2. Jansen R, Wang SQ, Burnett M, et al. Photoprotection: part I. Photoprotection by naturally occurring, physical, and systemic agents. J Am Acad Dermatol 2013;69(6):853.e1–12.
3. Yam JC, Kwok AK. Ultraviolet light and ocular diseases. Int Ophthalmol 2014;34(2):383–400.
4. British glass. Flat glass manufacture. Available at: http://www.britglass.org.uk/. Accessed November 6, 2013.
5. Glass for Europe. The float process. Available at: http://www.glassforeurope.com/. Accessed November 6, 2013.
6. Duarte I, Rotter A, Malvestiti A, et al. The role of glass as a barrier against the transmission of ultraviolet radiation: an experimental study. Photodermatol Photoimmunol Photomed 2009;25(4):181–4.
7. McCurdy T, Graham SE. Using human activity data in exposure models: analysis of discriminating factors. J Expo Anal Environ Epidemiol 2003;13(4): 294–317.
8. Kimlin MG, Parisi AV, Carter BD, et al. Comparison of the solar spectral ultraviolet irradiance in motor vehicles with windows in an open and closed position. Int J Biometeorol 2002;46(3):150–6.
9. Hampton PJ, Farr PM, Diffey BL, et al. Implication for photosensitive patients of ultraviolet A exposure in vehicles. Br J Dermatol 2004;151(4):873–6.
10. Foley P, Lanzer D, Marks R. Are solar keratoses more common on the driver's side? Br Med J (Clin Res Ed) 1986;293(6538):18.
11. Foley PA, Marks R, Dorevitch AP. Lentigo maligna is more common on the driver's side. Arch Dermatol 1993;129(9):1211–2.
12. Butler ST, Fosko SW. Increased prevalence of left-sided skin cancers. J Am Acad Dermatol 2010; 63(6):1006–10.
13. Paulson KG, Iyer JG, Nghiem P. Asymmetric lateral distribution of melanoma and Merkel cell carcinoma in the United States. J Am Acad Dermatol 2011; 65(1):35–9.
14. Almutawa F, Vandal R, Wang SQ, et al. Current status of photoprotection by window glass, automobile glass, window films, and sunglasses. Photodermatol Photoimmunol Photomed 2013;29(2):65–72.
15. Bernstein EF, Schwartz M, Viehmeyer R, et al. Measurement of protection afforded by ultraviolet-absorbing window film using an in vitro model

of photodamage. Lasers Surg Med 2006;38(4): 337–42.
16. Moehrle M, Soballa M, Korn M. UV exposure in cars. Photodermatol Photoimmunol Photomed 2003;19(4): 175–81.
17. European Window Film Association. Window film manufacturing process. Available at: http://www.ewfa.org/. Accessed November 11, 2013.
18. Boye C, Preusser F, Schaeffer T. UV-blocking window films for use in museums: revisited. WAAC Newsletter 2010;32:13–8.
19. Sasaki H, Sakamoto Y, Schnider C, et al. UV-B exposure to the eye depending on solar altitude. Eye Contact Lens 2011;37(4):191–5.
20. Moran DJ, Hollows FC. Pterygium and ultraviolet radiation: a positive correlation. Br J Ophthalmol 1984; 68(5):343–6.
21. Taylor HR, West SK, Rosenthal FS, et al. Corneal changes associated with chronic UV irradiation. Arch Ophthalmol 1989;107(10):1481–4.
22. Taylor HR, West SK, Rosenthal FS, et al. Effect of ultraviolet radiation on cataract formation. N Engl J Med 1988;319(22):1429–33.
23. Sui GY, Liu GC, Liu GY, et al. Is sunlight exposure a risk factor for age-related macular degeneration? A systematic review and meta-analysis. Br J Ophthalmol 2013;97(4):389–94.
24. Taylor HR, West S, Munoz B, et al. The long-term effects of visible light on the eye. Arch Ophthalmol 1992;110(1):99–104.
25. Dain SJ. Sunglasses and sunglass standards. Clin Exp Optom 2003;86(2):77–90.
26. Wang SQ, Balagula Y, Osterwalder U. Photoprotection: a review of the current and future technologies. Dermatol Ther 2010;23(1):31–47.
27. Dain SJ, Ngo TP, Cheng BB, et al. Sunglasses, the European directive and the European standard. Ophthalmic Physiol Opt 2010;30(3):253–6.
28. Sakamoto Y, Kojima M, Sasaki K. Effectiveness of eyeglasses for protection against ultraviolet rays. Nihon Ganka Gakkai Zasshi 1999;103(5): 379–85 [in Japanese].
29. Rosenthal FS, Bakalian AE, Lou CQ, et al. The effect of sunglasses on ocular exposure to ultraviolet radiation. Am J Public Health 1988;78(1): 72–4.
30. Australian and New Zealand Standard AS/NZS 4399:1996 – Sun protective clothing – Evaluation and classification. Sparkle 30 Aug 2012;633.
31. Hoffmann K, Laperre J, Avermaete A, et al. Defined UV protection by apparel textiles. Arch Dermatol 2001;137(8):1089–94.
32. Wang SQ, Kopf AW, Marx J, et al. Reduction of ultraviolet transmission through cotton T-shirt fabrics with low ultraviolet protection by various laundering methods and dyeing: clinical implications. J Am Acad Dermatol 2001;44(5):767–74.

33. Menzies SW, Lukins PB, Greenoak GE, et al. A comparative study of fabric protection against ultraviolet-induced erythema determined by spectrophotometric and human skin measurements. Photodermatol Photoimmunol Photomed 1991;8(4): 157–63.

34. Gambichler T, Hatch KL, Avermaete A, et al. Ultraviolet protection factor of fabrics: comparison of laboratory and field-based measurements. Photodermatol Photoimmunol Photomed 2002;18(3): 135–40.

35. Hatch KL, Osterwalder U. Garments as solar ultraviolet radiation screening materials. Dermatol Clin 2006;24(1):85–100.

36. Gambichler T, Altmeyer P, Hoffmann K. Role of clothes in sun protection. Recent Results Cancer Res 2002;160:15–25.

37. Das BR. UV radiation protective clothing. Open Textil J 2010;3:14–21.

38. Davis S, Capjack L, Kerr N, et al. Clothing as protection from ultraviolet radiation: which fabric is most effective? Int J Dermatol 1997;36(5):374–9.

39. Sarkar AK. On the relationship between fabric processing and ultraviolet radiation transmission. Photodermatol Photoimmunol Photomed 2007;23(5): 191–6.

40. Crews PC, Kachman S, Beyer AG. Influences on UVR transmission of undyed woven fabrics. Textile Chemist and Colorist 1999;31:17–26.

41. Srinivasan MG, Gatewood BM. Relationship of dye characteristics to UV protection provided by cotton fabric. Text Chem Color & Am Dyestuff Reporter 2000;32:36–43.

42. Veatch KD, Gatewood BM. Influence of light exposure on the UV protection of direct, reactive, acid, and disperse dyes on cotton and nylon fabrics. AATCC Rev 2002;2(2):47–51.

43. Gorenšek M, Sluga F. Modifying the UV blocking effect of polyester fabric. Textil Res J 2004;74(6): 469–74.

44. Stanford DG, Georgouras KE, Pailthorpe MT. Sun protection by a summer-weight garment: the effect of washing and wearing. Med J Aust 1995;162(8): 422–5.

45. Gambichler T, Hatch KL, Avermaete A, et al. Influence of wetness on the ultraviolet protection factor (UPF) of textiles: in vitro and in vivo measurements. Photodermatol Photoimmunol Photomed 2002;18(1): 29–35.

46. Ferguson JD, Jeffrey S. Photodermatology. London: Mason Publishing Ltd; 2006.

47. Edlich RF, Cox MJ, Becker DG, et al. Revolutionary advances in sun-protective clothing–an essential step in eliminating skin cancer in our world. J Long Term Eff Med Implants 2004;14(2):95–106.

48. Menter JM, Hollins TD, Sayre RM, et al. Protection against UV photocarcinogenesis by fabric materials. J Am Acad Dermatol 1994;31(5 Pt 1):711–6.

# Index

*Note:* Page numbers of article titles are in **boldface** type.

Dermatol Clin 32 (2014) 449–456
http://dx.doi.org/10.1016/S0733-8635(14)00052-7
0733-8635/14/$ – see front matter © 2014 Elsevier Inc. All rights reserved.

derm.theclinics.com

Printed and bound by CPI Group (UK) Ltd, Croydon, CR0 4YY

03/10/2024

01040381-0001